Everything You Never Wanted Your Kids to Know About Sex (But Were Afraid They'd Ask)

"For parents who've spent hours agonizing over how to talk with their kids about sex, only to find themselves stumbling, fumbling, and mumbling, help is on the way!"—*Today*

"A cradle-to-adulthood guide for parents who have come to the harsh realization that they're not nearly as hip and broad-minded as they thought they'd be. . . . Deals with the full range of sexual development issues . . . with a combination of frankness and sensitivity."
—*Washington Post*

"Richardson and Schuster have taken on what perplexed parents may regard as impossible: unraveling the secrets of surviving their children's interest in sex. The authors do so admirably, with wit and wisdom, covering a variety of topics, including . . . the 'junior Olympics of sexual desire' and the time 'when you and her blankie will no longer be at the top of the list.' "—*New York Times*

"The essential guide to managing the vast array of challenges involving kids and sex. Simultaneously wise and funny, this highly accessible book will help parents safely through what might otherwise seem like a thicket of anxiety and confusion. A must-read for every thoughtful and caring parent."—William Pollack, Ph.D., author of *Real Boys*

"A sensible, open-minded book for parents who want their kids to have a healthy attitude toward sex—but not have any. . . . [A] particularly hysterical primer."—*Salon*

"Richardson and Schuster bring extraordinary expertise and scintillating intelligence to this guide. . . . Thoroughly researched, extremely well written and chock-full of personal stories from parents, this 'survival guide' should be required reading for any parent who believes in being open about these touchy issues."—*Publishers Weekly*

"So entertaining that parents might actually read it. . . . Highly recommended."—*Library Journal*

"As the parent of a toddler and an educator of teens, I really appreciate this book's concrete, nonjudgmental, useful information and how it reflects a wide array of parents' opinions and beliefs. . . . I will use this excellent book in my home and the classroom."—Rosalind Wiseman, author of *Queen Bees and Wannabes*

"Filled with stories from parents that range from helpful to hilarious. More hilarious, of course, when it's someone else's kid."—*Daily News of Los Angeles*

"[A] medical guide no home should be without. . . . Thanks to their thorough and open-minded discussion, when your little one asks, 'Where do babies come from?' your response will be coolheaded, thoughtful, and aligned with your own values."—*Town and Country*

"Packing their book with the latest studies and information about children's sexual development, Drs. Richardson and Schuster . . . argue that the best way to help kids develop a healthy attitude toward sex is to talk with them early and often."—*Child Magazine*

"Drs. Richardson and Schuster have done a great service for today's parents by providing them with comprehensive and up-to-date tools for helping their children negotiate through all the stages of sexual development in a positive and safe way. This warm and rigorous book is bound to give the next generation the healthy start that all children deserve."—Laura Berman, Ph.D., coauthor of *For Women Only: A Revolutionary Guide to Overcoming Sexual Dysfunction and Reclaiming Your Sex Life*

"For parents whose tots are playing doctor in the garage and whose teenagers are pleading for coed sleepovers, here is some help. With wry humor . . . Richardson and Schuster combine experience in pediatrics and psychiatry to lend a helping hand."—*Booklist*

"A comprehensive and factual resource on a very delicate subject presented in a humorous and entertaining style. The authors cover all the bases . . . with a light and sensitive touch. I would not hesitate to recommend this book to the parents of my patients."—Joe M. Sanders, M.D., executive director, the American Academy of Pediatrics

"When this book arrived, we set it aside, thinking we'd donate it to charity. . . . Luckily, we glanced at it before we gave the box away. It's a funny, intelligent, user-friendly, creative guide to dealing with the subject that can make even the most loving and confident parents squirm."—*Arizona Republic*

"A sensitive and intelligent look at sexuality written with candor and creativity, this book will open the discussion for all the important issues."—Wendy Wasserstein, Pulitzer Prize–winning author of *The Heidi Chronicles* and *Shiksa Goddess*

"I thoroughly enjoyed this book! . . . Warm, nonjudgmental . . . with the perfect mix of humor, wisdom, and straightforward information. I highly recommend this book for every parent."—Ruth Bell, coauthor of *Changing Bodies, Changing Lives*

"This entertaining and mind-bending book is definitely a keeper."
—*Vancouver Sun*

Also by Mark A. Schuster

Child Rearing in America:
Challenges Facing Parents with Young Children

Everything you NEVER wanted your kids to know about SEX

(But Were Afraid They'd Ask)

The Secrets to Surviving Your Child's Sexual
Development from Birth to the Teens

JUSTIN RICHARDSON, M.D., AND
MARK A. SCHUSTER, M.D., PH.D.

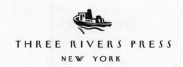

THREE RIVERS PRESS
NEW YORK

Grateful acknowledgment is made to the following for permission
to reprint previously published material:

Laura Greenfield: Excerpt from "Being 13" by Laura Greenfield (*The New York Times Magazine,* May 17, 1998). Distributed by *The New York Times Special Features.* Reprinted by permission of the author.

Irving Music, Inc. OBO Itself & Buggerlugs Music Co.: Excerpt from the song lyric "I am Woman," words and music by Helen Reddy and Ray Burton. Copyright " 1971 by Irving Music, Inc. OBO Itself & Buggerlugs Music Co. (BMI). International copyright secured. All rights reserved. Reprinted by permission of Irving Music, Inc. OBO Itself & Buggerlugs Music Co.

Sophie Radice: Excerpt from article by Sophie Radice (*Guardian,* November 10, 1999). Reprinted by permission of the author.

Radio National and the Australian Broadcasting Corporation: Excerpt from the show "Early Childhood Masturbation" by Bill Fleming (*ABC Health Report,* July 13, 1998). Reprinted by permission of Radio National and the Australian Broadcasting Corporation.

Maurice Sendak: Excerpt from *Where the Wild Things Are* by Maurice Sendak. Reprinted by permission of the author.

Published by Three Rivers Press, New York, New York.

Member of the Crown Publishing Group, a division of Random House, Inc.

www.crownpublishing.com

THREE RIVERS PRESS and the Tugboat design are registered trademarks of Random House, Inc.

Originally published in hardcover by Crown Publishers, a division of Random House, Inc., in 2003.

Printed in the United States of America

DESIGN BY LENNY HENDERSON

Library of Congress Cataloging-in-Publication Data

Richardson, Justin, 1963-

Everything you never wanted your kids to know about sex (but were afraid they'd ask): the secrets to surviving your child's sexual development from birth to the teens / Justin Richardson and Mark A. Schuster.

Includes bibliographical references and index.

1. Children—Sexual behavior. 2. Teenagers—Sexual behavior. 3. Child rearing. [DNLM: 1. Sex Behavior—Child—Popular Works. 2. Sexuality—Child—Popular Works. 3. Parent-Child Relations—Popular Works. WS 105.5.S4 R523e 2003] I. Schuster, Mark A. II. Title.

HQ784.S45 R53 2003

649'.65—dc21   2002011351

ISBN 1-4000-5128-2

10 9 8 7 6

First Paperback Edition

For my parents,

Mary Ann Richardson

and John J. Richardson

—J.R.

For my grandmother

Irene F. Schulman

—M.A.S.

Acknowledgments

At the top of our list of those without whom this book would be no more than a bright idea are the many, many parents and children who agreed to tell a (sometimes) virtual stranger some of the most intimate details of their family lives—and then let him write about them. This book is filled with their wisdom, their worries, their jokes. We wish we could thank them all by name, but because we promised them anonymity, we'll leave it at this: To all of you who shared your stories with us, whether through in-depth interviews (which always lasted longer than we said they would) or casual conversations, we thank you sincerely. You played an essential role in the creation of this book. You know who you are.

Parents and their children were not the only experts who helped with this book. Many authorities generously answered questions, read sections, or shared information. Thanks to Martin Anderson, Michael Broder, Willard Cates Jr., Heather Cecil, Deborah Cohen, Pinchas Cohen, Rebecca Collins, Allison Diamant, Patricia Dittus, Marc Elliott, Karen Fond, J. Dennis Fortenberry, John Fricker, Leslie Kantor, Mark Litwin, Michael Lu, Muriel McClendon, Jeffrey Merrick, Kim Miller, Robert Morris, Anna-Barbara Moscicki, Howard Reinstein, Ted Russell, Narayan Sastry, Wendelin Slusser, Loraine Stern, Susan Tortolero, Joseph Triebwasser, James Trussell, Susan C. Vaughan, Claudia Wang, Heide Woo, and Gail Zellman.

This book would not exist without the hard work and insight of a few key publishing professionals. Special thanks to our agent, Eric Simonoff, who managed to create two actual children in the time it took us to write this book. Thanks to our first editor, Betsy Rapoport, for embracing this book with such enthusiasm; to our second editor, Kristin Kiser, for warmly adopting it and making all obstacles to its production melt away; and to our assistant editor, Claudia Gabel, for helping in countless essential ways. Thanks to Tina Constable and Jason Gordon for expertly getting the word out.

Thank you, Christopher Keyser, for giving us our title.

—J.R. & M.A.S.

My psychotherapy patients have deepened my understanding of so much of what's covered in these pages. Because of the private nature of our work, their stories do not appear in here, but the knowledge they have given me surely does. I thank them all.

The heads, teachers, students, and parents of the schools I have worked with over the last several years have been an extraordinary source of learning and inspiration, which I have tried to return to them in the form of countless talks and, now, one book. For their trust, their insights, and their example, special thanks to a few particularly outstanding schools: The Brearley School, The Chapin School, Collegiate School, Ethical Culture Fieldston School, The Nightingale-Bamford School, The Packer Collegiate Institute, Shady Hill School, and Trinity School. Thanks also to the Association of Independent Maryland Schools and the New York State Association of Independent Schools.

My teachers at Harvard College, Harvard Medical School, the graduate department of social anthropology at Harvard, McLean Hospital, and the Columbia University Center for Psychoanalytic Training and Research have profoundly influenced my understanding of this book's subject. My sincerest thanks goes to all of them, especially Stephen Jay Gould, Jerome Kagan, Richard Lewontin, and Edward O. Wilson; Allan Brandt, Byron Good, and Arthur Kleinman; Bruce Cohen, Stephanie Engel, Shervert Frazier, John Gunderson, Len Glass, Leston Havens, Phillip Isenberg, Arthur Klein, Trude Kleinschmidt, Jonathan Kolb, Alex Sabo, Richard Schwartz, and Joan Wheelis; Richard C. Friedman; Karen Gilmore, Jonathan House, Nate Kravis, and Ellen Rees.

My conversations with three teachers in particular during the writing of this book have been enormously illuminating—I am particularly grateful to them: Betsy Auchincloss, Susan Coates, and Humphrey Morris.

Robert A. Glick has prepared me for this work and contributed in ways I may not completely understand but for which I will be forever grateful.

Thanks to my friends who encouraged me all the way through, who endured countless embarrassing dinner conversations, who tried always to seem interested, and who did without my attention more than they should ever have to, without ever once complaining. Among those whose ideas, assistance, and warmth were invaluable to me are Keith Bunin, Rachel Cohen, Doug Hamilton, Tom Hulce, Betsy Klein, Beth Schachter, and Eric Schorr. A special thanks to the endlessly generous Chris Keyser, Susan Sprung, Madeline and Benjamin Sprung-Keyser, and, of course, Puddleby, in whose delightful company a good bit of this book was written.

Thanks to my sister, Martine Sacks, who helped unlock some of the secrets of womanhood and motherhood that are written about here, and to my niece Lita Sacks, for being such a wonderful person.

Thanks to my parents who, as with every other endeavor of mine, supported me unstintingly through this process and who, among many other essential attributes, are the very best next-door neighbors a guy ever had.

Finally, I would have to be a much better writer than I am to express in words my gratitude for all that has been given to me by Peter Parnell.

—J.R.

Throughout the years, my patients and their families have given me a sense of purpose, taught me, and kept me connected to the challenges parents face. I am very much in their debt.

My colleagues, fellows, residents, and students at UCLA and RAND and particularly at the UCLA/RAND Center for Adolescent Health Promotion have challenged me to think in new ways about many topics covered in this book. Several collaborators with whom I conduct research on sexual development and parent-child communication have especially shaped my thinking about these complex subjects: I have gained much from the wisdom, insights, and support of Rosalie Corona, Karen Eastman, and David Kanouse.

This book highlights the importance of parents in raising healthy children. But there's another group that plays a critical role, both supplementing the work of involved parents and filling in for parents who might be unable to attend to their children's needs: teachers. Teachers have been especially important throughout my life. I wish to remember, among the many who have made a huge difference in my education, the following teachers and mentors: Miss Cooper, Miss Fagan, Mrs. Marks, Mrs. Morrell, Mrs. Moskowitz, Mrs. Kandell, Larry Moses, Mr. Finney, Mr. Grimes, Mr. Merrick, Mrs. Davison, Mr. Downs, Father LaPointe, Mr. Lay, Mr. Neale, Mr. Schloeder, Gerald Burns, Phoebe Ellsworth, Jeffrey Merrick, Mary Poovey, Rachel Wizner, John (Jeb) Boswell, Judson Randolph, Penny Chaloner, Suzanne Churchill, David Blumenthal, Mark Schlesinger, Tom Schelling, Edith Stokey, Mike Stoto, Grace Caputo, Alan Ezekowitz, Lewis First, Gary Fleisher, Holcombe Grier, Maribeth Hourihan, Fred Lovejoy, Ken McIntosh, David Nathan, Bob Bell, Sandy Berry, Tora Bikson, Lester Breslow, Bob Brook, Naihua Duan, Phyllis Ellickson, Jonathan Fielding, Neal Halfon, David Kanouse, Arleen Leibowitz, Rob MacCoun, Ed McCabe, Linda McCabe, Elizabeth McGlynn, Sally Morton, Al Pennisi, Linda Rosenstock, Mary Jane Rotheram-Borus, and Martin Shapiro.

A strong support network of friends cheered me on, checked in regularly to see how the writing was going, and kept me updated with the latest anecdotes about their kids. I thank them for their help and enthusiasm.

My partner, Jeffrey Webb, patiently watched and waited as I spent vacations, weekends, and nights working on this book. His thoughtful advice, wise criticism, endless encouragement, and ability to make me smile made the book possible. He also shared with me his large extended family, who have not only taken me in as one of their own but whose talent for raising such amazing kids has shown me just how effective good parenting can be.

Finally, I would like to thank and remember my parents, grandparents, and brothers, who were the first to reveal to me how profoundly important families are. I'd especially like to acknowledge my grandmother, who is so thrilled every time I am interviewed for an article or news program about teens and condoms, or teens and oral sex, even when, as she explains, "I didn't know people really did things like that."

—M.A.S.

Contents

Introduction

LET'S SAY YOU'RE A PARENT. And let's say that, like most kids' parents today, you came of age sometime after 1960. It would be tough to characterize such a diverse group, but we're willing to risk one generalization about parents like you.

Our hunch is that by the time you finished high school, you felt you knew more about sex than your parents knew. You talked more about sex than they did. And you believed, with a little luck, that you would have more sex than they had. In fact, of all of the differences that you felt separated you from your parents' generation, this one may have been the plainest. When it came to sex, you were cooler.

Then you had a son. Or a daughter.

And when your daughter, who just turned sixteen, finds you in the kitchen and asks if she can invite her boyfriend to sleep over next Friday, and you say you mean in the guest room, and she says no in my room, and you say what exactly are the two of you planning on doing in that room of yours, Tamara Louise—frankly, you don't feel so cool anymore.

What happened?

Well, like we said, you had kids. And, as it turns out, the sexual fumblings of adolescents look a teensy bit different when viewed from the other end of the kitchen table, even to someone who once had a tube top. Or pot plants growing in her dorm room. Even to someone who once ordered a drink called a Long Slow Comfortable Screw Against the Wall from a bartender with a bushy mustache.

Oh, your parents had it easy. When they panicked because you touched your little self in the high chair, or turned up naked with another five-year-old in the tree house, they had an answer. Their parents, and their parents before them, had handed down a universally embraced, one-size-fits-all method for managing every child's sex life: pretend it isn't happening. Failing that, say it's wrong or it's perfectly normal, tell her to stop, and pass the potato salad.

Our guess is, that's not going to work for you.

No, you're in a tighter spot than your folks, because just like them, your kid's sexuality is bound to make you squeamish, but unlike them— and here's the hitch—you think it shouldn't. You think sex is a good thing and you should be poised and nonjudgmental as you watch its first glimmers flicker across your toddler's cherubic face.

You think—and good for you—that the moment you stumble upon your three-year-old rubbing against her stuffed panda, you should say something genuinely helpful, something . . . *upbeat*. And that, friend, is a gauntlet your fine parents, devoted though they were, never had to run.

So here's the question. If you don't do what they did, if you don't want to tell your daughter to stop but secretly you really, really wish she would, what do you do?

A father who looked to be about forty-five recently asked one of us a question, and as he spoke, it seemed as if he was voicing the dilemma of an entire generation. "How can I give my daughter a healthy attitude toward sex," he asked in earnest, "but prevent her from having any?"

If you know where this guy is coming from, this book is for you.

We Hear You

It has been distressingly apparent that parents want and need help in learning how to address their children's sexual development. You can see it in the letters they send to advice columns. You can hear it on the radio call-in shows. It shows up on surveys.

You can find it in the great societal debates about sex ed at school, sex in the media, sex on the Internet. The one thing—perhaps the only thing—on which all sides seem to agree is that parents want to play a role in their children's sexual development. But they're not sure how to do it.

We hear it from parents in the clinic, in the office, and in the school auditorium. When a school announces that the next guest speaker for parents' night will be a physician talking about sex, it's not the usual ten or fifteen regulars who show up. It's more like a hundred parents, with lists of questions and a willingness to stay all night until the last one is answered.

We can't make it through a barbecue without being pulled aside, usually by an apologetic parent at her wit's end. What do I say when he asks me how to make a baby? Or when she asks if she can marry Daddy? What about when he says he wants to have sex for the first time, and he wants to do it in his bedroom? The questions go on. My child is downloading porn from the Internet. . . . My daughter wants to start taking the Pill. . . . I'm sure you've never heard this before, but my two-year-old is humping my retriever. . . . What do I do?

Actually, we *have* heard it before.

And so, after years of being asked, "Is there a book I can read to really understand this stuff?" we decided to write one.

Attack of the Ninety-Foot Teenagers

Do we need to point out that there are a lot of teenagers around these days? With a forcefulness that one newspaper recently dubbed the "Attack of the 90-Foot Teen-Agers," teens are making their presence known across the United States. Paired with an exploding generation of teens is an exploding generation of parents like you, anxious to do the right thing and not entirely sure what that is.

Some of what may perplex you, if you've got a teenager at home, will undoubtedly have to do with sex. Maybe you've decided your teenager isn't ready for sex, but if he were to have sex now, you'd want it to be safe. So, maybe you'll give him a box of condoms. But if you do that, will you be encouraging him to have sex before he's ready? When exactly will he be ready? And how well do condoms really work, anyway?

As the study of teenage sexuality expands, it becomes both more important and more impossible for parents like you to keep up with the facts. Which is why we've put them all here.

Steady Now

Then again, if facts were all you needed, this would be a much simpler business.

Imagine it's been half an hour since your six-year-old daughter and her friend Cecile went upstairs to play with their dolls, and you haven't heard a peep from them. You head up there to see if anyone wants some lemonade. You open the door.

Prancing gaily on the puppet stage under Cecile's guidance are two Barbies, wearing spiky heels and Day-Glo bathing suits pulled down to their waists. Your daughter's got one of her brother's action figures high in the air, egging them on, chanting, "Take it off, baby! Take it off!"

You say . . . what, exactly?

Or, the locker room at the pool is a little crowded, but you've found a spot on the bench for your four-year-old. He has agreed to sit there quietly while you get dressed. You slip out of your suit and reach for your underwear.

"Mommy," your son asks in his sweetest voice, "can I touch it?"

"Touch what, jelly bean?"

"Your woo-woo."

"My . . . ?"

"Down there."

Managing your kids' sexual education, you may have realized by now, would be a whole lot easier if it were just a matter of telling them the facts. This is what sex is. This is how not to have it. This is how to make it safer, and so on. No question, your kids need this kind of information.

But you're also giving your kids something more powerful and less planned than lessons like these. Especially in their earliest years, the bulk of your children's learning about love and sex comes from the way you relate to them, to their bodies, and to their curiosity about sex, and the way you let them relate to you.

When the noted psychoanalyst and pediatrician D. W. Winnicott wrote about sex education half a century ago, he said every child, if she's going to learn about sex in a healthy way, needs three things. She needs a reasonable person to talk to, she needs to hear the biological facts, and she needs "steady emotional surroundings" in which she can discover sexuality on her own. In short, she needs a home with parents whose response to her emerging sexuality is not anxious or puritanical, but one of mature, benign support.

If you are like a few other parents we know, you may find that there is one small obstacle in the way of your good intentions to provide "steady emotional surroundings" when your kid is asking to touch your woo-woo: dread.

Or maybe not dread; maybe just ordinary nervousness, uncertainty, and fear. You know, that feeling you get when your parents are over and your three-year-old son asks, "Grandma, when you rub *your* weiner, does it feel good, too?"

We have written this book because we know you're trying to make it through tricky moments like these.

Your Survival Guide

Our goal here is to help you survive your child's sexual development, to learn how to live comfortably enough with it, so that you can play your crucial role of fostering its natural, healthy growth—even cheering it on—in the way that only parents can do.

In writing this book, we have drawn on our education in science, medicine, and psychology. We have turned to Mark's research on sexual development and on the role parents play in that development and to Justin's work as a sex educator and a psychotherapist. We have built on the foundation of Mark's expertise in pediatrics and Justin's in psychiatry. But we also decided that in writing a book like this, we should take a step back. So we took a page from the Nobel Prize–winning physicist Richard Feynman and approached writing this book as if we were Martians—Martians who had never before heard of parenting, and had to figure it out by asking around.

We reread all the studies on children, parents, and sexuality that we've been quoting for years. We quizzed experts in the relevant fields about what they thought. We revisited the relevant disciplines—anthropology, biology, developmental and social psychology, epidemiology, pediatrics, psychoanalysis, sociology, and so on—and read the memoirs of parents who wrote about their kids and of kids who wrote about their parents.

And then we listened. You will notice that this isn't simply a book of statistics; it's filled with the personal stories of parents like you. Some are from the many interviews we conducted with parents and kids specifically for the book. Others are from parents who stopped us in the hallway or called us with a question or two. In every case, we have disguised the details to protect the confidentiality of the speakers and their family members.

This Is What We Found

The following pages contain what we have learned about parenting, children, and sex.

In Part I, we start with an overview of the natural history of your children's sexual development to help you find just where along that path your kids are right now and what lies ahead (Chapter 1). After nature, we go to nurture, examining what is actually known about how you can influence your child's development. We look at the outcomes of certain styles of parenting and specific parenting practices, letting you know what works and how. And we take up the knotty question of what should your kids know and when should they know it, which we answer by introducing the four sex ed lessons you can teach your kids (Chapter 2).

Part II of the book (Chapters 3 through 10) tracks your child's development in detail from high chair to high school. We start with some questions from the homes of little kids (Chapter 3). Whom can they see naked? Who can bathe together, and until when? We explain just what we mean when we write that the seeds of a child's sexuality germinate during these early years, under the warmth of a healthy, loving relationship with you. We don't have to teach you how to love, but you'll teach your kid. And you'll do it before he hits kindergarten.

Next comes the junior Olympics of sexual desire, as we take up the kinds of pleasure little kids seek out (Chapter 4). What should you do about masturbation, which can start in infancy, and the sexual games little kids play with their friends? Your responses will introduce your child to the dueling twins of sexuality—pleasure and responsibility—a lesson best introduced now, while he's still talking to you. Speaking of sexual desire, in Chapter 5 we go on to consider how your child arrives at his sexual orientation. We encourage you to explore the possibility that your child could turn out to be gay and, given that chance, to create a home environment that will allow him to make a smoother transition to adulthood than he could without your help. The lessons in this chapter will also help you encourage any child to grow up with a greater understanding of human sexual diversity.

Then we hit puberty. Chapter 6 lays out all of the changes you can expect of your child as she reaches this exciting but daunting milestone, complete with information about how to talk with your daughter about menstruation before it begins and how to give a heads-up to your son about the new trick his penis is about to pull.

There is something a little melancholy about the events that start to unfold next. Soon, when your little one muses about whom she loves most, you and her blankie will no longer be at the top of her list. You've been beaten out by a spindly middle schooler with braces. Chapter 7 prepares you for the eventuality of your child finding love elsewhere and suggests an effective approach to the practical dilemmas posed by a teenager in love, like what if you hate the guy.

Once she starts dating, the sex question is soon to follow. Chapter 8 explores the decision on which so much seems to be riding: Will she have sex? We analyze the abstinence decision and address the question, What should you be rooting for, and how? But before anyone has sex, you want to have a talk about safety. Chapter 9 is your education in the mechanics of sexual protection and how to encourage it, before your child's first sexual encounter.

What follows is up to your kids. The last chapter in Part II begins with your child's first sexual encounter. What will it be like for her? And what will it be like for you, as you gradually assume a more peripheral role in your child's sexual world? Here we take up the issues you'll face now that you've got a kid who's having sex, like, what will you do if she asks how to give a blow job?

In Part III, the book ends with two chapters devoted to two of the major risks of teenage sex: sexually transmitted diseases (Chapter 11) and unintended pregnancies (Chapter 12). In them, we will give you the information you need to teach your child why it's so important to prevent these all-too-frequent outcomes, and if she is unfortunate enough to experience them, what she can do.

Our Bias

Treat them [children] as though they were young adults. . . .
Never hug and kiss them. Never let them sit in your lap. If you
must, kiss them once on the forehead when they say goodnight.
Shake hands with them in the morning. Give them a pat on the
head if they have made an extraordinarily good job of a difficult
task. Try it out. In a week's time you will find how easy it is to
be perfectly objective with your child and at the same time
kindly. You will be utterly ashamed of the mawkish, sentimental
way you have been handling it. . . . [W]on't you then remember
when you are tempted to pet your child that mother love is a
dangerous instrument?

—JOHN B. WATSON, PH.D.,
Psychological Care of Infant and Child, 1928

Parenting books have a checkered past.

In the long history of the genre, experts have developed an irksome habit of changing their minds. They told us parents should feed their babies on a strict schedule, for example, and then extolled the values of feeding on demand. The breast was out; now it's in. Circumcision went from yes to no to maybe. And as for discipline, the prevailing wisdom seems to reverse itself with each new presidential administration.

We suspect that some of what we write may be passé before it hits the bookstores, some of it may be out of fashion in a decade, and some of it may remain standard parenting practice for years to come. Positions sometimes get reversed because we learn more; but often, it seems to us, parenting advice ages poorly because it was never based on data in the first place. It was opinion dressed up as fact. We have worked very hard not to fall into that trap, which means that in some cases we'll explain the (often ambiguous and rarely definitive) data, but we won't give you a definitive recommendation.

We intend this book to be used in the context of your own values. We have tried to write it in a manner that is open to all perspectives. Instead of declaring what you should do, we tend to say what you could do and, when we can, give you enough information so you can make the best choice for you and your family.

You may believe that sex during adolescence is fine, even advisable. Or you may prefer that your kids wait until they are out of high school, or over twenty-one, or until they have been involved with a partner for quite a while. Or you may believe that your kids should wait until marriage.

Some believe that masturbation is morally wrong; others consider it a way of life. We think everyone will benefit from understanding how it develops and the possible impact on your child of the way you react when you find her in the sandbox with her hands down her pants.

Think of this book as a compass, not a road map. You know the general direction you're going—guiding your child through infancy and the middle years, then into adolescence and beyond, all aimed at producing a healthy adult—but there are many ways to get there, and you don't always need to stay on the main road.

Lest we mislead you, let us admit up front that we are not without opinions. We've got plenty, and you will come across them in here, too. But we have tried to present them for what they are—opinions, albeit educated opinions—but not facts.

First and foremost, we are physicians, and we believe in promoting children's health as a leading principle in deciding how to deal with their sexuality. Our definition of health includes physical health, by which we mean the absence of sexually transmitted disease and unintended pregnancy, and safety from sexual abuse and violence; and emotional health, by which we mean the ability to take pleasure in sex, the freedom of mind to make choices about love and sex, the possession of a meaningful value system to guide those choices, and the presence of strong self-esteem.

We don't expect you'll agree with everything we recommend. You know yourself and your family, your values and your needs, better than anybody. If nothing else, we hope to give you a chance to reflect a bit more on what you do, to learn some different approaches, and to consider some new techniques. The bottom line is that you are the parents. You decide.

And please let us know what you think. Let us know your stories—what's worked and what hasn't. You can reach us at our e-mail address (comments@richardsonschuster.com) or through our website (www.richardsonschuster.com). Share your voice with us so we can broaden the reach of the book in the future. Or you can just vent.

As Good As It Gets

By the time you finish this book, you will have figured out how to respond should you discover that your daughter is producing a strip show in her puppet booth, or should your four-year-old ask to touch your woo-woo in a locker room full of women. You may even have found a way to reply confidently should your teenager inquire of you how best to give a blow job. In fact, you should come away having formulated responses to many, many other situations as well.

Of course, even if you do figure it all out, and you put your ideas perfectly into practice—even if you do everything right—this won't necessarily result in a trouble-free sexuality for your child. Child development is just too complex a process for us to predict or control any of its outcomes, particularly one so mysterious as sexuality.

So you won't get that guarantee. But you will get something nearly as good, or at least as good as it gets. You'll get a way of thinking about every sexual issue that may come up at home—an understanding of what's at stake in any of your decisions—that will help you manage them in your own way with confidence, with a sensitivity to your child's needs, and with an awareness of your own needs.

As you work out the questions of modesty and pleasure, responsibility and freedom, and spontaneity and danger that start spinning around your home once you've got a kid in the house, you may also get something you hadn't anticipated.

Our guess is that your sexual development hasn't stopped. Although you may have your sights fixed on your kid, you are growing, too. And working out all these sometimes embarrassing details of how you'll describe sex to your child, what you'll say if he walks in on you, what you'll let him do, and what he does anyway, it's all bound to move your own relationship with sex a bit further.

You may find you're developing a deeper understanding of your own sex life. You may discover you have some inhibitions you weren't aware of, or that you have been living with assumptions about what you want sexually that you have never really explored.

Believe us when we say that if you pay attention to what your kid is going through, you are bound to change, too. You will learn something about sex and love and your own life, just as the simple act of becoming a parent, however long ago it may have been, unalterably deepened your appreciation of what it means to be human and to be alive.

Welcome to the next step in your child's development, and in your own.

Part I

The Nature and Nurture

of Kids and Sex

Chapter **1**

How did this happen?

THE NATURAL HISTORY OF YOUR CHILD'S SEXUALITY

YOU ARE FLAT ON YOUR BACK. Your shirt is pulled up over your belly, and your pants are down around your hips. Someone has just squirted a glob of cold jelly below your navel. This is one of those miraculous moments in life that doesn't always live up to its billing in terms of physical comfort. The ultrasound.

Your main concern is whether the baby will be normal. But you are hoping for a little fun. "I want to see a face," you say, craning up from the table. And you want to know if it's a girl or a boy. The last time they said they couldn't be sure.

The radiologist starts sliding the probe over your belly.

"There's the head."

"The head? Where?" She bends the monitor in your direction.

"See, right here."

You see something that looks like a blizzard being broadcast on a 1969 Magnavox.

"Where?" (Is she pressing harder?)

"Here, right here, see that?"

She is definitely pressing harder. You consider humoring her. Then a ghostly face appears in the snow. It is tiny, but it is a face. You can make out a delicate profile: an eye, and a nose, and cupped up near its open mouth, a tiny . . . something.

A burger?

"That's its left hand."

A left hand! The baby looks so sweet and tranquil, as if it's asleep. A sleeping angel. A staticky sleeping angel.

"It's a boy."

You are now in a new part of the blizzard.

"Are you sure?"

"Pretty sure. See, here? Between the legs?" Now she is pressing with real excitement.

"Oh yeah, those are legs. I *definitely* see them."

"Well, if you look right between them, you can just make it out."

"Make what out?"

"His penis. You see? He's got an erection."

"A what?"

An erection.

Your Child Is Already Sexual

We know two things about children's sexual development: Children learn about sex from the world. And children are inherently sexual.

We have all easily accepted the first idea. The second one gives us a little more trouble.

At least since the Enlightenment days of John Locke, the idea of a child as a blank slate scribbled on by the world has been a favorite. Nowhere has this idea held more sway than in the area of sexuality: We like to think our children are born without it.

A hundred years ago, the Victorians, who perfected the idea of the innocent child, made a science out of sheltering children from knowledge about sex, going so far as to clothe suggestively nude piano legs with ruffled skirts. Children were innocents. Adults were sexual. If children became sexual, it must be through the influence of adults. Just as we worry about the effects of the Internet today, Victorian heads of household feared the nursemaid might kindle randy thoughts in their children while Mother and Father were away.

Little wonder the world considered Freud's theories of the inherent sexuality of children about as welcome as salmonella at a state dinner.

We have learned a lot about the sexual development of children since

Freud first alarmed our ancestors. Many of the specifics within his theory have been discarded. But the core of his heretical idea remains. Sexuality, we understand, develops naturally in all children. Its seeds can be found in infants, and it unfolds into mature sexual feeling in children as they grow, whether we tell them what it all means or remain resolutely silent.

How does this happen? How does an erection on an ultrasound evolve into the complex mating ritual practiced in a school stairwell by a nervous eleventh grader and his best friend's girlfriend's sister?

We are going to answer this question in a moment, to the extent that it's possible, by walking you through the sexual development of one girl and one boy. By the time these two are approaching adulthood, you will have learned all you need to know about the way a child becomes sexual. Throughout the book, we will revisit each of the issues these two lives raise. But before we start inspecting those particular trees, we want you to have a clear view of the forest.

As you will soon discover, sexuality isn't created in a child by her first sex education class. Nor is it turned on by a single hormonal switch that gets flipped at puberty. Instead, try thinking of sexuality as something assembled by each developing child over a period of years out of component parts. Some of the components a child will use for this job are on hand at birth, such as her genitals. When you get a baby girl, the vulva is included, and even before she can speak she will discover that touching her genitals feels good. It looks like there's something sexual about that act, but full-fledged sexuality requires more than sensitive genitals.

With time, this element will connect with other elements not available during infancy. Fantasies of being close to another person may come along several years later. When they do, a child will find that having these fantasies makes her genitals especially sensitive. The pleasure of touching them increases, and from then on, that pleasure is linked with thoughts of being with other people. Now something that resembles our grown-up image of sexuality is beginning to take shape.

In every child's life, several basic elements will grow and combine to form her nascent sexuality. Consider them sexuality's wheels and gears. They are:

- Spontaneous genital arousals
- Pleasurable genital self-stimulation
- Exploratory "sex play" with peers
- Attractions to others
- Fantasies of sex
- The ever-maturing ability to love

To make a long story very, very short: Over the course of a childhood, arousals that were once spontaneous start being cued by attractions to people. Arousing attractions then get linked to fantasies of sexual behavior. And when fantasies stimulate sexual experimentation with peers, an adultlike sexuality is born—at an age young enough to make the average parent gasp.

Obviously, someone needs to learn how to drive this thing. And so, as she is assembling these components, a child will also be developing the intellectual understanding, the moral structure, and the psychological maturity necessary to steer her burgeoning sexuality.

Whatever her childhood experiences, whether she's raised at a nudist colony or learns to sound out the word *abstinence* in preschool, every child will fashion and refashion some kind of working sexual scooter as she grows. Of course, how it is assembled and how it looks will differ depending on her particular temperament and life experiences. As you may know from your own experience, your child's sexuality will be added to and altered throughout her life. Sexual development never ends.

But we are getting ahead of ourselves.

Let's take a visit to a sleepy community hospital where, side by side in the nursery, are two infants, one a wriggly little newborn—a girl— and one a tiny bald boy, silently sleeping.

Welcome Eloise and Max.

Infants and Toddlers (Birth to Age Two)

Max is born with all the equipment a little boy needs. Before he leaves the hospital, something alarming will be done to his penis. Eloise, who is born with all the equipment a little girl needs, will not suffer any such surprise. They are bundled up and swept off to their new homes. Once there, they will get a lot of action going simply by crying. That action will include a good deal of diapering.

As with other newborns, at diaper time Eloise's and Max's parents may be able to observe that they have spontaneous arousals. Max will develop an erection. Eloise—although it will be much harder to see—will lubricate. It is unclear what causes these arousals at this age, whether they are responses to physical stimulation or to an internal signal in the baby's mind or body. Some consider these arousals a kind of reflex. They represent the earliest functioning after birth of a child's sexual apparatus.

Being held and caressed are among the greatest pleasures of infant life. So is having your chin stroked and your back rubbed. And so is playing with your genitals. In her eighth month, Eloise coos when her diaper is changed if she feels a breeze on her labia. Max, at ten months, likes to play with his penis, especially in the bath when the water is warm.

It is not clear at what age children begin to find genital stimulation more pleasurable than gentle touching elsewhere on their body. But infants certainly do seek it out, often before their first birthday. Can they have an orgasm if they stimulate themselves? No one really knows what an infant is feeling, but responses that look like orgasms (without ejaculation in boys) have been observed in children during their first year.

Early Childhood (Ages Two to Six)

At age two, Eloise has acquired a vocabulary of 197 words. Modesty is not one of them. There is little she loves more than trotting around the house with nothing on and being chased by her father with a diaper on his head. When she accompanies her mother to the office, she seems to have no problem finding her way into her pants at dull moments. Like at staff meetings.

Ultrawet, the name Max's parents have given his nightly bathtime aquatics show, typically features Max delighting his evening's guests with amazing feats of splashing, prancing, and grooming frivolity.

Like most two- and three-year-olds, these two enjoy being naked, and they have an uninhibited curiosity about bodies—their own and other people's. They will poke, peek at, and squeeze any family member or little friend who gives them a chance. They want to see what people are up to in the bathroom.

Max takes this curiosity with him to nursery school, where, at the age of four, he and his friend Timmy are discovered giggling under an arts-and-crafts table with their pants down. Casual, silly games like this one mark the very beginning of what is commonly called sex play. At Max's age, sex play is usually limited to showing and looking and is inspired by a desire to explore. As best we know, sexual attractions are unusual in preschool and probably don't play a major role in the fun of early sex play.

Before strong attractions emerge, children will also begin rehearsing for romance. In their choice of friends, beginning as early as age three or four, they will begin to limit their inner circle to peers of the same sex. The older they get, the more this will be so. But there may already be some special attention given to the other sex.

Although she rarely plays with him, Eloise has claimed a boy in her preschool class as her boyfriend. He is the only boy she wants at her fifth birthday party. She is talking about marriage. Eloise does feel a special affection for her friend, but theirs is a kind of playacting rather than a true romance. Eloise and her friend are imitating the way they have seen adults behave.

Imitation also seems to be behind the mock-sexy performance Eloise, now in kindergarten, puts on for her favorite uncle at Thanksgiving. She slips two tangerines under her sweater, pulls it up to show her belly button, and performs what she calls a Pocahontas dance before running away into her room. That, her mother announces with confidence, she did not learn at home.

Middle Childhood (Ages Six to Ten)

One year later, Pocahontas has skipped town. Eloise, now in first grade, rushes into the kitchen on her way to a playdate, stops dead, and gasps. "Oh my God, my underwear is showing!"

Something has happened: Modesty is in. Sometime after the age of six, most children's attitudes toward their own nudity change noticeably. The change seems to be linked with children's new comprehension of social mores. They begin to internalize adult attitudes toward sex and privacy. Even in homes where open sexuality has always been accepted by parents, children tend to absorb the taboos about nudity and sex they learn from peers.

Not all children become as scrupulously modest as Eloise. Max, for example, remains content to march around the house in his underpants at age seven. Still, most children do change, girls more so than boys. Their new modesty probably helped popularize the Freudian concept of latency.

An undeniably appealing notion, latency meant that after the years of wacky nudie shows, masturbating in the supermarket, and giggling in the bathroom, children (at age six or thereabouts) would give up on sex play and pour themselves into sorting marbles and collecting stamps.

A lot of people could get behind a theory like this.

It now seems that children's sexual behavior doesn't stop at six; it just drops out of sight. Kids learn to close the door, and their sexual behavior goes on developing in relative secrecy.

Eloise, at the age of eight, has a favorite place in the woods behind her house where she and her friends hide out. Occasionally they play "husbands," a game they invented together. One gets to be the husband, another plays the wife, and a third gives the instructions. The husband and wife pretend to come home from work and then take off their clothes. (This game is better played in the summer.) The director, Eloise's favorite role, tells the husband which part of his wife's body to touch. All the girls find this game pretty exciting.

As they grow through middle childhood, children are more likely to have had this kind of sex play with peers. The quality of their play is different from before. It is not only much more covert than it was in preschool; a new feeling of physical excitement and arousal may enter the picture. Yet, children this age still don't seem to pick sex-play partners because they are attracted to them, and they don't feel that they are having a romance.

At age eight, Max has a way with woodies. They come and go throughout the day, but Max hasn't yet had to give his erections a lot of thought. They seem to do fine without much input from him. Woodies just happen.

In 1943, one research group interviewed 291 boys to find out what it was that gave them erections. The boys dutifully provided an exhaustive list. It included, among other highlights, sitting in class, sitting in church, sitting in warm sand, and setting a field on fire. The national anthem was also responsible for a few erections. So was finding money (understandable) and, for a few unfortunates, being asked to go to the front of the class.

Good grades and hurricanes do indeed give Max erections, but at age ten, there are some new items on his list. Like underwear ads.

A new component of Max's sexuality has arrived. In middle childhood, children like Max who have been getting physically aroused more or less indiscriminately since infancy start to respond physically when they feel an attraction. Boys see someone naked, or think of someone's body, and they get erect. Girls do the same, and they lubricate. This new kind of sexual response has been recalled by adults as beginning anywhere from ages four to thirteen. But on average, it seems to start at about ages nine or ten. Those who have been asked tend to remember the first of these attractions occurring spontaneously while looking at a person or at someone's picture.

Attractions like these form the basis of crushes, which begin during these years. They also lead to a child's first erotic fantasies, and when fantasies begin, masturbation gets a major boost.

As they go through middle childhood, kids—especially boys—are more and more likely to masturbate. Their masturbation is not quite like it was a few years earlier. Modesty makes them less likely to do it over dinner. And their new fantasies—which vary considerably in their degree of detail—can turn the event into much more than a few desultory tugs.

These days, after she gets into bed, Eloise will sometimes rub herself on a throw pillow. When she does, she pictures a playground she once visited. She is standing by the swings wearing her best blue dress when an older boy from her swim class arrives. He is handsome. He smiles and walks towards her. Then he lies down beside her, and finally he kisses her.

Max rubs his penis thinking of *Baywatch*.

This is not to suggest that Eloise and Max are actually talking to members of the other sex. Fourth-grade society doesn't quite work that way. In fact, between the ages of eight and eleven, gender segregation reaches its lifetime high. Boys and girls will almost invariably cluster in single-sex groups whenever given the chance.

Eloise and her friends Gita and Claire eat at the same lunch table every day with a few other girls in their class. They seem utterly indifferent to the goings on at the boys' table. Ask Eloise why, and she will explain, "Basically, the problem with boys is, boys are loud and they will take your stuff and get it dirty."

Today Max's teacher has asked him to share a library book with Claire.

"Huh?"

"You can just give it to her at lunch." In Max's ears, this sounds like "Walk until you reach the great pyramids of Egypt. You will find Claire in the lap of the Sphinx. Be back for recess."

In the cafeteria, Max makes the drop by focusing his mind on other things and refusing to look at Claire. He tramps stiffly back to the boys' table.

"Hey Max, did you give Claire a love note?" Everett has seen him.

"What did you do, Max?" Timmy asks, almost looking up from his lunch.

Aware somehow that a few years ago when he was just a kid he would have cried at a time like this, Max punches them both in the arm. Hard.

Eloise and Claire poke at the book and giggle.

"You like him, don't you? That's why you asked for his book." (A senseless accusation from Gita.)

"What's that on your turkey sandwich, Gita?" retorts Eloise cannily. "A booger?!" They burst into giggles.

Ah, the refined courtship rituals of middle childhood. If romance were a planet, this would be its Cretaceous period. "Liking" and "hating," and fighting and wooing are difficult to distinguish during these years and are not always mutually exclusive. Boys chase girls and threaten to steal their things. Girls chase boys and threaten to kiss them. Anyone who gets too friendly with a member of the opposite camp will almost certainly be teased. In grade school, there is a name for the allure of the other sex. It is "cooties."

Such is the state of sexual relations in middle childhood. There is sexual play, but it has little to do with attraction. There are sexual attractions and crushes, but they don't translate into romantic relationships. And there is nothing yet like love. Playing at sex and playing at relationships, which have been developing independently, are not yet well connected. But they are about to be.

Preadolescence and Puberty (Ages Nine to Twelve)

Tonight is the night of the seventh-grade dance.

At the far end of an empty dance floor, Max and Timmy are hanging with the deejay and a cluster of boys. Max is doing his air guitar act for the guys.

They are aware that there are girls in the room.

In the preadolescent years, boys and girls still tend to congregate in single-sex groups like this, but those groups are now mixing in public. Birthday parties often have both sexes on their guest lists, and there is a general consensus among preteens that boys and girls are supposed to start dating. Dates, such as they are, actually start to happen.

Eloise, for example, is going to the dance with Everett. They have had two dates, both involving other friends, and Eloise has Everett's key chain in her backpack. Under Gita's definition of going out, Everett and Eloise qualify. They haven't kissed, but Everett has hopes for tonight.

The pairing off that begins for some at the start of middle school is more a response to peer expectations than to love or desire. A girl may have a passing crush on the boy she decides to go out with, but their actual contact is typically minimal. With dates arranged through intermediaries, they may barely speak to each other, and when they meet it will often be in a group of friends. But being able to say that she is going out is exciting and confers a certain status on a girl among her peers—even if the relationship doesn't last past fourth period.

The deejay puts on a slow song. Eloise and Everett step together, tentatively put their arms around each other in a tingly, loose embrace, and rock. This is the most they have ever touched.

Timmy is trying to figure out where to hold Claire. His curiosity about how hard or soft her breasts are is becoming irresistible. His right hand accidentally brushes her bra strap, as his mind reels.

Max sticks with the deejay.

However fleeting, the preteen contacts among children will move their sexual development one important small step forward. For the first time they may experience sexual arousal in a romantic context. Any sexual experimentation that takes place now will have a substantially different quality from that of earlier preadolescent sex play. Three key elements of sexuality—sexual arousal (attractions leading to erections and lubrication), sexual behavior (looking, touching, and showing), and romantic relationships—have begun to link up.

Social forces, while perhaps the most important factor, are not the only stimulus for the new erotic adventures of preadolescence. Hormones are also beginning to have their say.

At twelve, Eloise is one and a half years into puberty. Her peers, on average, began puberty at age ten (with a typical range of six or seven to thirteen). Eloise's puberty started with what is called breast budding and then the arrival of pubic hair. She shot up a few inches and began to use deodorant. Over the last several months, her breasts have been growing a bit. Eloise has considered wearing a bra largely because Claire told her about her own. As the most noticeably developed girl in the seventh grade, Claire has received some distinctly unfunny attention from the boys. Eloise quietly considers Claire's endowment both enviable and unfortunate.

Still, Eloise is some months away from the Saturday afternoon when, alarmed but composed, she will call for her mother through a closed bathroom door. Menstruation typically begins about two years after the onset of puberty, on average just before a girl's thirteenth birthday.

Staring blankly into the punch bowl, Max is not too far into puberty. Boys tend to start puberty about a year after girls, at an average age of eleven (the typical range is nine to fourteen). Max is already developing larger testicles—which he hasn't noticed—and body odor—which Tim has (especially tonight).

Over the next year or so, he will get the first signs of pubic hair, a larger penis, and the great surprise of his first ejaculation. Max will reach this last milestone when masturbating in his room with a page of a magazine Timmy tore out for him. Nearly a head shorter than a few of the girls in the class, Max won't hit his peak growth period until he is thirteen, two years after his puberty began.

Once puberty is well under way, both Max and Eloise will experience an increase in their sex drives and, with the development of their genitals, a maturing of the physical pleasure of genital stimulation. For reasons variously attributed to nature and nurture and likely contributed to by both, the sexual drive and behavior of boys get more of a kick in puberty than that of their female classmates.

The quality of children's sexual fantasies during these years is likely to change, too. While Max once masturbated conjuring the vague image of a girl in a bathing suit, he now pictures actual sex acts, like intercourse.

Lingering by the pretzels, Max is thinking about that picture Timmy gave him of a naked woman. He watches the back of Eloise's head. Her hair looks so soft. Max slips a hand into his front pocket to try to hide his bulge. His nose feels strange.

Everett and Eloise lean in, she closes her eyes, he keeps his open, and they kiss (mouths closed). "Is that it?" Eloise wonders as she smiles at him.

Everett smiles back, thrilled that the one thing everyone will remember about the seventh-grade dance is that it was the night he kissed Eloise. In fact, what they will remember is that it was the night Max got a nosebleed at the snack table.

Adolescence (Ages Thirteen to Twenty-one)

There is something undeniably rudimentary about the preadolescent's forays into mating. From here on in, though, things get less rudimentary pretty darn fast.

The slick patch of road in a child's development we call adolescence is about to lurch into view. And when it does, the distant crushes and dating games of middle school will begin to remodel themselves into something that for the first time actually approximates an adultlike sexuality.

"Why? Why? WHY!?!" a parent occasionally inquires.

The prime forces behind this development are two of the teen years' greatest inventions: romantic love and interpersonal sex.

An early adolescent's search for a boyfriend or a girlfriend is partly driven by puberty's increase in sex drive. It is also driven by the typical adolescent's struggle to feel attractive and popular. The social status and the psychological reassurance a teenager gets from a romantic relationship are among its most compelling rewards. In fact, for a while, at least, these may be the most important aspects of dating.

Then, as the song says, the moon hits your eye like a big pizza pie.

Yes, little children feel love. But that special brand of pillow-hugging, you-hang-up-first-no-you-hang-up, falling-in-love kind of love is an exclusive product of adolescence. Teens spend much of their waking hours looking for it, and when they find it, the stick-figure romances they sketched during preadolescence morph into heavyweights.

Suddenly, an adolescent's view of the kid he loves and their future together looks about as realistic as an image in a funhouse mirror. His emotions run five-minute laps around rapture and gloom. And his ability to concentrate in class? What class?

Meanwhile, something new is happening to sex. What was previously a fantasy, a pleasure-seeking game among pals, or a solitary pursuit is now delivered into the setting of a charged, intimate relationship.

When that happens, a teenager is confronted for the first time with the adult ramifications of sexual behavior: responsibility, heartbreak, contraception, and begging.

The complexity of sex just keeps getting cranked up.

This afternoon Max is over at Eloise's. Her parents are both at work. Eloise invites Max up to her room, which he's never seen before, although they have been going out for nine weeks.

At seventeen, Max and Eloise are in love.

They started talking at a party earlier this spring and ended up kissing next to a pile of coats. Now they see each other whenever they can and think about each other the rest of the time.

Max goes to sleep every night picturing Eloise. He masturbates daily with her (and a few other women) on his mind. His friends are cool about his dating Eloise, especially since it hasn't yet interfered with their usual conversations about who's hot and who's not.

Timmy isn't seeing anyone, but Everett says he had sex with two different girls at the same time, a claim that Max actually believes. Perhaps Max believes it because he himself usually tells the truth about what he does. Max told Timmy that after they had been together for a month, he managed to unbutton Eloise's pants. They both undressed a little and touched one another. He didn't mention to Timmy that he was too nervous to go further and stopped before having an orgasm.

In class, Eloise's mind wanders into romantic fantasies in which Max tells her he loves her and the lighting makes her skin look flawless. She also thinks about making out. Max's stopping that night was a relief to Eloise, who has some reservations about semen. This is a matter about which Gita is sympathetic. Gita, who has shown Eloise her birth control pills, had sex twice last summer at tennis camp. Gita thinks Eloise has waited long enough to have sex with Max.

Eloise and Max make their way upstairs into her room. No one else is around. The only sound is the rumbling of a lawn mower next door. Max and Eloise start to kiss.

They are juniors in high school. Eloise is the captain of the math team. Max is going to visit colleges next week. Eloise just got her driver's license. Max wants to be a writer. They haven't yet taken the SATs. They are an average American boy and an average American girl born seventeen years ago in the same hospital on the very same day. They have intercourse.

How is it?

Do they use contraception?

Will he tell his friends?

Could she have gotten pregnant?

Did she feel pressured?

Did he?

Will they stay together?

Did You Say, "An Erection"?

All of this lies ahead of you, stretching out into a hazy future that for the moment remains completely irrelevant. All you know right now is that your belly is sticky, you have to pee, and your little fetus, who doesn't even have a name yet, is already having an erection.

You pull up the elastic waistband of your pants. You slip the ultrasound pictures of the face and the erection into your backpack and head out to the car, wondering what kind of a mother you will be.

One thought settles in: The horse is out of the barn.

Your child, who at this point measures only slightly larger than a sneaker, is already somehow sexual. As the days pass, he will only become more so. His biology will see to that.

It's a strange feeling, not to have had a vote in something this important. Weren't you supposed to determine when your child would discover the world of sex? Wasn't there supposed to be some kind of chip to install in the TV?

Do not despair.

You may not be able to control the inevitable unfolding of your child's sexuality. But your child will still have a lot to learn. Someone is going to have to teach him the words for his penis and what it's up to.

He'll need to know what those feelings are and what to do with them. You can't have a heart-to-heart with a hormone.

Your child will become a sexual person with or without your intervention. But a sexual child isn't enough. You want your child to be wisely sexual, to be healthily sexual, to be happily sexual.

That's where you come in. You are going to teach him.

Chapter **2**

What can you do about it?

GUIDING YOUR CHILD'S SEXUAL FUTURE,

AND THE TROUBLE WITH TALKING ABOUT SEX

RAISING KIDS ISN'T ROCKET SCIENCE. If only it were. At least we know how to aim a rocket.

There's a formula for the mechanics of rocket launching, and it's as plain as force equals mass times acceleration.

What, we would like to know, are the scientific laws that tell you how to raise a child? Say you want to instill in your daughter a healthy regard for her own attractiveness, or postpone her first sexual intercourse until marriage, or reduce the risk that she will get pregnant in high school. How do you know what to do? Is there anything you *can* do?

Science has obligingly opened a small window into the workings of parenting and sex, and a good deal can reasonably be deduced from what shows through it. We'll lay it all out for you in good time, but for the moment we'd like to point out one fact for which there is firm support— a notion to which you may have been optimistically clinging for some time. Parents really can guide their children's sexual development.

Here's what you've got covered.

You have a strong hand in establishing some of the basics of your child's sexual life, like the nature of his self-esteem and the likelihood he'll take risks with his health. Your parenting can improve his sexual knowledge, shape his moral views, and mediate his peers' influence over his decision making. There's even some evidence that you can play a role in delaying the age of his sexual initiation, improving the chance that he will use condoms, and limiting the number of sexual partners he'll have in adolescence. And you're bound to have other realms of influence out there waiting to be proved.

We just can't print the formula that explains how you do it. The hard truth is that there is no Newtonian law of parenting. The best research may explain the effect of a certain intervention averaged out over a large group of families, but the closer you look at how a single parent influences a single child, the murkier the picture gets. Why? Because parenting is the product of a relationship, not a physical law, and while physical laws are coolly consistent from case to case, relationships are wonderfully unruly, idiosyncratic things.

In this chapter, we will take you through the uncertain science of how parents influence their children, sketching strategies for dealing with the issue of sexuality at any age. As you will soon discover, few matters are more ambiguous than the conundrum of talking to your kids about sex. We have devoted most of this chapter to helping you formulate an approach that works for you and for them. When the data run out before the answer is in—as they often do—we will lay out your options, show you what some other parents have done, and give you our best guess as to how to proceed.

What can we say? Shepherding your child through his sexual development will never be as predictable a process as getting a three-thousand-ton space shuttle into an interplanetary trajectory. But look at it this way. At least it doesn't cost $1.7 billion.

What Do You Want?

I've made clear to them that the sequence of events is love, then marriage, then baby. You won't be doing this unless those other things have been fulfilled. Premarital sex? N-O. I want them to at least hold off until they are eighteen. I think that they have to hear that from me.

—*Caroline, on her ten-year-old daughter and eight-year-old son*

I never say you have to wait until you're married, because to me that's not reality. I emphasize the need to be respectful of each

other, and how it is a beautiful thing to share. And I talk about
needing to be old enough to take on that responsibility.

—Monica, on her seventeen-year-old daughter

As you begin to ponder the various ways to parent your child, it makes
good sense to start by wondering what you want to accomplish. There are,
to be sure, a few goals all parents agree on. You don't want your child to contract a sexually transmitted disease (STD). When sex happens, you want it
to be a positive experience. But beyond a few narrow islands of consensus,
you and your fellow parents probably have widely divergent plans for your
children's sexual lives. You might consider an adolescence of celibacy a
missed opportunity. Or you might want to mandate it. Your partner, who
continues mysteriously to possess a will independent of your own, may disagree. And if you're like Caroline, above, who believes both that premarital
sex is always wrong *and* that it may be okay for her children to have it after
they are eighteen—if indeed you are like most healthily complicated people—you may well be harboring a few conflicting aspirations of your own.

So it seems to make sense to pause here, before we jump into the
mechanics of parenting, to answer the not-so-simple question, "What
do you want for your child's sexual future?"

When I got married, I hadn't had a whole lot of sex. But some.
I was active enough—like a typical young woman in the seventies. Well, maybe less than typical, but still I wish it had been
even less. That's one message I will definitely pass on to my kids.
Do less than I did.

—Jennifer, on her twelve-year-old son and seven-year-old daughter

On the one hand, I've told my son, Ollie, he can't force himself
on girls. On the other, I've encouraged him to do *something*
with them. In between that, I leave it up to him. I actually feel
he should do a little more than his parents feel comfortable
with. He should experiment and take his knocks.

—Guy, on his fourteen-year-old son

Much of the health research on parents, children, and sex assumes your top goals are to delay your child's first experience of intercourse (quaintly called the "sexual debut") and to ensure the faithful use of condoms if he or she debuts outside of marriage. From a straightforward public health perspective, the cardinal sexual virtues are not getting sick and not getting (unintentionally) pregnant. These may sound like pretty easy goals to endorse. Then we remember the health educator who would stand up in front of a room full of parents and pose two questions: "What if I could promise you that by the end of your sexual life, you would never have had an STD or an unintended pregnancy, how many of you would take it?" All hands go up. "And what if that was all I could promise about your sex life?"

Obviously, safety isn't the only worthy goal.

Perhaps, like Monica above, your first wish is that your children learn to be emotionally responsible toward their partners, or that they come to see sex as a beautiful act of love. Or maybe you don't want to organize your parenting around any particular outcome at all. Take Guy, for example. Within a fairly broad range of possibilities, he hasn't specified the kind of sexual experiences he wants his son to have or when he hopes he'll have them. What he wants is that Ollie face his sexual decisions in a way that fuels his desire to explore the world and grants him a sense of authorship over his increasingly grown-up life.

Martin, a father with two daughters, doesn't have his eye on any particular sexual outcome, either. For him, maintaining the quality of his connection with his children comes first. "I like to think I will be pretty nonjudgmental about the fact of the kids having sex," he explains. "But the thing that would drive me crazy would be having a feeling that we could no longer talk in the way we do now. I will try to prevent that by being very accepting of boyfriends, and girlfriends, and whatever."

None of these values is absolute. A wish for a certain kind of relationship with your daughter doesn't always trump your hope that she'll avoid a certain type of boy. Nor will your goals as the father of a fifth grader necessarily be the same when he gets to high school. You're developing, too, and your views may well remodel themselves as your children grow. The best you can do is to strive, at any given moment, to articulate to yourself what it is you most want to achieve. And then, of course, you try to achieve it.

How do you accomplish that?

The Nature of Nurture

Over the last several decades, researchers have pieced together a body of knowledge intended to crack the mystery of just how you influence your kids. Among the various elements of parenting that they have studied for clues, one has gradually emerged as a major player in the story: parenting style—or the nature of nurture.

In their efforts to define parents' styles, researchers have focused on two traits all parents express to differing degrees: demandingness and responsiveness.

Demandingness refers to setting high standards for children's behavior, making those expectations clear to them, watching closely to see how they behave, and enforcing the rules when kids slip. As Cora explains, "I'm a big one about raising the bar of expectation. If you set it low, that's where they will go. But if you set it high, I think kids will rise to the expectation."

Responsiveness, on the other hand, refers to tuning in to your children. Responsive parents listen carefully and recognize their kids' individual qualities, involving themselves in their kids' lives. They are loving, warm, and supportive. Take Stan, whose daughter is in high school. "I would say I have much more of a friendship with her than my parents had with me. We do things together that I only do with her. I talk with her about problems I am having with people at work, and she tells me about people who are difficult for her in her life. There's a lot of love and affection and cuddling."

If you accept the proposition that demandingness and responsiveness are two essential elements of parenting, then it's not so hard to get to the notion that there are four kinds of parents: those who exhibit a lot of one or the other, neither, or both.

Let's look at the four styles.

What Is Sex For?

Reviewing some simple questions may help clarify your wishes for your child's sexual future. Consider answering some of these questions for yourself, and then see how your answers compare to your partner's.

- What is sex for?
- How do you feel about your own sex life so far?
- Would you like your child's sex life to be different from yours? How?
- What makes for a good love relationship? For good sex?
- Can you describe the attitude you would like your child to have toward sex?
- Is it acceptable to have sex outside of marriage?
- If yes, when is the right time to begin having sex?
- In what kinds of relationships should sex take place?
- Do you feel the same about your daughter's sexuality as you do about your son's?

First are the parents who are highly demanding but not very responsive. These parents—all rules and little warmth—are described as *authoritarian.* Communication in these families runs principally in one direction, from parent to child. Expectations may be high, but because the parent isn't well attuned to the child's experience, the rules may be a poor fit for the child's abilities and may be rigidly maintained when they ought to be allowed to bend. The children of authoritarian parents tend to be quite obedient, but their self-esteem is generally low relative to that of other children, they are more prone to emotional problems, and their moral reasoning is less advanced than their peers'.

On the other side of the coin are so-called *indulgent* parents, mothers and fathers who are highly responsive but not particularly demanding of their kids. In indulgent families, a child is warmly attended to, but his misbehavior may pass by without comment, and kids' half-hearted efforts to achieve may garner as much praise as earnest striving and even accomplishment. Children of these parents tend to be social kids with seemingly good self-esteem, but they also can be more impulsive and aggressive than other kids, and they are more likely to cause trouble at school, leading or following their peers into risky activities.

Then there are *neglectful* parents, who offer little in the way of expectations or warmth and seemingly sow as they reap. Their kids are typically the least well adjusted of all.

And finally, at the top of the heap, are the *authoritative* parents, high in both their demands and their responsiveness. Authoritative parents make their expectations clear to their kids, but they also listen carefully to what their children have to say about the rules, giving them a voice in important matters and a certain degree of independence. They definitely step in when a child isn't living up to his side of the bargain, but they remain a warm and comforting presence.

In study after study, the children of authoritative parents outperform all the others in almost every area that matters to parents. They tend to be mature children with high self-esteem who follow the rules but are also self-reliant. As a group, they get along better with their peers than other children, are good at resolving conflicts, and adjust better to school than any of the other three groups of children. It gets better. They earn higher grades, they are less angry, and they are less likely to smoke or drink.

Authoritative parenting is about as close as science has come to offering a recipe for healthy kids.

We don't actually know why this style of parenting is so successful, but it does make sense. Children whose parents love and respect them sense that they matter, and so they take care of themselves. They know what their parents expect, and they try to please them by delivering it, not because they have no choice, but because they sense that that's how the relationship works—through reciprocity. They get good at relationships. And as they do right by their parents and others, they feel even more strongly that they are good people, which further reinforces their instinct to take good care of themselves. You can see just what a power-fully reinforcing system authoritative parenting creates.

What does all this have to do with sex? Well, we don't yet know how the sex lives of these children differ from those of other kids. But it is reasonable to expect that authoritatively reared kids' high self-esteem and ability to negotiate conflicts would serve them well in romantic and sexual relationships. Their maturity may translate into a more thought-ful approach to the responsibilities that go with sexual behavior—like the responsibility to prevent pregnancy or to protect a partner's feelings. It's even possible that their avoidance of practices their parents consider dangerous, like smoking and drinking, could extend to a greater caution regarding sexual risk.

Keeping an Eye Out

I think I know all his friends. I decided to make it easy for them to use our house as their hangout. I'd rather him be home with friends than out roaming the neighborhood. I give them privacy when they're here—they're usually in the basement or the back-yard—but I also bring them food. That's my way in. If I haven't heard from them in a while, I just take a snack to them down-stairs.

—Marivar, on her fourteen-year-old son and his friends

There is another way to look at what works in parenting. Rather than examine an entire style of parenting, you might look at some specific parenting practices that seem to make a difference in the way kids grow up. Watchfulness, or monitoring, is one of these. As it turns out, simply keeping track of where your child is, whom he's with, and when he's coming home can have a fairly substantial impact on what he does while he's there.

Closely monitored children are more likely to do things that please their parents and less likely to do things that don't. In particular, they seem to take fewer risks: They drink less alcohol, they are less likely to smoke, they have fewer disciplinary problems at school, and they get better grades.

The relationship of monitoring to children's sexual behavior is no exception to this rule. The children of watchful parents tend to wait until they are older to start having intercourse and, when they become sexually active, have sex less frequently and have fewer sexual partners.

Watchfulness may be an easy concept to understand, but putting it into practice has its challenges. First and foremost, it takes a lot of work. The ongoing vigilance required can be tough to sustain.

And then there is the booby trap of intrusiveness. In some ways, too much monitoring is as bad as not enough, and various problems are found among kids who experience either extreme. The research on sex hasn't been done yet, but some think overmonitoring may have the opposite effect on sex of what's intended: Children who experience their parents as too intrusive may start having sex at younger ages, perhaps as a kind of rebellion.

You probably can't know in advance how much monitoring is too much, but you should be able to tell along the way. Kids who feel intruded upon generally grouse about it. They don't want to answer your questions about who was on the phone or what everyone was talking about out there in the parking lot (although sometimes it will be important to press for an answer when the stakes are high). If you have a sensitive ear, and the will to work on it, you should be able to tailor your level of watchfulness to your child's evolving needs. As a rule of thumb, it's always fair to ask, as long as you don't require an answer on those occasions when you sense you've trodden upon the tender sprouts of your little one's independence.

Younger children, of course, tolerate closer monitoring, but that doesn't mean adolescents should be cut loose. Watchfulness works well into the teenage years.

The Tie That Binds

Children can also tell you how parenting affects their sexual lives. Imagine sitting down with a group of adolescents and asking them about their parents: Do they like the way their parents relate to them? What do their folks think about sex? And so on. Then ask them if they've had sex, and try to see if the ones who are sexually active feel differently about their parents from the ones who aren't. Do this with about, oh, ten thousand kids, and you have some pretty good data.

When a group of researchers did just that, they found support for one more insight into the way parents influence their children's sexual development. Adolescents who are more satisfied with their relationship with their parents—or who feel closer to them—have less sex.

There have been a number of these inquiries into the relationships between parent-child closeness and teens' sexual choices, and although the question has been asked many different ways over the years, the results have been fairly uniform. Adolescents who feel close to their parents or satisfied with their relationship tend to become sexually active later than children who don't. When they start having sex, they have it less often and with fewer partners. Closeness works for mothers and for fathers, and it has similar effects on boys and girls.

The quality of the parent-child bond may even influence a teenager's use of contraception. In the large study we mentioned, teens who were very satisfied with their relationship with their mother were almost twice as likely to use birth control during sex as those who weren't. A year after they told interviewers how they felt about their parents, the least satisfied teens were four times likelier to have gotten pregnant than the most satisfied. That's a big difference.

How does it work?

As with parenting style and monitoring, it is easier to say *that* closeness works than to answer precisely *how.* But a good guess would pin the effect on your values, specifically the fact that as an adult, your ideas about sex are likely to be more carefully thought out than those of the kids with whom your child hangs out.

The daughter who feels close to you will identify with you more strongly than will, say, her sister who feels distant. Identifying with you means modeling herself, at least in part, on your example. And so your close daughter may base a greater part of her value system on yours, including, for example, your belief that sex is a pleasure that should be tempered with responsibility. Her sister, who feels less close, may give the opinions of her friends greater weight. As she enters middle school, she may be more likely to see sex through their eyes as a novelty, or an adventure, or a ticket to popularity.

Of course, it's also possible something else is going on that explains the research findings—for example, parents may simply feel closer to kids who happen to follow their rules.

If closeness were something you could simply give your child, like a hot lunch or mittens, no kid would go without. Closeness doesn't work that way, because unlike monitoring or even style, it isn't a thing you do. It's a quality that emerges in a relationship through the ongoing interplay of two personalities. In this case, one of those personalities belongs to your kid, so closeness isn't solely up to you. Some kids are easy to feel close to, some are hard, and some pairings just seem to work for no discernible reason other than pure chemistry. Then there's your partner's personality, and your other kids and the roles they play in the family as they compete for closeness and configure the possible routes to achieve it. That warm feeling of closeness with your child, as desirable as it is, can't be dialed up. But it can be worked toward.

Say What?

So: high standards, responsiveness, monitoring, and closeness. All of these sound like good, plain, Norman Rockwell parenting. If there's anything surprising about them, it's that these seemingly generic practices could have such specific effects on your child's sexual behavior. What about more targeted efforts that specifically address your children's sexuality, like talking to your kids about sex?

At first glance, discussing sex with your children would seem to be the most obvious route toward influencing their sexual ideas and habits. For example, it stands to reason that if you thoughtfully discussed contraception with your teenager, she would be more likely to use it and less likely to get pregnant. But, friends, this is where what is reasonable and what we know with certainty part company. At least according to the research that's currently available, the sensible practice of talking about contraception doesn't consistently produce kids more likely to use it. In fact, if for a moment you decided to put aside your common sense and reviewed all of the research into the effects of talking with your kids about sex, one impression would emerge. With some studies supporting it, and others finding no real impact, we don't have conclusive evidence that talking works.

What's going on?

Part of the problem has to do with the difficulty of measuring communication in a survey. When you ask parents if they enforce a curfew for their child, and they say yes, you have a pretty quick and straightforward indicator that they are monitoring him. But when you ask parents if they discuss sex with their child, things get a little murkier. It's harder to know what a "yes" means.

Take a study that tries to connect teenagers' sexual choices with whether they have discussed sexual morality with their parents. It's not too surprising that such a study is inconclusive when both the mother who said, "Sex can be a beautiful thing when shared with someone you love," and the one who said, "If you do it, you're a whore," both get to check "Yes, we discussed morality." Only a detailed interview has a chance at ferreting out the subtle meanings contained in your communications with your children, which makes studying the effect of talking among large-enough numbers of parents to generate solid data terribly, terribly difficult to do well.

Also working against us is the fact that the studies, which focus on outcomes like delayed sexual debut and lower pregnancy rates, have not focused on other potential benefits of talking to your child. If careful discussions about sex with parents made children grow up to be more comfortable with their sexuality, or enabled them to enjoy sex more than their friends, or have healthier relationships or happier marriages, we wouldn't know it. The questions just haven't been asked in a major study.

We confess, we'd *really, really* like to offer you ironclad evidence that talking to your kid about sex works. And when all is said and done, we still think it's an extremely good idea. We just can't prove to you that we're right. And so, if you want to base your parenting choices only on hard-outcome data, we can't give you much indication of what to tell your kids about sex or when to tell them.

So what do you do? You can't exactly wait for science to get around to answering this question, especially if your youngest is raising his reedy voice from the backseat in an insistent query—"How are babies made?"—and you want to give him an answer before he cashes in his IRA.

We're going to construct a responsible answer for you by piecing together what we know about talking to kids about sex with what we believe and what we can logically deduce. To give ourselves a running start, we might as well begin with the parts we are most sure about. And there is at least one thing we can say about discussing sex with your kids with a deep and unswerving certainty:

You Don't Want to Do It

A few years ago, to celebrate Father's Day on the radio program *This American Life,* host Ira Glass gave a college freshman and her father a chance to ask each other anything they wanted to know but never had the guts to ask about before. Chana was filled with questions for her father. Her dad had only one.

"Of course, you know, Dad's . . . one of Dad's mainest concerns is . . . uh . . . is your love life."

Chana laughs uncomfortably. Her father goes on.

"Your . . . uh . . . your situation, you know, with sex and how that situation is . . . uh . . . I don't know how to put it, coming along I guess, you know, or is it a problem, or are you just handlin' it?"

"No it's not a problem . . . um . . . 'course, I'm sure you can just kind of . . . [long pause] . . . I . . ."

"My major concern is your being safe."

"Yeah, definitely."

"Okay."

End of conversation.

Let he who has had an easier time cast the first stone.

Overhearing a sputtering exchange like this may make you squirm, but it doesn't really surprise you, does it? We've spoken with lots of parents on the subject of talking to kids about sex, and we hardly know a soul who actually considers himself good at it. Most people get very uncomfortable, and for many, that fact is reason enough not to do it. Maybe they are right.

Maybe the obstacles that get in the way of these conversations should be respected; maybe your inhibition is a gut instinct that you should obey, and the prudent choice is not to push yourself into deeper discussions about sexuality with your children.

On the other hand, maybe the discomfort that holds you back is a kind of irrational fear that you ought to stare down in the interests of educating your child. Maybe your hesitation to talk about this or that subject at this or that age is no more than trepidation masquerading as insight.

One way to decide whether and when to discuss sexuality with your child is to look carefully at what causes you to hesitate in the first place. If your reasoning seems sound, you may be doing the right thing by keeping quiet. If not, if your inhibitions are based on fears or beliefs you can't entirely explain or defend, well, then you might decide you have some talking to do. Let's look at what holds you back.

Breaking the News

Now, there are different kinds of discussions you can have with a child about sex, and the different talks come with different reasons for not having them. It's an oversimplification, but for the sake of clarity we would break the whole set of sex talks you and your child might have into two main categories: fact-focused talks with younger children and feeling-focused talks with older ones.

In the first category are those talks in which you tell your child some fact about sex or reproduction you suspect he doesn't already know: This is how babies are made. This is what a tampon is. Breaking the news about various aspects of sexuality tends to be the focus of the sex talks you might pursue with preschool-age or elementary school–age children.

Talks of the second sort feel more personal, because they touch on your child's actual sexual feelings and choices: Whom are you attracted to? Have you been talking about having sex with her? Are you remembering to use condoms? These are the conversations you either have, try to have, or avoid having with older children, in middle school and beyond, whom you suspect have begun to explore or at least desire love and sex.

Let's start with the first category—talks about the facts of sex with little kids. Conversations like these typically get sparked by a question about procreation. Your daughter sees a picture of the family before she was born and asks, "Where was I then?" Or you are six months pregnant, dressing for work, and she asks, "Did the baby go in through your mouth?" Quickly, you decide how detailed an answer to give, if what happens in those tense few seconds can properly be termed making a decision.

"When Sarah asked me how babies were made, I told her everything up to the point of how the sperm from the father gets into the mother. I stopped before I got to that. When she asked what happened next, I froze. I looked her straight in the eye and said, 'I forget.' " Peggy is a biology teacher. "I can't believe it! This is an intelligent person talking. I'm sure I just panicked, and I was thinking, 'I have to talk to your father before I answer that question.' But what actually came out of my mouth was, 'I forget'!"

We hear this a lot. However uncertain they may be about answering sex questions, most parents don't consider active deception a viable option (the stork and the cabbage patch are history, it seems). These days, vagueness has taken the place of deceit, and that vagueness seems to hover over one particular part of the baby-making story.

The penis goes in the vagina.

Nina finessed it in the parking lot of a liquor store when her five-year-old daughter and seven-year-old son decided they had to know where babies came from. "I finally told them. I said, 'Well, when two people are married, they get very cozy under the covers. The man has sperm in his penis. And the woman has eggs inside her body. They get very close, and the sperm meets the egg. And together they grow inside the woman's body to make a baby.' That was it. They were satisfied." Nina's kids apparently were in a mood to let their mother off a little easier than Sarah was.

Now, Peggy thinks she was nuts to "forget" about penetration. But Nina definitely believes she was right not to tell her kids about the fact of intercourse. Why? Nina explains: "I think that at this age you don't need to be so specific and graphic. Because, I think that can be a little upsetting." And that's a fairly common belief. Many parents imagine that finding out just how the sperm meets the egg would be disturbing—maybe even damaging—for their children. Sometimes that impression is based on how things went with the last kid.

Tonja explains: "My oldest daughter, Kiki, is shy and reserved. But she's also my little Einstein. She asked me at eight years old when I was pregnant, how does the baby actually get inside my stomach. I was tucking her in. I said, 'Women are born with eggs in their bodies and those eggs can only grow into babies if they are fertilized by sperm from a man.'

" 'How does the sperm get in there?'

" 'The man has sperm in his penis and it goes into the woman's vagina and the sperm come out and go to fertilize the egg.'

"A veil came over her face. It seemed to sort of confirm her worst fears. That was the look I got, so I stopped. I felt I maybe told her a little more than she wanted to hear."

Two years later, when her next daughter turned eight, Tonja asked her if she knew about having a baby. "She was like 'Yeah I know all about it, and it's really disgusting, so you don't have to tell me.' And so, you know what? I didn't. I just said, 'When people love each other, it isn't disgusting.' "

Kids really react this way to hearing about intercourse. They get that look Kiki got. Or they make loud gagging sounds. Some seem to work on it over days, asking a few times, "Did you really do that to make me?" If you're trying to decide whether to relate the penetration part of the story, you have to wonder what these responses mean. Why do kids say it's gross?

It *Is* Gross

Until it's erotic, it *is* gross.

First of all, in their elementary school years, as we explained earlier, children may become particularly modest about their bodies. The idea of showing their genitals to another person is embarrassing. At the very same age, you'll remember, gender segregation is at its lifetime peak. Many girls Kiki's age want to keep far away from boys, and boys feel similarly disinclined to cozy up to girls. Intercourse? When these kids see a man and a woman kiss, they threaten to barf.

Then there is the act itself. If you haven't eroticized the idea of penetration, which most school-age children have not, it presents at the very least an unappetizing image. A person sticks a part of his body into you and then squirts a fluid from the inside of him into the inside of you. Without its erotic sheen, intercourse probably sounds something like: "Well, Billy, when a man and a woman really love each other, they get together very close and the man puts his nose inside the woman's mouth and blows some snot out of his nose into her mouth." If your kid doesn't think it's gross, he wasn't listening.

This is probably what that look on Kiki's face meant. From her eight-year-old perspective, the image of being naked and getting close to a person of the opposite sex is unappealing, and the idea of intercourse is icky. That's all. Gross though it may be, as long as it is something only other people do, she doesn't have to worry about it. And so most children deal with their momentary disgust by vowing aloud or to themselves, "I'm never going to do that." Fine. You can support this idea by telling your little one,

> "As long as you think it's gross, you never have to do it. The grown-ups who have sex only do it because they decided they want to, because it isn't gross to them anymore. Maybe your feelings will change someday, too. But that is a long way away."

Then she has to reconcile the fact that you, who are ideal, had intercourse, which is gross. Some children who get the news from a friend insist that their parents would never do such a thing and leave it at that.

But if your child hears it from you, she may have to think a little harder. Still, there's no reason to think the education is harmful. Depending on her age, she will either work on developing a more mature image of you or of intercourse (hence the questions over the next few days: "Did you really do that?") or she'll table the whole matter until it makes more sense. She will take care of deciding which approach is best for her.

But Will She Get It?

> ARNIE: *I know where the baby comes out. It comes out through the vagina.*
>
> LUKE: *No, it's the bagina.*
>
> ARNIE: *Uh-uh. It's the vagina.*
>
> LUKE: *Bagina. I know, because my mother told me.*
>
> ARNIE: *Well maybe that's what it is on her, but my mother's penis is called a vagina.*
>
> *—Overheard in the backseat of a first-grade carpool*

While you're considering whether your little one can stomach the facts of life, it also makes sense to wonder, "Will she get it?" Perhaps, some parents suggest, if she isn't yet capable of understanding the details, it may be better to wait to tell her.

Let's take a look at this idea as it applies to the mystery of making babies.

Your child's level of cognitive development definitely determines what she will glean about reproduction from a talk with you. For example, children as young as two or three can't yet grasp the idea that something that presently exists might not have existed in the past. They can't wrap their minds around the concept of creation, so when they ask where a baby comes from, they mean *where.* What place was it in before it got here? Your tummy? The freezer? Kmart?

As they get a bit older, preschoolers catch on to the notion that babies are created. Typically, they start by imagining procreation as an assembly process in which infants are pieced together from their parts by grown-ups, just like cars or birthday cakes. By the time they reach kindergarten, children usually understand that babies grow into being like other natural creations. As their ability to think and reason develops during their elementary school years, their comprehension of just how that natural process takes place deepens, until, by age eleven, most American children understand that babies are the result of a developmental process kicked off by the union of an egg and a sperm.

Importantly, while children in all cultures are thought to go through the very same process of cognitive development, and therefore theoretically should be able to understand procreation at the same rate, in some parts of the world children seem to get the facts straight much more quickly. A study of children's sexual knowledge found that while the majority of North American children could give a reasonably accurate explanation of how babies are made by age eleven, the majority of British children surveyed could do so at nine, and the Swedes, famous for their openness regarding sexual education, had the answer down at seven.

Apparently, waiting to tell your child about procreation until you think she will fully understand only delays her ability to grasp the facts. The sooner children hear about the facts of life, the sooner they will be able to understand them.

Timing your talks about sex suddenly becomes much simpler if you accept one basic principle of how children's minds grow. Learning takes place at the edge of understanding. The best way to stimulate your child's intellectual growth is to present him with ideas that require him to stretch his understanding of the world a little. You needn't worry about those facts that are too far over the edge for him to grasp. He will either let them go or reconfigure them to fit his present conceptual abilities. The capacity to ignore information he can't appreciate is one of your child's talents you can count on.

Cognitive science has one other helpful hint for you. When choosing your words, keep in mind that preschool-age and early school-age children don't do metaphor. Little kids' thinking is literal, which means that if you tell them a diaphragm is "like a little wall" between the sperm and the egg, they picture Sheetrock. Animal analogies fare equally poorly; hence the child who had learned about the birds and the bees and who answered a query as to how to make a baby with a helpful,

"Um, get a rabbit." Speaking as literally as your child thinks will give her a better chance of getting your point.

Thou Shalt Not

If you are like some parents, this kind of logical reassurance may not entirely soothe your misgivings. Behind the spoken concern that discussing sex could upset or confuse your child may lie a deeper, unarticulated sensation that sharing these facts is just inappropriate, or wrong—perhaps morally wrong. Where does that feeling come from, and should you respect it?

Recently, in an elementary school assembly hall filled with parents eager to learn about sex and parenting, the first question came from a woman sitting alone near the front of the room. "I want to talk to my first grader about where babies come from, but I'm afraid she will discuss it with the other kids. What should I do?"

What was this parent worried about?

She explained that she was afraid that if her daughter told her friends what she learned, they would then tell their parents, and their parents would be angry at her.

Did she have any particular parents in mind?

No, no one in particular.

Did any of the other parents share her worry?

Absolutely. It was a popular fear.

Was there anyone present who would actually get angry if this woman's daughter told their children where babies come from?

No hands went up. In fact, heads were shaking all over the room.

This concern surfaces again and again in diverse settings. Yet where are all the censorious mothers and fathers so many of us are afraid of? Who are these parents?

It may be that they are our own, and we may fear their disapproval, because we learned long ago how our parents felt about children and sex.

If you are like many parents, you grew up as a child with sexual feelings and curiosities and parents who made it clear such things would not be discussed. It may only have been an inhibition passed on to her by

"Maybe We'll Wait Until He Asks"

Timmy had been asking for a brother or a sister for months. Finally, we said "Guess what?" We told him it was in my belly. He never asked how the baby got there. No, he never asked, so we haven't had to deal with that one! I've been surprised that he hasn't been interested.

—Jean, on her six-year-old son

If you can't decide when it's best to tell your children about sex, or even where babies come from, you might find yourself wondering, "Why don't we wait until he asks?" Waiting for an invitation is, in fact, a popular strategy, albeit one that seems to make more emotional than intellectual sense.

From a pedagogical standpoint, having your child structure his own education is sort of a curious notion. Yes, experimental classrooms had their day in the sun, but these days most parents wouldn't consider waiting until their child asked about spelling or fractions or long division to have his school teach those lessons. It's even harder to imagine waiting for your child to ask what crossing lights are for before telling him to stop at the don't walk sign. Generally, you decide what subjects your child should know, and when, and then you tell him.

Given that there is so little definitive information available on talking about sex, it's not surprising that many parents fall back on the waiting method—especially when saying nothing at all (which is a typical result) can seem safer than speaking too soon. This strategy's popularity is even more understandable when you consider the sense of prohibition that many parents feel about speaking to their children about sex. However old he is, if he's the one who brings it up with a question, you feel you have permission to answer.

The problem is that some kids never ask—or never ask

directly enough to give hesitant parents the unambiguous clearance they feel they need to talk. Moreover, if you feel uncomfortable responding to your children's sexual questions, it's easy to miss them, or to unwittingly deflect them, rather than react in a way that encourages the very asking you feel you need to wait for. In many families, the waiting method can easily turn into a pocket veto of childhood sex talks.

Better to decide what you would like your kids to learn and when, and if they haven't asked by then, teach them.

her own parents that kept your mother from discussing sexuality with you, but as a young child you don't experience your parents' silence on a subject as a sign of inhibition. You experience it as a moral commandment: Parents must not talk to children about sex. However much you may consciously disagree with that position today, commandments from childhood have a way of sticking.

This old inhibition may be one of the sturdiest obstacles to talking about sex comfortably with your children. It is so much easier to surrender than to fight it and speak. But if you stop for just a moment and think about it, without your four-year-old peering up at you and asking how the baby got *in*, you might agree that, as a reason not to talk about sex, the fact that your parents wouldn't probably doesn't deserve the power it wields.

Our Suggestions for Young Children

Having looked carefully into the various objections parents raise about sex talks with young children, we haven't come across one we would endorse. While a certain reluctance to talk about sex with young children is understandable, and the many reasons parents give for avoiding such talks may be heartfelt, there really isn't a clear, objective reason not to tell your children the facts of life in their preschool or early school years. You should feel free to do it without worry.

On the other hand—although it may reflect a lack of research on the topic—we haven't turned up any proof that not teaching young children about sex is harmful. As far as we know, you don't *have* to do it.

But we would. Why? Well, first, we just value learning too much to feel good about withholding information from genuinely curious children. At least from the age of three, your kids are busy formulating their own personal explanations about where babies come from. And if you develop an ear for it, you can hear them asking a stream of questions about bodies and sex. That native curiosity, if it thrives, is capable of transforming their world into a place urgent with wonder. What better way to reward and stimulate it than with a complete, fascinating answer?

Then there is the matter of closeness. Closeness is not only one of the great tools of effective parenting, it is its chief reward. As we see it, the efforts you make, from the toddler years on, to figure out how to talk about potentially tense topics like sex help pave the way toward a deeper and sturdier connection to your child.

So we suggest you push yourself to say a few direct things about sex to your kids. Reading through the chapters that follow will help you address almost any sex-related issue that comes up at home. But to make things simpler, here is an overview. We've divided up your child's home sex education into four lessons, each of which concentrates on one type of learning, and we've assigned each lesson to an age range we think best suits it. Any of these lessons can be started earlier than we've indicated, but we don't recommend starting them much later. While the following outlines summarize the minimum you should consider discussing with your child, you can certainly talk about much more.

The first three lessons focus on the relating of facts and attitudes about sex to preschool-age and school-age children. We will have a few more things to say before we get to the fourth and final lesson, for older kids.

Lesson One: Your Body (Birth to Age Four)

We have had many erection talks. It is still shocking to see a tiny little baby with an erection. Recently, he said, "Hey, what's that?" He had never seen it get hard. I said, "That's when your penis gets erect. It feels good to touch it. The same thing happens to Dad." I find when we are really honest with him, he doesn't worry about it.

—Bess, on her two-and-a-half-year-old son

Think of the first four years of your child's sex education as his introduction to his body, with an emphasis on its goodness, on the pleasures of touch, on trust, and on closeness.

Give your children names for their genitals. A boy should learn to name his penis and testicles (or scrotum), a girl her vulva and vagina. Both should learn the difference between boys' bodies and girls' bodies (easy: *"A boy has a penis and testicles, a girl has a vulva and a vagina"*).

The loving way you name and touch your child's body can teach him that all of his parts are good, that physical closeness is both safe and wonderful, and that he is lovable. In all of your child's sexual education, this is the single most important lesson.

Chapter 3 discusses this lesson in detail.

Lesson Two: What Is Sex? (Ages Four to Eight)

Ages four to eight is a good time to teach your child where babies come from. Your lesson should include intercourse, the egg and sperm, pregnancy, and the birth process. For example:

> "When a man and woman (or husband and wife) love each other and they want to have a baby, they get very close. The man puts his penis inside the woman's vagina and when they rub together, sperm come out of his penis and travel into her body. If one of the man's tiny sperm meets one of the woman's tiny eggs, together they start to grow into a baby. The baby grows inside the mother's body in a place called the uterus. When it is big enough to be born, it leaves her uterus through her vagina. That's how you came into the world."

You can clarify that this is something that they won't get to do until much, much later:

"Making a baby is something you only do once you're older/married/grown up and ready for it."

You can explain what having sex is, and include the fact that it's pleasurable:

"When a man and woman rub their penis and vagina together like that, it is called having sex. People do that even when they are not trying to make a baby. Grown-ups who are in love do it because it feels really good, and it's a way of saying they love each other."

If you still have a gnawing feeling that you will be accosted by an angry mother in the school parking lot because your son enlightened hers, we grant you that there are indeed some parents who may not thank you for sparking a sex ed chat in their own home. Should these parents determine how you parent your child? You have to decide. But, as we see it, if you teach your child factual information about a natural life process, you don't have anything to apologize for.

During these years, if you discover your child playing with her genitals, you can acknowledge her pleasure and introduce the notion of the responsibilities that go with this kind of pleasure:

"This part of your body, your vulva (or your penis), feels good when you rub it. That's something you can enjoy, but in private."

Chapter 4 takes up the matter of talking to young children about sexual pleasure and responsibility in depth.

Lesson Three: Expect Puberty (Ages Eight to Twelve)

I have prepared China for things that are going to happen to her body—that they are normal. The other day when we were getting into the car she said, "I don't know why, but I just feel like I am going to cry." I told her to rest and close her eyes. And when we got home I told her, "Your hormones are changing, and they have a very big role in your emotions." I told her about how that happened to me when I was her age. I told her if she is having that, her breasts may start to get sensitive and then she can wear a training bra. She asked about tampons versus pads and how much blood comes out and how many days. I'm trying to explain it all to her in advance. Then I'm hoping she'll just tell her sisters.

—*Janet, on her ten-year-old daughter*

At eight, puberty may be a few years off for your little one, or it may be just around the corner. The less it comes as a surprise for all of you, the better. This third of the major lessons in your child's home sex education is no great mystery. Your task is simply to describe the changes your child can expect from puberty in a positive light before they happen.

The key topics to cover are:

- Menstruation and what to do about it
- Erections and ejaculation, including wet dreams
- What to expect for breast development
- New hair in new places
- Feelings of attraction and other swells of emotion

In speaking of the development of your child's attractions, allow for the possibility that they may be directed toward people of the opposite sex, the same sex, or both. If by this time the opportunity hasn't come up naturally, explain to your child what the words *gay* or *lesbian* mean. Chapter 5 details how to address the facts of sexual orientation with your child. We take up the matter of preparing your child for puberty in depth in Chapter 6.

Which Brings Us to the Older Kids

Your sixteen-year-old has just said goodnight to the last of her friends. Not coincidentally, the last one to leave after an evening spent watching

Some Other Ways to Make a Baby

They don't ask Dave and me too much about sex. The con-
nection between sex and our being their parents is not such
an obvious one. When they've asked where they came from,
we generally say something like, "There was a woman who
was good at growing babies in her body. She started growing
you but wasn't able to be a mommy yet. We were ready to be
daddies, and we really wanted a baby, so she let us become
your parents."

—Richard, on his three- and five-year-old adopted sons

Obviously, not all children come into the world in the same
way. If you didn't use the Daddy's-penis-Mommy's-vagina
method, you should craft an answer to your child's "Where did
I come from?" that fits her particular situation. She can find
out later how other kids are made.

There is little agreement on just how and when to broach
the subject of a child's adoption, surrogate birth, or techno-
logical conception. When it comes to adoption, some experts
have encouraged parents to begin discussing the matter while
their child is still an infant, others have argued for the preschool years, and still others have suggested waiting until the
child can fully comprehend the meaning of his adoption, such
as after the age of eight. As an adoptive parent, you balance
the desire to wait until your child is old enough not to misin-
terpret what you say, with the importance of acting early to
avoid creating a potentially hurtful family secret.

Because it can affect a child's sense of his belonging in a
family, his identity, and his view of his own desirability,
answering the where-did-I-come-from question obviously has
greater ramifications when parenting an adopted child than
simply breaking the news about sex. Much more has been writ-

ten about these discussions than we can do justice to here. The website of the National Adoption Information Clearinghouse (www.calib.com/naic) offers a clear summary of the research with helpful advice for parents and a host of resources for teaching children of all ages.

The issues at stake in families with children born via in vitro fertilization (IVF), gamete intrafallopian transfer (GIFT), donor insemination, egg donation, surrogacy, and so on have been much less well studied. In the case of a technology that uses both parents' gametes, many parents are inclined to leave out the medical details when answering their child's questions. Some parents who use donor eggs or sperm are inclined to do the same, although it seems to carry a greater risk of creating a potential bombshell of a secret. What do you say, though, to a four-year-old who is the product of one of her mothers' eggs, an anonymous donor's sperm, and her other mother's uterus? Here's an explanation offered by the mother in one such family:

"It takes three things to make a baby. A woman's egg and a man's sperm to start the baby, and a woman's uterus for it to grow in. You have to get all three things in order to make a baby."

This sensible introduction seems adaptable to a variety of gameto-uterine permutations. When best to begin the discussion is anyone's guess. As with every other aspect of making a family through unconventional means, you will have to make good use of your creativity. What we can say is that as with the standard way of making babies, our bias is to favor openness over secrecy. With all the various reproductive technologies, telling a birth story before a child can fully understand it seems preferable to explaining things after your little one has assumed from your silence that her birth was just like her friends'.

Casablanca in her room for history class is Fernando, undeniably this season's heartthrob. You are fine giving the two of them a little time alone in her room. And you're not particularly troubled to notice as she walks him to the door that their ears are unmistakably pink, and her hair is sticking up in the back.

Hey, a little exploration is okay with you. But that doesn't mean you aren't in the least bit concerned. So you decide to get a little conversation going, and just lightly touch on her thoughts about what it means to her to get intimate with this guy. You stick your head in her door.

"Hey, how's it goin'?" You're cool. You've actually got a kind of Bogart thing going.

"Fine."

"How's Fernando?"

"Fine."

Talking Points

Some of the little exchanges that, cobbled together, make up these three lessons will fly along smoothly. Some will sputter and die. A few tips on talking may help improve your chances of success.

- If your little one starts things off by asking you a question, give her a pat on the back. A simple *"Good question!"* may help encourage her to keep sharing her curiosity with you.
- Start by clarifying just what it is your child is asking, so you can be sure of answering the right question. Try to get a sense of how much she already knows. For example, if your daughter asks, "What is sex?" you might try:

  "Sure, I can answer that. Sex can mean a lot of different things. Tell me what you heard about sex, so I know which one to talk about."

Or:

> *"Okay. That's a good one. Why don't you tell me what you know first, and then I can fill in the rest?"*

- If, when you bring up a subject for discussion, your child tells you she already knows all about it, don't assume she does. This is an infamous technique used to deflect sex talks with parents. You might ask her,

> *"How would you feel about discussing it again with me?"*

Then listen for her response. If she says she would rather not, talking about *that* may be even more interesting than discussing the point you originally wanted to make.

- Remember that young children's thinking is concrete. Avoid using metaphors that your child might take literally. For example, to the question "What is an orgasm?" try:

> *"An orgasm is a really good feeling you can get from having sex or masturbating."*

It's a better answer than

> *"It's a great feeling you get from sex, like scratching an itch, only better."*

The latter comment may lead your child to believe that all orgasms require scratching (when, in fact, only some of them do).

- You don't always have to know the answer to your child's question. If you don't, say so and make a plan to look it up together. Use a book, search the Internet, or call her clinician. Do so as soon as you conveniently can, before her curiosity evaporates.

- You may know the answer but not be sure you want to give it. If so, tell your child,

  "That's a good question. I want to take a little time to think about what to say, so I can give you a good answer."

  Set a specific time when you will give her your answer, preferably by bedtime that night or the next morning. Remember to follow through.

- Feel free to be authentic in these conversations. If you feel uncomfortable, it's okay to say so. Sometimes a simple statement like the following can actually make it easier to proceed:

  "Wow, for some reason talking about this gets me tongue-tied. I think I get embarrassed sometimes. Do you ever feel that way?"

- Your child may have a harder time recognizing and commenting on her feelings than you. She may feel she has to continue a conversation even if it is uncomfortable—which, of course, she doesn't. If you sense she's freezing up, it may help if you put her feelings into words:

  "Do you feel a little bothered by what I just said? Maybe this is tense to talk about. What do you think?"

- If your child isn't asking you about the sexual topics you want to discuss, try to create a setting that will spark her curiosity.

Visiting a pregnant friend can be helpful. So can looking at pictures of the family shortly before your child was born. A natural "Where was I then?" can get the ball rolling.

- Many books have been written for parents and children of all ages to help teach these lessons. Try them. We recommend *It's So Amazing* for children in preschool and the early years of elementary school and *It's Perfectly Normal* for children ages ten and up. Both books are by Robie Harris and Michael Emberley.

- As the conversation is winding down, check to see if you got your point across. *"Did I answer your question?"* sometimes works. If you really want to check for comprehension, you might try:

    "So if you had to explain this to your sister, how would you say it?"

- Even if your child seems to have understood, expect to revisit any topic a number of times. Many of these lessons need to be repeated often to allow your child to master them.

- Remember in all of these conversations that one chief goal, aside from teaching a fact or two about sex, is building a relationship in which your child feels sexual questions will be accepted and explained.

Yep, you've got a nice light touch. A little dry. A little hip. You're in the room.

"And you two guys, how are you two doin' these days?"

"Dad. Would you mind your own business, if I, like, ask you nicely?"

"Baby, you are my business."

"Dad. I am *not* a baby. Please!"

"Figure of speech! Figure of speech!" You are now walking backward out of the room.

"I have to write in my film journal, okay?"

"I . . ."

Slam.

If anything could make you nostalgic for dilemmas like "Is she too young for the word *uterus*?" this would be it: talking to a teenager about sex. Sex talks postpuberty are just as difficult as they were before, only now the reasons have changed. Now the reasons for not talking seem better.

First, there is the challenge of what you actually should say. At least with a question like where did I come from, or what is this hair doing here, you know the answer. But conversations about sex now are no longer so simple. The focus isn't on easily knowable facts anymore, but on feelings, and rather private feelings at that. Up for discussion is your teenager's tender sense of her own attractiveness, the reactions she's having to the boys or girls she likes, the sex she may be having or turning down, and how she feels about that. If you fall into a discussion of any one of these topics, you may not know just what it is you want to say.

And then there's the matter of how you get the talk going in the first place.

At least with your five-year-old strapped into the backseat of the car, you've got a captive audience. You talk. He listens. But enter the teen years, and the dynamics have shifted.

"The couple of times that I tried to have a meaningful discussion, it's not clear that it really went any place," says Alex, a father with two teenage boys. "In their teenage years, one of the things we've had to reckon with is our inability to construct the conversation. It was easier when they were younger. Now they are controlling the conversation as much as we are."

But you're the parent. Can't you just . . .

"Not unless you want to rant and rave or make a speech. And that's not at all what you want. What you're aiming for is a dialogue, which is not so easy if they refuse."

Now, teens are not globally oppositional people. But when it comes to discussing sex with their parents, they do shut a lot of doors. Why?

Good Fences

Consider your own reactions to the prospect of discussing sex with your teenager.

It's one thing to say, "Sex can be wonderful," to your six-year-old, who is making puke sounds about it in the backseat. It's another to say it to the sixteen-year-old seated up front next to you. You know and she knows that you didn't just read about this in a book. As your child grows older and more sophisticated in her thinking, you may begin to sense that when you talk to her about sex, she sees through to this little truth: what you say is informed by your own sex life.

Suddenly, you feel a little shy.

It's hard to talk about sexual matters authentically without at least acknowledging that you've been there. And that's something some parents just don't feel comfortable sharing with their teenager. Indeed, you may find you have a natural inclination to keep your sexual feelings out of the room when talking to your kids. They may feel the same way.

Paul fielded some personal questions recently from his daughter about his participation in the Summer of Love. But when the fact that he and her mother still have sex leaked out, "she was aghast. We were kind of mouth open about it. What have we raised here? It wasn't just that at sixteen, Kellen seemed shocked to find out. It was that her tone was actually kind of reproachful."

There is a theory about this.

It holds that a parent and a child will try to keep their sexual feelings private from each other, because to share them would raise the fear that something in the way of arousal could pass between them. As children grow older and more sexually developed, and as their sexual appetites strengthen, efforts to prevent this worrisome possibility get stepped up. Talking about sex feels riskier.

Taboo

The nearly universal (some think it's genetically preprogrammed), strongly felt aversion to sexual feelings between parent and child is called the incest taboo.

Parents and kids, the theory goes, conduct their lives in ways to minimize stirring up these troubling feelings of arousal. When was the last time, for example, you tried to picture what your parents did in bed? Habits of modesty and privacy (like the ones we describe in Chapter 3) probably owe a lot to the endeavor to keep any stray arousals away. In fact, the thought of being stimulated by your kids or your parents can be so uncomfortable that those who glimpse even the shadow of such a feeling may well keep it a secret even from themselves. But does that mean the feelings never come up? Psychoanalysts, who spend hours upon hours with patients slowly creeping up on their unwanted ideas, say they do.

Gail, talking about her family of three adolescents, herself, and her husband, puts it this way: "You have to understand, when all of us are in a room together there is a massive incest taboo. I think I could educate someone else's kids much better than my own, because I'm trying to protect my kids from my sexual interest in them. Which is genuinely there. I am awfully aware of that. And so I have to steer away from it. It's a very heated erotic situation."

Gail can express her feelings about this heated situation because she has accepted them as normal and knows she can have her feelings and yet never act on them. But they still affect how she approaches talking about sex with her kids.

"You don't want to talk as if you are seducing your child and telling them stories that will turn them on, and turn you on," Gail says. "You are constantly choosing between being too stimulating on the one hand and being artificially clinical on the other. It's hard to find the way that doesn't feel too puritanical or too prurient."

Your kids may be working under the weight of their own incest taboo. Their aversion to confronting your sexuality may protect them from being aware of their own possible interest in it. This is one way of interpreting Kellen's reproach to her father.

This is not a boundary you want to break down. Your teenagers need to be able to keep a distance from your sexuality, and you should be allowed to keep yours from theirs. One of the lessons you want to teach about sex is that your kids can hold a firm boundary around sexual issues. They can keep their own feelings private, and they can fend off sexual stimulation that they don't want. So sometimes you let them rebuff you if they need to.

A Little Mystery

Passing up detailed sexual discussions with your teenagers may not only help preserve healthy boundaries. It's a speculative idea, but at least a few parents we know feel that keeping a bit of mystery about sexuality may make sex sexier for their kids.

"I always feel that there is some important mystery between us and the kids about sex," Wanda says. "I think it makes the world more erotic. I feel nervous around people who give their kids too much information. It shouldn't be like an anatomy lesson. I think there should be some mystery."

Now this sort of musing is a luxury for those who have completed Lessons One through Three with their children. At those young ages, the compelling need to get a hold of the basic facts runs rings around the possible allure of a little mystery, but come the teen years, some strategic ambiguity may have a place.

This is an idea you've become familiar with through arguments about our seen-it-all society and the lost excitement of a once titillating secret of sex. Author Daphne Merkin recently revisited the subject in the *New York Times Magazine,* writing, "The power of secrets is that they are natural aphrodisiacs, conjuring rooms we have not yet entered, erotic mysteries we can only guess at."

You see parents tiptoeing around sexual topics all the time, of course, although we doubt many parents intend it as an aphrodisiac. Sex is discussed at home with a wink and a nudge. "There is a huge amount of code," one father says of his own family. "We joke constantly about sex and in the jokes are embedded the family expectations." And the family secrets.

Our Suggestions for Preteens and Teens

At some point, you may decide that the boundary around your teenager's sexuality, whatever its benefits, should be crossed. Because at some point you start to worry about STDs and pregnancy and your child's tender feelings. Or you want to make sure she's heard your views of right and wrong.

Once middle school begins (and even a little sooner if you like), we believe you should have some talks about sexuality. In these talks, you might try to set a course between, as Gail put it, the too prurient and the too puritanical. Your discussion needn't be the somber anatomy lesson that lays everything bare. Nor should it be a steamy thumbing through of your own sexual stories or theirs.

Be clear about the dangers you want them to understand and the means of protection you expect them to use. In the interests of monitoring, ask your kids if they are being safe, but try also to leave them their privacy. "Are your condoms made of latex?" is fine. "Do you prefer the ribbed ones?" may be a bit much.

"With Ryan I went through a truncated version of what I thought he needed to know," Christian recalls, "truncated because it was clear he was just waiting for me to get done. 'Do you know the dangers, and do you know what you need to do to avoid them?' was the main thrust of it. I found a way to let him have the conversation without him having to commit to whether or not he was already sexually active. I thought he wasn't, and I didn't want to wait until he was."

The mounting aversion to talking about sex that many kids feel as they grow older, whether due to the incest taboo, their need to assert independence in many aspects of their life, or a sense that their parents will be judgmental, is one reason we encourage you to teach them about sex early. Do it when they're younger and your comments about guys who might try to manipulate your daughter aren't taken as a verdict on her actual boyfriend. If you start early, you'll also have a foundation on which to build that may make occasional conversations as she ages more natural and less charged.

If perspiration has begun to bead on your forehead in anticipation of the talks that will constitute Lesson Four, you might console yourself by considering what you don't have to discuss with your teenager. You don't have to tell him about your own sex life, even if he asks. You don't have to describe the details of sex acts and how best to perform them.

Who Does the Talking?

(a) Mom, (b) Dad, (c) none of the above

My husband, Sam, is so sweet with the girls. He is such a hands-on Dad. But when it comes to talking about sex, he's of the talk-to-your-mother school. I used to dream that he would go out and buy them a bouquet of flowers or make a beautiful toast when they first got their periods. But, I've got to say, I don't think it's going to happen. He would just want to crawl under the table.

—*Sheryl Lee, mother of three girls*

When it comes to talking to their children about sex, mothers are much more likely to talk to their daughters than to their sons, while fathers more often teach the boys.

One study found that while 78 percent of mothers discussed birth control with their daughters, only 35 percent took up the topic with their sons. But fathers didn't make up for their sons' sex-ed gap—only 31 percent of fathers in the study had discussed contraception with their sons. Even fewer had discussed it with their daughters. The figures were similar for discussions of sexual morality.

As a result of this division of labor, boys are much more likely than girls never to have discussed numerous aspects of sex with a parent.

You don't even have to find out the details of what your kids are doing sexually or, as Christian discovered, if they've even had sex—unless troubles arise, in which case you might well press for them.

When you talk to your teenager, you don't have to sound like a sex educator. You don't even have to appear entirely comfortable, if you aren't. All you need to do is get the key points across, show you care, and make yourself available to listen and respond to your child's thoughts.

Lesson Four: Safety, Responsibility, Pleasure, and Choice (Ages Twelve and Up)

Now is the time to pull out your answers to the value questions we asked at the beginning of the chapter. The object of this lesson is to find a way to let your children know what you consider the standards by which they should conduct themselves sexually. At a minimum, hit these two key topics:

- *Sexual ethics.* You'll need to say a little about your philosophy of sex, such as what you think it's for, and what is good about it. If you feel there are certain conditions under which sex is or isn't acceptable (before a certain age, outside of marriage, and so on), explain them. Make it a discussion and invite your children to tell you their thoughts. Let them know that you expect all of their sexual behavior to be respectful and consensual.

- *Sexual protection.* You'll need to express your concerns about the risks of STDs and unintended pregnancy. Say that you expect them to use a latex (or plastic) condom every time they have vaginal or anal intercourse outside of a long-term monogamous relationship. Make sure they know how to get condoms and how to put them on, and that condoms sometimes fail. Tell them there are alternatives to intercourse that are much safer. Tell them that oral sex is indeed safer than intercourse, but not risk-free, and tell them how to reduce the risk from oral sex. You needn't walk them through the details of sex beyond that.

Of course, if you are invited in, there is much, much more about sex and love that you may profitably discuss during these years. You may find your way into conversations about your teens' dating dilemmas, their feelings about particular boys or girls, their opinions about what other kids are doing sexually, and more. Perhaps you know these discussions. They are the very fabric of a close parent-child bond that makes this whole enterprise meaningful.

The subjects of this lesson are covered in depth in Chapters 7 through 12.

Sexual Abuse Prevention

Part of me worries we're going a little crazy about all this sexual abuse stuff, and part of me worries that thinking we've gone a little crazy is burying my head in the sand. You tell me.

—*Sylvie, mother of two*

We can't end a chapter on how to pursue your parenting goals without addressing an aim all parents share: You want to protect your child from sexual abuse.

Childhood sexual abuse is a genuine risk, though exactly how great a risk is hard to say. A 2001 U.S. government report estimated that one hundred thousand children are sexually abused each year. Can you protect your child?

If you are like many parents, the question probably triggers thoughts of a good touch/bad touch talk with your little one. Chances are you've been informed that teaching your child to recognize and refuse sexual advances will lower her risk of being abused. This seemingly straightforward assumption was popular enough to have led by the early 1990s to the implementation of school-based prevention programs in the majority of American public elementary schools. A generation of children has been taught, starting in preschool, what sexual abuse is, how to stop it, and how to report it.

Unfortunately, we don't know if these programs work. While some research has been done on the matter, no one has yet been able to demonstrate clearly whether teaching kids about sexual abuse reduces the likelihood that they will be abused. There are some good reasons to doubt that it does. However much they know, for example, little kids just don't have that much power over abusive adults. Short of preventing abuse, it could be that these programs reduce the distress of kids who are abused, but the best chance they have of helping children seems to be in the area of reporting. There is some evidence that teaching kids about abuse increases the chance that they will tell someone if it happens to them, which can get them removed from the situation and treated faster.

We also don't know what other effects these classes have on the sexual future of the children who take them. Some worry that when young children's principal introduction to their genitals is through a lesson about dangerous bad people, their relationship to their own sexuality may be contaminated by fear. We simply don't know whether these classes affect a child's feelings about his body and his own sexuality, his experience of physical affection from adults and peers, his youthful sexual play and exploration, or the unfolding of his sexual relationships in adolescence and early adulthood.

If your child's school is going to provide an abuse prevention program and you haven't already taught him about his genitals, it's a good idea to do so before the program begins (we'll say more about this in Chapter 3). You can also go to the school to check out the curriculum and see if you're comfortable with it. Talk to the teacher if the lesson seems overly alarmist. And if you think the class would be too disturbing for your child, have him sit it out. If he takes the class, talk about it at home before and after the fact and minimize any fears that may have resulted.

What should you be teaching your child about abuse? Our recommendations follow.

Words about Abuse

One thing I say to them is any grown-up who tells you to lie to me is a bad guy, and that kind of covers a lot of things. It's always okay to tell on a bad guy, I say.

—*Dana, on her seven-year-old daughter and six-year-old son*

Once in a blue moon one of them will grab my penis when I'm in the shower with them or dressing. I'll say, "That's mine. You don't touch someone else's unless you ask them first, and it's got to be a friend. And if an adult ever does that to you, you say no, and come and tell us."

—*Stuart, on his three- and six-year-old sons*

When they're seven or younger, you don't need to give your kids a specific talk on sexual abuse. Sexual abuse is thought to be less common during these ages than later, and if there are negative effects of these talks—teaching your kids, for example, to fear adults or their own genital play—we would expect those risks to be higher for the younger ones.

You can address the subject without much detail as Dana and Stuart did above. Any lessons, like theirs, are probably best done in a fairly off-hand manner without urgency or fear in your voice. You can start with Dana's lesson that people shouldn't tell them to lie to you. Then explain that if anyone other than Mommy, Daddy, or their other caregivers touch their genitals, they should tell you.

By the time they're eight, when sexual abuse may be a greater risk and kids' relationships to their own bodies are better established, the potential benefit of improved reporting seems to better outweigh the risk of frightening your child. During these years, we suggest you teach a few lessons focusing not on your children protecting themselves from abuse, which they still aren't likely to have the power to do, but on recognizing and reporting it when it happens.

Tell them about abuse:

> "It's wrong when an adult, even someone you know, touches your vulva/penis or asks you to touch his penis/her vulva. It's also wrong if another child touches you this way and you don't want it to happen. The only exceptions are if your father/mother or I are washing you or checking you when you're not feeling well or if the doctor is examining you."

(If there is someone else—like a nanny—whom you trust with your children, you can include her as an exception, too.)

Does your child understand? You can check with some follow-up questions:

> "Is it wrong if a grown-up like a neighbor asks if he can give you a bath and wash your penis?" "Is it wrong if another adult wants you to touch his penis?"

And so on. Then focus on reporting:

Sex Ed at School

Of course, abuse isn't the only sexual subject your children will be learning about at school. What you will probably want to do, and what we recommend, is to look over your kid's entire sex ed curriculum, reading the syllabus and flipping through the textbook, even talking with the teacher.

If you find the program is excellent, breathe a sigh of relief, but don't stop there. Going over your child's homework and asking what the teacher talked about will reinforce the material. It will also give you a chance to share your values and perspectives on sexuality. You can provide a personal context for the basic facts taught at school. If the school presents information and options in a nonjudgmental manner, leaving it to students to determine the most appropriate choices for themselves, you can play a big role in helping your child figure out what is best for her.

But what if you find the program omits important material or presents views you disagree with? Then you've got your work cut out for you. You can teach your child about sex, love, decision making, responsibility, and any number of topics, as we've recommended throughout this chapter. You can also share why you disagree with what the school is teaching, and use the opportunity to teach him to question what he learns and to think for himself. You can give your kid books and videos to supplement the school's, and you and your child can surf the Internet together to find additional resources.

You can also advocate for changes at your kid's school. You may be able to convince a teacher to adjust the lessons, but for any significant change, you will probably have to talk with the administration. Keep in mind that the teacher and the principal may agree with your concerns but lack the power to implement a change. Sex ed policies may be decided at the school district or state level.

"If anyone ever touches you like this, I want you to tell me. I promise never to be mad at you if you tell me. It is never okay for someone to tell you that you have to lie to me or keep a secret from me about something like this. If you tell me, I will take care of you no matter what they say."

Finally, lessons on abuse can be repeated and linked with other less troubling points about sexuality, in the way Stuart reminds his boys in a few sentences to report abuse, respect others' boundaries, and keep sex play among friends. Reassure your child that it is very unlikely that she will ever be sexually abused. Because she can't prevent it, there is no clear benefit to having her worry about the possibility.

Then keep your eyes open.

If someone in the family is going to worry about sexual abuse, we'd rather it be you. There are no data on whether your caution can actually reduce your child's risk of abuse; the common sense intervention of careful monitoring just hasn't been tested. But we recommend it.

Talk with the adults who take care of your child. Make surprise visits. Listen carefully to your kid's comments about the grown-ups in her life. If you turn up anything suspicious, investigate it to your complete satisfaction.

Bear in mind that adolescents can be sexually abused as well. When your children are older you can refresh this lesson with them.

Parenting by the Book

We recently noticed a public service announcement that put a caption like "If only they came with an owners' manual" under the photo of a young girl with the words "Tell me you love me" or some such phrase printed on her arm. Have you seen it?

This ad raises a lot of questions, such as who would write this manual? How would they know what to say? And if it took a tattoo on her arm to remind you to tell your kid you love her, would she think you meant it?

What would prevent her from crossing it out and writing "Raise my allowance"?

If someone could work out these bugs, a good set of operating instructions would be such a relief. If you could know what actions of yours led to which outcomes for her, it would be much easier to decide what to do at any given moment with your child. We've been on the lookout for information like this for a long time. This chapter and all those that follow record what we found.

But, of course, they're not enough. Research can never completely answer the question "What should I do now?" because research doesn't address the specifics of your five-year-old, and the struggle you two have been having, and the fact that you're pregnant by his stepfather when he asks, "Where do babies come from?" (which in this case may mean, "Are you getting a replacement baby like you got a replacement husband?"). Scientific predictions of parenting effects must be general by nature. But your choices of what to do or say will always be exquisitely specific, and those specifics will determine how your responses work out. Which is why there never will be a scientifically certified owners' manual for parents.

The good news? You get to decide what to do.

The bad news? You get to decide what to do.

We intend to help. In the chapters that follow, we will walk you through as many parenting challenges related to sex as these pages and your interest will allow. We will explain as best we can what's known about your child's behavior, lay out the various options for your consideration, and help you understand the possible ramifications of those choices. As a strictly scientific primer, this book is no match for, say, NASA's space shuttle manual. But suppose it was. Suppose a vast leap in the scientific understanding of parenting enabled us to draft a complete set of instructions for raising your child. Imagine that you could have those instructions at just the perfect moment, with the answer you need neatly written on your kid's left arm.

What sort of parent would that make you? A parent who never made a mistake? Who never learned a better way of doing something than the first time she tried? Who didn't have to discover by relating to her child what he actually wanted or needed, but knew already?

Now *that* would be a perfect way to really screw up your kids.

A Special Note to Grandparents

If you are a grandparent or some other member of the family with a close relationship to the little ones, much of what appears in this book applies to you, too. You can provide your grandkids guidance, love, support, and wisdom.

Share your values. Although your grandchildren may laugh at your "old-fashioned" view of the world, they might later be amazed at how remarkably contemporary you sound. If relations with their parents grow strained, you may be able to serve as a safe haven. (It has been tartly observed that children and grandparents get along so well because they share a common enemy, the generation in between.) They may turn to you one day as the only one they want to cry to.

"My grandmother taught me about sex. My mother never said a word," Maeve says. "My grandmother sat me down one day and taught me the birds and the bees. It was so interesting hearing it from her perspective. She spoke from the perspective of someone looking back over her life who understood what was important and what wasn't."

Part II

Your Child's

Sexual Development

Chapter 3

All in the family

NUDITY, MODESTY, LOVE, AND SEX AT HOME

IN YOUR CHILD'S EARLIEST YEARS

YOU HAVE JUST STEPPED OUT of your first long shower in a week. The kids are downstairs with their father, and no one seems to be screaming. Peace in our time, you think, closing the bedroom door behind you.

You stand in front of the mirror, toss your towel on the bed. How are those breasts doing?

Not bad. A few months after weaning, and they are back to their old selves. In the past, the word *pert* has been used, not inappropriately, to describe them. ("Pert and Ernie," your mirthful husband once dubbed them.)

You swivel to check on your behind. Oh, well. At least it's in the back, so you don't have to see it.

The sun is pouring through the window, and strains of Helen Reddy begin to filter into your mind. As you inspect your thighs, you start to hum "I Am Woman." You get louder when you reach the "Yes, I am wise" part where Helen really opens up.

You let it rip.

YES I'VE PAID THE PRICE, BUT LOOK HOW MUCH I'VE GAINED.

IF I HAVE TO, I CAN DO ANYTHING!

You are prancing in the mirror now.

I AM PERT. (PERT.)

I HAVE A SAGGY BUTT. (A SAGGY BUTT.)

I AM WOMAN!

There is a rustling in the blankets. You spin around to two wide eyes blinking at you from under a sheet. You pluck back the covers and reveal your uncharacteristically speechless five-year-old son, grinning uncertainly.

"Boo?" he says.

"But It's Wisdom Born of Pain"

Some people think matters of sex first enter family life when kids hit puberty. These people have not recently tried living with a five-year-old. If you have, you know that during your children's first several years, from infancy to the middle of grade school, there is a lot going on at home that involves sexuality—theirs and yours.

Will the kids bathe together? What if they walk in on you? What do you say when your son squeezes your breast, and how much of what you don't say shows on your face anyway? If you have little ones at home, you confront questions like these every day. And your decisions, added up over time, help shape your children's development. Over the years, encounters with you will teach your children how to interpret their bodies, how to understand their evolving sexuality, and how to love.

In this chapter, we will examine the aspects of home life that involve your young child's sexual development. We will look at some of the decisions you face, and we'll lay out, as much as science permits, the possible effects on your child of various choices. As for those situations that don't seem to offer a choice, we'll fill you in on what's happening so that you can at least maintain some degree of composure.

Because, as we see it, if you get caught naked talking to your breasts and singing "I am pert" into a hairbrush by a startled five-year-old, you're going to need all the composure you can get.

Very Touching

When I was a little girl, I watched a mother cat give birth. I remember watching her lick the kittens clean. She licked them into life. That's what I think you do for your kids. You wake them up into their body and into life.

—*Eleanor, mother of a twenty-month-old son*

You have just given birth. What's the first thing you want to do?

Okay, after you vow never to let yourself be talked into doing this again, what's the next thing?

You want to touch your baby.

Getting to hold a baby is one of the great all-time perks of parenthood. In fact, the wonderful feeling of cradling an infant in your arms probably helped lure you into the birthing room in the first place. Lucky thing cuddling your baby is a pleasure, because it also happens to be essential to his physical and psychological development. Babies who aren't touched can't grow.

But what does touching have to do with your child's sexual development?

Well, the moment you first take him in your arms, you invite your baby into his first physical relationship, his first experience of love, and broadly speaking what passes between you two will set the stage for all of the loves that follow. When you cuddle and tickle him, you teach your baby that he can take in pleasure through his body and through close relationships with other people. If all goes well, he will continue to seek out experiences like these for the rest of his life. If not, as in the case of babies who are terribly deprived of human touch and warmth, there can be trouble. There may be no need to say it, but we'll do it anyway: you will be doing your little child a great service if, in the first months and years of his life, you enjoy him. Playing sweet games with each other and gazing into each other's eyes turns out to be a big part of the sex ed of infancy, and boy, is it easy to teach if you simply let yourself go.

There is also a more specific lesson about love and sex you can give through the way you touch your baby.

Answer this if you can: Do you feel the same about touching every part of your child's body, or does it feel a little different to touch his penis? Perhaps, like some parents, you are slightly less at ease when touching your infant daughter's vulva than, say, her tummy. If you are, you might find that you tend to limit the times you touch, or refer to, or even look at your child's genitals. That's another way touching turns into sex education. For some children, their parents' tendency to touch or not to touch their genitals teaches them the first lesson they'll learn about their sexuality.

Eleanor caresses her twenty-month-old son a lot. And when they are playing, she makes it a point to name and touch his penis as often as she does his other body parts. "I want him to get to know his own body," she says. She bases her practice on the notion that small infants and toddlers like Nate are busy constructing mental maps of themselves and their bodies. To selectively ignore one body part such as his penis might deny it a well-deserved place on that map. To treat it with tension or discomfort could affix the label *bad* to that particular location.

Many of those who study child sexual development would agree with Eleanor. It is no small feat for an infant or a toddler to make sense of his genitals. They are usually hidden under a diaper, and he generally doesn't get to see other people use theirs. This challenge may be greater for girls, who have more difficulty than boys in seeing all of their genitals. Some scientists maintain that to habitually guide a girl's exploration away from her vulva, or to avoid touching or referring to it yourself, risks distorting her body image.

Naming Names

If touch teaches your infant that she has a body, words teach your toddler what you and the world—the world of rules and language—think of it. During her first few years of life, as your child learns the names of the objects around her, they come into existence for her in a new way. This is as true for her body parts as it is for the animals in the alphabet book and toys on the shelf. So, you might want to give some thought to the words you'll use for her . . . thingy.

Most parents ultimately discover that language is not entirely cooperative in the effort to name a child's genitals. As we see it, the thoughtful American parent has several options to choose from. She can sling locker-room lingo, speak Latin, offer general directions ("down south"), or resort to one of a host of terms that sound better suited to snack foods.

"Hi, honey, did you wash your woowoo? Your hoho? Your winkle?"

Some parents, out of genuine discomfort with these four options,

Privates on Parade

vulva

In common usage, vagina has come to mean the whole female genital. If your daughter says vagina, she will no doubt be understood by others. But, if you don't mind bucking the trend in favor of anatomical accuracy, consider teaching her vulva. It has a nice ring to it, and it happens to be the correct term to describe the entire collection of labia, vagina, clitoris, and mons pubis—the small pad of flesh that sits looking down on it all from its perch on the pubic bone.

vagina

Shaped like a collapsible tube, the vagina runs from the cervix (the neck of the uterus) on the inside to the labia on the outside.

Sure, it's hidden, and it's dark down there, but let's not forget that it's through this prodigiously elastic organ that most of humanity has passed (a *much* better record than the Bermuda Triangle).

labia

This is the word for the vulva's inner and outer "lips." Anyone who says a girl's genitals aren't visible isn't looking at these. The outer labia are referred to as the labia majora, the inner as the labia minora. Both sets of labia contain erectile tissue and swell during sexual excitement.

clitoris

She won't be able to see it without a mirror, but she can feel it. Your daughter can learn that her clitoris is the part that feels especially good, found just behind the place where her labia meet in the front. Only the top third, called the glans, is visible. The rest is submerged, looking like a tiny rocket with a narrow body, two long tail fins stretching back behind it, and only its nose poking up through the skin.

The clitoris varies in size among girls and grows as they grow. It also doubles its size with stimulation. With a higher concentration of sensory nerve fibers than the lips or the fingertips, the clitoris is famously the only organ in the body whose sole function is to feel pleasure. Nice work if you can get it.

penis

Well, the penis doesn't really need a publicist, does it?

After all, it seems to bear the one genital name that kids and parents commonly use. And, although it is sometimes derided as a bit of a numbskull, the penis is typically regarded with a mixture of humor and respect that seems just right for this bouncy pleasure seeker.

The penis has parts, which you can point out to your child if you like. They are, quite simply, the body and the head, or glans. (See our discussion of circumcision in this chapter for some thoughts on the foreskin.)

testicles (aka testes)

If you thought the male genitals were all about fun, consider the testicles, the slavish workaholics of the masculine endowment. Even before your son is born, these little organs have begun their lifelong chore of pumping out testosterone, the hormone responsible for growing male genitals in utero, deepening the voice in puberty, and pounding the dashboard in adulthood.

As if that weren't enough, the testicles, operating on the principle that more is more, manage to create millions of wriggling, blindly ambitious sperm every day from puberty to death. Millions! Every day! At 40 million sperm per cubic centiliter, semen is so packed with this testicular bumper crop that if sperm were people, one good orgasm could populate Japan.

scrotum

This is the sack in which a boy's testicles reside, but it is no mere passive receptacle. It has its own muscle, the cremaster, which serves to pull the testicles up and out of harm's way. Dads: Remember the last time you waded into cold water?

urethra

Tell your children that this is what their urine comes out of. Boys will have no trouble seeing its opening in the glans of their penis. A girl will be able to see hers with a mirror—it's between the clitoris and the vaginal opening. Her urine, you might point out, does not come out of her vagina.

If you want to be really precise, "urethra" is the name for the narrow tube that carries urine from the bladder to the world outside. The proper name for the opening itself is "urethral meatus."

Please call us if you can get your kid to say this.

anus

Both boys and girls should be able to use the word anus to refer to the narrow, muscle-lined passageway out of (or into, depending on your point of view) the large intestine. ("Rectum" actually refers to the very last part of the intestine that ends as the anus begins.)

buttocks

There are so many fun names for this amiable body part. We all know buttocks is correct, but who can resist the sassier "butt," or the more endearing "tush"? Even the geographic "bottom" will get you to the right location. Unlike the other, perhaps subtler, private parts, whatever you call the back-of-your-front, it's hard to miss what it's all about. So why not let your kid go?

plead the fifth. They avoid naming their children's genitals at all. Girls, it seems, are especially at risk for receiving the silent treatment. A recent study of children between fifteen and thirty-six months of age found that while 95 percent of the boys had been taught the word *penis,* only 52 percent of girls had been given a specific name for their genitals. Forty percent of girls were given no word at all. In fact, girls were more likely to have been taught the name for boys' genitals than for their own.

Of the available ways of referring to your child's genitals, not naming them at all is one we would strenuously advise against. Young children need words not only to talk about themselves but, perhaps more importantly, to think with. Wordlessness significantly limits a child's ability to understand her body.

What about the other options?

After silence, our least favorite are the mysterious location euphemisms. Words like *bottom* or *down there,* when used to refer to genitals, cloak a girl's entire sexual and excretory endowment in a dense fog (the Bermuda Triangle comes to mind). The popular but vague *private parts,* when it's the only term she learns, seems to us similarly unhelpful in unveiling for her the secrets of a child's body.

Locker-room language at least has a kind of earthy directness to recommend it, but frankly, despite their appealing barnyard referents, we can't quite imagine teaching our children to say cock or pussy, let alone some of their coarser companions. This is really the language of hot sex talk, on the one hand, and of open aggression, on the other.

Which leaves us with *Gray's Anatomy* or Twinkies.

Cute words for genitals, breasts, buttocks, and so forth are fine as long as they are used alongside a thorough education in their "official" names. Pet names, like wiener and willie, have the distinct advantage of making genitals sound like fun things you wouldn't mind having attached to you. Still, these words can be awfully misleading. *Milkers* drains breasts of their sexual feelings, while *hooters* suggests that when you grow up you could teach them to call a square dance.

Which is why, whatever pet names you occasionally use, you should also school your kids in the anatomical words that go with them. When should these words be taught? No age is too early to teach a child the names of his own body parts. We typically teach children language before they can use or understand it, and these words are no exception. As for the genital names of the other sex, you can teach them as soon as the subject comes up, such as when she asks you or when she sees someone naked at home.

In the accompanying list of the best anatomical terms to teach, you'll notice we don't stop at one word for a boy and one for a girl. We recommend you give your child names for each of the key parts of her genitals. Being able to distinguish these components is immeasurably helpful to your child as she tries to learn how her body works. The more specific the language you teach her, the more specific will be your child's appreciation of her genitals, their feelings, and their functions. At the least, toddler girls should learn vulva and vagina, and boys should learn penis and testicles (or scrotum).

The Naked Truth

Whose idea was it to invite your parents over for the Fourth of July weekend? Your husband's? The parakeet's? Satan's?

"Honey? Lorraine?" your mother intones. "You don't really want them eating right now just before we go to the pool. *Do* you? Lorraine?"

It is 102 degrees.

"How long have they been here?" you whisper to your husband, sounding like a delirious suburban woman who has been held in her kitchen at knifepoint by a wayward band of Brownies for nineteen days.

"One hour and forty-two minutes," he replies with a damp smile. "Hey kids!" He shouts in a desperate attempt to distract you from violence. "Let's turn on the sprinkler!"

The faucet creaks, the sprinkler gushes to life, and in a flash your four-year-old tosses his clothes into the shrubs and jumps into the spray, naked and squealing.

God bless him. He is still too young to hate weekends like these.

Sitting in a lawn chair, your father sets down his gin and tonic and wrinkles his brow at your wet little boy. In a well-practiced gesture, a pantomime that suggests a camper trying to light a fire, he begins to rub one

index finger over the top of the other. Even now, at thirty-seven, surrounded by the evidence of your upstanding, adult life, and wearing the
most conservative bathing suit seen in your neighborhood since the forties, you feel the cold fingers of humiliation on you.

"Shame, shame, Dennis!" your father crows, squinting and scolding. "Shame, shame."

Ah, yes. One only needs to mention sexuality for thoughts of shame
to sneak their way into the conversation. You learned long ago how the
one seems to travel in tandem with the other, and now your child may
get his own lesson about that pairing, through the world's reaction to his
naked body.

There are as many approaches to family nudity as there are families.
Some do not want to have their children naked anywhere outside the
bedroom and the bathroom. Others are happy to have a seven-year-old
cruise around the house nude except when friends are around. For their
part, children from birth until somewhere between ages four and nine
are eager to see and be seen and are, generally, unaware of any reason to
keep their pants on. What should you do? Should you have them cover
up, and if so, when and where? How will your decisions about nudity
affect your child's feelings about his own naked body?

Your own reactions to your children's nudity probably derive from
a hodgepodge of rational and emotional influences, some recently
learned, some picked up in your childhood, some you're aware of, some
you'll probably never know. Beware: Unconscious motives are rarely reliable instructors. For the sake of your child's sanity, and your own, you
should take some time to consider what norms you would like to establish, and why. The specific rules you make about nudity at home are
probably less important than the way you choose to convey them.

Whatever norms you choose, consider following these three guidelines.

First, try to be as consistent as possible with the norms you have
decided upon, but adapt them as your child grows.

Second, when encouraging modesty, be sure to explain your reasons
in a way that is not shaming. Any limit to a child's happy display of his

form should be conveyed in a way that remains admiring and respectful of his body:

> "Just like with grown-ups, your body is special. Only people who are especially close to you should get to see it now."

The goal is to distinguish your attitude toward his body (always favorable) from your opinion of his showing it in certain situations. Keeping this principle in mind will help you raise a child who is modest about public nudity but not ashamed of his body.

And third, however much modesty you endorse, there should be at least one setting in which your child's naked body is accepted and enjoyed.

With You

As Samantha gets her two little boys ready for their nightly bath, she announces tonight's game: the tickle zone. Samantha's three- and five-year-olds, two rambunctious gigglers, squeal with excitement, and the game begins.

Samantha strokes her chin in mock contemplation. "I've got it!" she says. The two boys start slowly exploring the room, eyeing their mother carefully. Nicky's hand delicately tests the dresser as if it were a hot oven door. "Tickle zone!" Samantha calls out, and chases her shrieking Nicky, delighted to have stumbled into the place Samantha had fixed in her mind. She lifts him up, tickling his little chest to his vast excitement, and yanks off his shirt.

"It's a game I invented to get their clothes off and get them into the bath. They love it."

They sure do. As the game goes on, the boys show more and more skin, and the shivery anticipation of who will find the next tickle zone (they are never sure if they do or don't want to touch it, but they can't resist trying) gets almost dizzying, until, finally, everyone lies in a hilarious heap on the floor and the boys are naked. They toss their clothes in the hamper and slip into a long, warm bath. Partly because of the water and partly because they are exhausted from the day's last and best game, the mood turns gradually, blissfully peaceful.

If you ever heard it said that the seeds of sexuality germinate in the first few years of life under the warm sun of a parent's love, this is what was meant. Samantha's boys are learning about the joys of physical pleasure, by getting naked and being tickled by a mom they adore who looks out for just how much excitement they can hold onto without being overwhelmed. This is how the kind of silly play parents and kids naturally invent starts children on the road that will eventually lead them to grown-up physical love.

Samantha, in a moment of uncertainty, asks, "Do you think it's okay?"

It's more than okay. It's what kids thrive on.

In their toddler and preschool years, if you find yourself setting limits on the time your children can be nude in private around you, if you are unable to play comfortably with them in this way, give it some thought. Your reservations may be a signal of a general unease addressing issues relating to sexuality with your child. Perhaps they are a holdover from the way you were raised. If so, you might not want to pass this inheritance down to the next generation.

Circumcision: Keep the Tip?

We promised we would say something about the foreskin, and since we're on the subject of giving your boy a bath, this seems like a good time to do it.

How do you decide whether to circumcise your sons?

For the most part, circumcision remains a cultural and religious rite. If your beliefs about circumcision are strong, they will probably outweigh any information you can find about the physical or psychological risks and benefits of the procedure.

In reviewing these risks and benefits, the American

Academy of Pediatrics found some health advantages to circumcision and some risks, but they did not find that either was strong enough to argue for routinely circumcising all children or for calling for an end to the practice.

Here are some of the advantages: During their first year of life, uncircumcised boys are more likely to develop a urinary tract infection (UTI) than circumcised boys. The risk of a UTI for both drops greatly after the first year. Uncircumcised males may be more susceptible to acquiring certain STDs and more likely to transmit them (including HPV, which can cause cervical cancer). They may also be more likely to develop penile cancer, although penile cancer is rare (affecting only one in one hundred thousand men in the United States). Minor inflammations appear to be more common in the uncircumcised male as well, although properly cleaning the penis and foreskin reduces the risk.

Cleaning beneath the foreskin, the anticipation of which is sometimes a motivation for circumcision, is actually rather simple. By the time most boys reach age five, although it takes longer for some, the foreskin separates from the glans and becomes easy to retract for washing. Before then, there is no need to try to wash beneath it.

It is commonly said that if a father is uncircumcised (or circumcised), his boy should be as well so that they look alike. We have our doubts about this argument. If you were ever a little boy who once looked up and saw his father's penis, you can vouch for the fact that circumcised or not, that big swinging organ looked *nothing* like yours. There may be a case to be made for being similar to other boys in the locker room, although you can only guess now whether most will be circumcised or uncircumcised.

As for sensation, it is not clear how removing his foreskin

affects a male's sexual pleasure. Some say that circumcision doesn't have any effect. Some say that there are sexual advantages for the male and his partner. It has also been said that without the foreskin's protection, the glans becomes less sensitive. There isn't as much known about all of this as we would like. Still, it is hard to get around the fact that a circumcised male is missing one very sensitive part of his penis.

If you opt for circumcision, it is best performed during the newborn period and with appropriate local anesthesia (it hurts). This is the most common surgical procedure performed in the United States, and you can take comfort in knowing that complications (which occur in about one in five hundred cases) are usually minor. Bleeding is the most common, and it's typically easy to treat. Infections, the next most common, are also usually minor. Serious complications are rare.

Whether or not you choose to circumcise your son, you might let him know that not every boy looks just like him in this department, and you can explain your reasons for why he does or doesn't have a foreskin.

Two Kids in a Tub

During these immodest years, you may wonder how familiar your little ones should get with their naked siblings. Bath time may bring this question most strongly to mind. "It's all very casual and fun," you may wonder, "but at six and eight, are they getting too old for this?" "Is it inappropriate?" "Will they get aroused?"

Cobathing among siblings is not uncommon. Older children are less likely to bathe with a sibling than younger ones, but some families continue it for years. When should it end?

Some parents end joint baths when practicalities demand it. The kids get so big and splash around so much that you can't keep the water in the tub. In other cases it is a child—usually the older child—who decides to stop bathing with her sibling when she becomes modest. Occasionally, parents separate their children when one of them becomes sexually aroused.

If your child asks for a separate bath, she's made your job easy. Say yes. Then consider asking her about the reason for her change of heart. She may tell you that her little brother is too dirty, or too silly, or that she simply doesn't want him looking at her. Here's a good opportunity for you to discuss her feelings about nudity and her body and to support her wish for privacy, if she expresses it, as a sign of growing up.

Her little brother may not understand, or he may be quick to jump on the modesty bandwagon, insisting that he, too, wants to bathe alone. In either case, make sure to explain to him the reasons for the change as honestly as you think will be helpful to him:

> "Your sister wants to take her bath alone now, because she wants her privacy. That's what happens when you get older. You may also feel that way someday."

Too Much

If your children don't ask for separate baths, you may still want to end cobathing at a certain point. The argument for separating children is usually expressed in terms of protecting them from overstimulation. Let's clarify just what that means.

A youngster in the preschool or early school years who is exposed to nudity may develop feelings of arousal. All such stimulation is not necessarily harmful. But it can become troublesome if the arousal is more than the child can understand and comfortably tolerate, or if the child is stimulated in a situation in which she believes feelings of arousal are unacceptable.

Both may be the case in cobathing. A young child who is aroused by seeing a naked sibling may have difficulty understanding her feelings. And she may also pick up implicit messages from family members that such feelings are wrong. As a result, rather than using you to help figure them out, she may try to hide or inhibit her reaction and end up feeling tense and anxious.

That is what we mean by overstimulation.

Overstimulated kids may request separate baths, or they may express their tension through their behavior. They may grow louder and more boisterous, or increasingly insistent in touching their sibling; they may get the giggles, or get cranky at bath time. A persistent change in the quality of your child's attitude toward cobathing may signal that it has become too arousing. If this occurs, consider a trial separation.

Tell your child:

"Now that you are older, we think you deserve a grown-up-style bath. You deserve to have a bath all by yourself."

Keep in mind that your overstimulated child hasn't done something shocking. She's just reacted naturally to her sibling. You are giving her a private bath to help her more comfortably contain her reactions until she matures. Someday she will be able to contain them on her own.

Take It Off, Daddy

Now that you're older, we think you deserve a grown-up-style bath, too. Unfortunately, you may be unlikely to get one these days, when five minutes of privacy seems like just enough time for your toddler to redecorate the dining room with a box of crayons.

Even if you do secure a little private time, you can never quite be sure you're in the clear, can you? One blessed day off, Alfie was soaking naked in the tub when his four-year-old daughter popped in on him. She took a long, wary look into the water, then rendered her decision. "I don't like it, Daddy. Take it off."

If there is a seriously underrated component of your kids' sex education, here it is. Catching a glimpse of you changing or in the shower may be their first and most potent lesson in how bodies look. Your children will learn what to expect of their own bodies by seeing yours, and like Alfie's daughter, they can use the experience to grasp certain salient differences between girls and boys. Moreover, your kids will absorb your attitudes about having a body, showing it, or hiding it as they watch you navigate the slippery bathroom floor. Here, then, is another way to transmit your attitudes of pride, modesty, or shame about your body to your child. How do you decide what they should see, and when?

Julie's parents, Teri and Ben, have never been big on getting into the bath with her. But when one of them is alone with their two-year-old and has to take a shower, Julie will join in. Teri doesn't mind the company, but she noticed that before Julie was twenty months old, Ben began to wear jogging shorts when he and Julie showered together. Teri hasn't asked why he decided to cover up, but she does know from her own experiences that Julie takes a keen interest in looking at bodies. Maybe she studied Ben more closely than he liked.

Rick occasionally showers with his six-year-old son, Seth, who appreciates the opportunity to collect data about the wonders of the world and, more specifically, about his dad. In a typical shower, Rick will field a stream of questions, from the challenging "Does sperm come out in your pee?" to the unanswerable "Why is there hair on your back?"

As for Seth's older sister, Cassie, Rick stopped showering with her before she turned six. Cassie is perfectly able to shower on her own, Rick points out, so there is no longer a practical reason to wash together. But more important to Rick, "it just feels like the wrong thing to do." Rick can't identify any event that told him it was time to change. Still, he feels fairly confident that he made his decision at the right time. "You realize she is approaching puberty," he explains. "She's just too old for that. It could be confusing for her."

Let's first observe that Rick, Ben, and Teri all fall well within the very wide range of bathing habits found in American households. At any child's age you can find some parents who think letting their child see them naked is fine and others who consider it awkward or just plain wrong.

There are some common themes to the modesty habits of American parents. In general, both mothers and fathers are more modest around children of the opposite sex. And parents become increasingly modest as their children grow older.

The Big Cover-up

In deciding when to cover up, parents seem to weigh two main factors: their own sense of comfort and their hunches about what seeing them naked means to their child.

Ben probably donned his jogging shorts in the shower because he was simply uncomfortable being seen by Julie. His own discomfort was reason enough for him.

We agree. Children's experience of their parents' bodies should take place in an atmosphere of calm and comfort. If you need clothing to provide that comfort, so be it. Stretching the limits of your own modesty to demonstrate to your child that nudity is fine can backfire. She's likely to sense your discomfort and end up feeling uneasy herself. Better to tell her nudity is healthy, and mean it, with your pants on.

But Rick is responding to more than just his own comfort level. He's also trying to follow Cassie's reaction. When Rick wonders if Cassie will find seeing him nude confusing, he is thinking about the possibility that she may experience feelings of arousal. As with sibling cobathing, we suggest you look for the signs of overstimulation we described above. Cover up if you sense your child becoming aroused by the sight of your body and offer an uncharged, nonblaming explanation for the change.

All right, you may be thinking, it's one thing to have to consider the idea of your little ones getting a bit randy in the bath together. But "your child becoming aroused by the sight of your body"? What's that about?

Perhaps we should say more.

A Tonka Truck Named Desire

Mona Gable, a writer and a mother, recently described her four-year-old boy's efforts to woo her in the essay collection *Mothers Who Think*.

"I'd go to sit on the couch and he'd slide his hand under me, grinning madly," she wrote. "I'd go to hug him and he'd burrow his little head into my breasts, lingering there a minute too long. I'd be taking a shower and suddenly the curtain would be flung aside by a pint-sized blond in Ninja Turtle briefs. 'Mommy's in the shower,' I'd say. 'Oh,' he'd say, holding his ground."

Sound familiar?

Children have been spying on their parents and inviting them into odd little assignations for centuries. Parents have been trying to figure out how to respond for just as long. Freud once reported treating an overwhelmed mother whose three-and-a-half-year-old girl suddenly clamped her thighs around her mother's hand as she was being changed. "Oh, Mummy, do leave your hand there," she is supposed to have said. "It feels so lovely."

Freud did not mention whether this event was solely responsible for propelling the woman to his couch. And we can only dream of what he may have told her. Chances are, however, that his explanation may have involved his great discovery (or invention, depending on your point of view)—the Oedipus complex.

For decades, the Oedipus complex was held up as the great psychic hoop we all had to jump through on our way to maturity and health. If it wasn't perfect science, it sure made a great story. Here are the Cliffs Notes for the boy's version. At age two or three a boy watches his parents' intimacy with jealous eyes, wishing he were the one his mother loved most. He woos her, fantasizes about her, and tries to edge his father out of the picture. But he doesn't get far, for at some point or other it becomes painfully clear to our little hero that his father is unbeatably bigger and stronger than he. And when that happens, anxiety spoils his reverie. If his father discovers his designs and gets angry, the little boy fears, he might just cut off his rivalrous little penis.

As Freud saw it, a healthy boy wants to keep his penis more than he wants his mother, and so, around the age of six, he pushes his wishes to win her into his unconscious, never to recollect them again, but never entirely free of their covert influence. He'll marry someone like her someday. And for years to come he'll work hard to fight off any thought that threatens to trigger the memory that it was his mother he wanted all along.

Freud's model does offer one possible explanation for some of the puzzling behavior we observe in children. Kids between ages three and six really do have a way of popping in on their parents in compromising moments (they're trying to interrupt them, Freud would say). They do behave in a curiously seductive manner with their parents. And little boys do answer innocent questions such as "Do you want Daddy to tuck you in?" with an emphatic "I want Daddy to go to Pluto, I want Mommy to tuck me in." Come age six or seven, all these behaviors seem to subside.

No one has ever proved the Oedipus complex to be the cause of these goings on. And when it comes to their actual feelings for their parents, children's experiences are probably more variable than the theory allows (we don't really know, for example, how many children experience romantic interest in a parent). In trying to understand your own child's amorous behavior, we suggest you take the approach favored by contemporary psychoanalysts. Rather than holding onto a particular theory and trying to fit your observations into it ("She's three. She's going to be after me any day now"), watch your child without expectations, and try to learn from her. And if you wake up one morning to find yourself the star of a five-year-old's bodice ripper, enjoy it.

Answer Your Fan Mail

How, you ask, are you supposed to respond to this fervent wooing? Our answer: Receive it with the innocence in which it's been offered.

Accept your child's adoration as the precious gift of a generous soul. Avoid translating his attentions into adult terms, calling him a Romeo or a lady-killer. But admire his courtliness as you would any of his efforts to win your praise and attention. Treasure his offerings of love.

When your boy hugs you and tells you he wants to marry you, hug him back and tell him you love him, too. But also tell him that he can't marry you because you're his mother. "Someday you may find someone else wonderful to marry," you might say.

To encourage your child's development in this area is to walk a fine line. Showing too little interest in his flirtation can communicate an aversion to affection and love, and, in particular, to his worthiness as an object of love. Too much involvement in a seduction can become intrusive and troubling for a child. Somewhere in between, you will find a way to encourage and endorse your child's earliest forays into the world of love.

If you want one guideline to keep in mind, it might be this: Let your child's desire unfold under its own logic. Try not to expect it, or to need it, to hasten its demise, or to keep it alive when it starts to fade. Your child's development is bound to be quirky and idiosyncratic. If you let it, it will follow its own rules, knowing better than you what it needs to mature.

Your Delicious Child

> But the wild things cried, "Oh please don't go—
> we'll eat you up—we love you so!"
> And Max said, "No!"
> —*Maurice Sendak,* Where the Wild Things Are

Whenever we give a talk on kids and sex, a few parents inevitably linger afterward to ask a private question or two. One spring evening after one of these talks, two mothers hovered near their seats. Tentatively, they made their way toward the front of the room, and when everyone had left, they began to ask the questions they didn't want the others to hear. They wanted to talk about hugging and squeezing.

One was explaining her concern that she was "too intimate" with her daughter when the other, Cecily, abruptly ended her circumspect silence. "And what about with a six-year-old boy?" she said. "He is just so delicious! How much cuddling is too much?"

We have heard this before: a parent describes how scrumptious her child is and then quickly expresses some sort of reservation about her feelings. Our reaction? Children *are* delicious. And there are good reasons to restrain your impulse to gobble them up. But there are also plenty of unfounded anxieties that can cramp your ability to delight in your kids.

Earlier we described the intimacy of caring for an infant. Let's not forget the fact that as your child grows and sheds by inches his need for close physical attention, your sense of his body doesn't vanish. We have spoken of the curious workings of your child's hunger for you. Let's not neglect the fact that within this precious bond, hunger flows in two directions.

You may sense this yourself as your five-year-old climbs onto your knee to whisper some confidence and breathes his warm breath in your ear, or as you stoop over his sister curled in her bed and stroke her cheek while she dreams.

Then you recall all you have learned about childhood sexual abuse, and suddenly you find yourself second-guessing your own pleasures. "Is this inappropriate?" you wonder. "What would someone else think?" Your commitment to honoring the incest taboo is righteous and ardent—this is a good thing—but the result is that sometimes you may question the natural expressions of your decent parental love.

George talks about his son. "His skin is so soft. It's so smooth. I could just hold him for hours. That's okay, right?"

Lisa says how delicious her baby girl is. She craves Kelly's soft hugs, but says she worries about hugging her too much. "Am I doing it for my own pleasure?" she asks without having to explain her assumption that taking pleasure in her child is necessarily a suspect activity. Speaking with caution about her uncertainties for the first time, Lisa reveals that admiring her little girl "has made me understand what pedophilia must be."

Well, Lisa doesn't really understand pedophilia. The desires of a pedophile hinge on fantasies of sexual acts performed with (or rather, upon) a child. Lisa's are nothing like that. But her mixing up of an adult's sexual urge with her motherly craving for Kelly's sweetness is not uncommon. It seems to be the secret fear of many a self-doubting parent.

The delights that George and Lisa and a world of other parents describe are not only ordinary and normal—they are essential. "When they were young, I called all my children 'sweet potato,' 'muffin,' 'cutie-pie,' " writes anthropologist Sarah Blaffer Hrdy in *Mother Nature*. "I'd say, 'You're so adorable I could eat you up.' " But Hrdy didn't eat her children. Instead, she explains, she fell into step with a great evolutionary chain of mothers for whom the deliciousness of their children has inspired the extraordinary sacrifice of time, energy, and resources all good Darwinian babies need to survive. The child's cuteness is cousin to the finch's beak. It's the best tool he's got for getting fed.

So, when you worry about your passion for your sweet potato, remember this. The tender yen you feel for your child will help you give her all that she needs. To feel it is to know that you have opened wide the door through which your nurturance will pass.

Cecily's question still hangs in the air. How much cuddling is too much? We would like to say something simple like "No amount of cuddling is ever too much," but that would neglect one crucial fact that many parents know. Children need to be hugged and caressed, but they also need to be let go. The cuddling that is too much is the cuddling that forgets your child's wish to be free of you, just for the moment. It is the cuddling that intrudes, controls, or demands—that eclipses a child's desire for her own little bit of autonomy. So, sometimes, you hold back.

Just as an infant turns away when he's had enough cooing for the moment, your youngster will do the same with your affection if you let him. When he's had enough, he'll squirm away, wipe your kisses from his cheeks, and go off for a breather. But, oh, to let him go . . .

One mother, overheard on the sidewalk, summed up the sweet pain of the beguiled parent's dilemma. She looked down delightedly at her little boy giggling in his stroller. "You're so delicious, I want to gobble you up!" she said as a melancholy note crept into her voice. "But then you'd be gone."

The Primal Scene

With all this talk about naked baths, breasts, and penises, you would think early parenthood is a time you'd be more in touch with your sexuality than any other time in life. Somehow, though, we don't often hear new parents saying things like "Since I had my baby, my sex life has sky-rocketed!"

Children present some practical challenges to your unfettered carnal enjoyment of your partner—like lack of time, lack of sleep, and lack of privacy. Happily, one year after their child's birth, most couples are having sex as frequently and enjoyably as they did before. But if you have reached this stage, you may find sex involves a challenge you haven't experienced since your roommate days: You want to have sex, but suddenly you discover there is *always someone else around.*

Jacob, a dad who installed a lock on his bedroom door before his daughter turned two, put his feelings this way: "Hey, I'm not in denial about my daughter's sexuality. I'm happy to have a sexual kid. But as far as her knowing about my sexuality? Not cool."

If you feel as Jacob does and you'd like to limit your chances of being walked in on, explain to your child that when your door is closed, she should knock and then wait until you say it's okay before opening it. Then get a lock. Unless you are an extremely light sleeper, keeping your door locked throughout the night may prevent your kids from waking you if they need you. But for the part of the evening (or morning or afternoon) when you are having sex, a lock works wonders.

And what if you didn't lock the door, because you don't have a lock, or you were sure the kids were asleep, or for once you were briefly able to forget that you are the steadfastly dependable mother of three and lose yourself in a moment of simply feeling sexy? What if in the middle of enjoying the full force of that feeling with the father of those three children, you and he discover that at some point—and for all the many times you two will later review this evening, you will never really know when—your four-year-old has wandered into your bedroom and is waiting at the foot of the bed for one of you to notice him.

You notice him.

What are you supposed to do now?

First, let us point out that no one can tell you what effect seeing his parents having sex will have on your child. There was a time when all manner of psychopathology—from headaches to hysteria—was traced back to the inadvertent viewing in childhood of what analysts called "the primal scene" (an apt description on a good night). Anthropologists disagreed, pointing out that in some non-Western societies, where people seemed to be no more neurotic than we are, children see or hear their parents having sex often. Even in the United States, a child seeing a parent having sex is common enough—about 20 percent of parents report being seen, most often by a child between ages four and six—that if it always led to psychological problems, we'd be a nation of loonies. . . . Okay, maybe that's not a good argument.

At any rate, we now believe that your child's reaction to an event like this depends in large part on whether he views what you were doing, or the fact that he saw it, as bad. A child might be upset, for example, if he interprets his parents' sex as a violent or angry act (which may be more likely if he lives in a home where parents are often violent or angry with one another). Likewise, a child who is yelled at by a parent for intruding, and who isn't capable of understanding why his parent would be so angry, would probably be more troubled by the event than a child whose parents adopt a calmer tone. A child whose parents help him understand what he saw as positive and ordinary will likely fare better than the kid left to figure it out for himself.

We still marvel at the composure of Jack and Simon. When their four-year-old boy walked in on them having sex, Jack managed calmly to say, "Oh, you found us doing the special thing that people in love do when they want to make each other feel good; now which of us do you want to put you back to bed?"

You don't have to be as unflappable as these guys to find a way out of this dilemma. If you discover your four-year-old standing at the foot of the bed when you're having sex, first, resist the impulse to pull the covers over your head or to pretend it hasn't happened. Instead, stop what you're doing, cover up enough to feel comfortable talking to him, and then try to find out what he wants.

Let's imagine it is the proverbial glass of water. You might tell him you'll get him one if he wouldn't mind waiting outside your door for a minute. (Stalling has an undeservedly bad reputation. We like it. It allows for thinking before talking, the preferred order.) Pull yourself together and take him for his water.

While you are doing so, even if he doesn't seem to have any curiosity about what he just saw, explain it very briefly. You might try:

> "When you came in, we were having sex. It's a way that grown-ups like us show that we love each other. Do you understand?"

Let him ask any questions he has. When you have answered them—and chances are there won't be many—you can make your second point:

> "When we close our door, it means we want to be private. Can you knock before you open the door from now on?"

And that's it.

You can now tuck your little one into bed, go back to your room, and perform CPR on your partner.

Who Told Thee Thou Wast Naked?

After the intense cuddling and skin-to-skin contact of infancy, after the impromptu peep shows of the toddler years, and after the impassioned wooing of your preschool suitors, the sexual rumblings in the average family have a way of quieting down.

In all the frenzy to coordinate the newly complex carpooling schedules and cheer on the harder homework assignments, you may not notice the change. But should you find the opportunity to pause for a moment of thought in the middle of your kids' grade school years, you may notice the one most striking aspect of this new order. Suddenly there's a lot less skin around the house.

Your children are becoming modest.

It came to Dan as a sudden realization: Sammy, who at seven, had confessed that he was Captain Nudie ("What are your special powers?" his father, Dan, humbly asked. "I am naked, and I wear a cape.") was now spending all day in his civilian clothes. Sammy banished his little sister Peg from his bath, and the morning ritual of getting dressed with her in front of the TV came to a halt. One afternoon Sam and Peg were playing tag in the park when Peg looped her finger into the former nudist's waistband. His shorts slipped, fleetingly baring his left buttock. Sam freaked.

Peg, for her part, once had a reputation as a garrulous pooper, inviting anyone who didn't have dinner burning in the oven, a car up on jacks, or some other equally urgent excuse to join her for a long chat while she sat on the toilet. But when Captain Nudie hung up his cape, Peg slammed the door on her poop talks. These days she regards any requests to join her in the bathroom as the preposterous ravings of a lunatic.

What happened to these two? Did they eat an apple? Was a snake involved? "Who told thee thou wast naked?" Dan might have cried into the outside of a double-locked bathroom door.

Well, a few factors may have been involved. For one, children may cover up in response to a new message from their parents. As your kids grow into their elementary school years, as they start to look less like muffins and more like males and females, you may become a little less comfortable with nudity around the house—and then show it. Children may also get modest under peer pressure. This was probably the case with Peg, whose modesty seemed to result from her imitation of her brother and her wish to avoid his teasing.

And then there's the theory of the Oedipus complex, which, you'll remember, holds that around age six formerly lusty children renounce their wish to seduce their parents (knowing they will fail) and swing to the other extreme, making sure their renunciation is easily maintained by morphing into little prudes.

Whatever the causes, researchers have shown that children tend to become modest in one or a few abrupt leaps during their early school-age years with timing that roughly fits Freud's model. Girls make their leaps towards modesty between the ages of four and six. Boys do it a bit later, between ages five and eight.

Newly modest kids aren't only shy about being seen. They don't want to sneak a peak at you, either. If they open the bathroom door while you're drying off, they whisper "Sorry" and disappear. And those professions of undying devotion to you? They start to lose some of their ardor. Author Mary Gordon sensed the change in her son, she writes in *Between Mothers and Sons,* when her erstwhile admirer casually reported, "My friend Johnny said he thinks you have a big butt, and I couldn't tell him he was wrong."

Comments like these can be a bit dispiriting. And as for the modesty, you may begin to wonder "Isn't Camilla a little *too* modest?" as your daughter limps from the bathroom bound in a fiendishly tight towel. Some kids do become much more rigid about nudity than their parents ever wished, but if your child's shyness troubles you, let it ride. There is no compelling reason we know of to try to lessen a kid's modesty.

Instead, take comfort in the knowledge that by the time your children reach the modest years they're less likely to barge into your shower or to hide in your room in order to catch a peek of you in the buff. Soon, once urgent decisions about who sees whom naked—and when—will slip into the foggy past and be forgotten as easily as the *Teletubbies* program schedule. Some day you may look back on these times with the soft ache of nostalgia.

Boo?

At the moment it's hard to think that far ahead.

Helen Reddy has flown out of your mind, and here you stand, shivering slightly, and holding your hairbrush like a fig leaf before your speechless five-year-old son.

What might you be thinking right about now?

To the extent that thought is possible, you're probably trying to think of what to say. "Don't yell, don't look ashamed, don't blame him, don't let him do it again," you may be telling yourself.

There are other thoughts, too, working their way through the back of your mind, thoughts that have very little to do with how this is going to affect your son's development, like "What must I have looked like?" or "I can't believe my son saw me enjoying my body. How could I have let myself go?"

"You caught me by surprise," you decide to tell your son. "Did I surprise you, too?"

Later, after your son has gone out to play, you find yourself remembering the time your mother opened your fitting room door and called to the sales girl, a girl who went to your school, for a larger size. Or the time years earlier, when you walked in on your father in the bathroom, and he looked so strange sitting there, reading the paper with his pants in a heap around his ankles. He laughed out loud when he saw you; you never knew why. Maybe, it occurs to you now, he was laughing at the perplexed look you must have had on your face. Or maybe he was just terribly embarrassed.

You've revisited such moments from your past before, but not quite in the way you have today.

And this, friend, is a secret about managing modesty, nudity, sex, and love at home with your children. All the wondering about baths and changing and who sees whom isn't just about your child's sexual development. It's about yours, too.

True, you're a grown person with children. You've been having sex with the same partner for eleven years, and it feels like a century since you went on a date. But your sexual development hasn't stopped. Raising these kids is pushing it along.

When you decided to have children, you made a choice destined to change your relationship to your own sexuality in ways you couldn't have predicted then, or now. Which is why, when it comes to sex and love, parenting your kids will never be simply a science.

Oh, no, it will never be less than a leap.

Chapter **4**

"Don't touch that—

it'll fall off."

MANAGING YOUR YOUNG CHILD'S SEXUAL BEHAVIOR

> *Look at my wiener! I can make it stand up. I rub it and it*
> *stands up and it feels good. Sometimes I rub it a lot and it feels*
> *very, very good.*
> —THREE-YEAR-OLD BOY IN THE MASTERS
> AND JOHNSON FILES

THERE ARE SOME THINGS you just would rather not hear your little one say, aren't there?

There are some things, just a few, you would really rather not have to know.

Now, you are a caring parent. You are a dad unlike any dad that your father's generation, God bless them, could have imagined on their monotonous commutes home from work.

Tonight, for example, you are a dad who is perfectly comfortable hosting his daughter's eighth-birthday sleepover while her mother is out of town. For her pioneer theme party, you have created an Oregon Trail treasure hunt featuring a note from the Donner party in the freezer. You have made individual pioneer pizzas that actually resemble little wagon wheels. You're wearing a cowboy hat. That's the kind of dad you are.

Still, there are some things you would rather not deal with.

The girls have gone upstairs to decorate their bonnets. You trot up there after a little downtime in the kitchen with some canteens of pioneer punch. There is giggling and merriment. You open your daughter's door to find six girls almost entirely naked except for brightly painted bonnets. They are . . . stripping.

"Here's the punch!"

And you're outta there.

This Is One of Those Things

Odds are you don't welcome the chance to confront your little one's sexuality. You might even prefer to imagine that it doesn't exist, and you would not be the first. Who hasn't wished, at one time or another, that our children were innocent of the appetites that are forever complicating our adult lives?

The trick is, of course, that little kids are sexual. Preschool and school age children have sexual feelings. They masturbate. And they pursue exploratory games of looking and touching with their friends.

No one has prepared you for the moment when this will become embarrassingly clear at your daughter's first slumber party. Caught by surprise, you may wonder, is this unusual? Is she . . . *abnormal*? Does this mean she's been abused? And in this moment of discovery, with these thoughts in mind, what will come out of your mouth? This is an occasion in a parent's life when cool reason may succumb to the fight or flight response. You might actually hear yourself blurt out a version of the time-tested "Stop that!" You might drop the pioneer punch and run. Or, if you are like one or two squillion other parents, you might pretend that nothing in fact has happened at all.

Which would be a shame, because moments like these are among the most potent opportunities you have to teach your child about the meaning of sexual pleasure and sexual behavior, about respect and responsibility, and to establish a role for yourself in schooling your child's later sexual decisions.

In the preceding chapter we described the way your responses to your young child's body and to her curiosity about yours can lay a sound foundation for her relationship to her physical self and nourish her sense of her own lovability.

In this chapter we are taking on something a bit trickier. We are going to look at the challenge of responding to your youngster's discovery of her own sexual sensations and urges—her first sexual experiments.

What follows is designed to help you make the most of the unexpected teaching moments your prepubertal child's early adventures present. Keeping an eye on your youngster's two main sexual pursuits—masturbation and sex play—we will explain what sexual behaviors we consider healthy and what we consider worrisome, and how to react to both.

The M Word

Do we detect a little discomfort about masturbation?

As far as we can tell, sentences that include both "masturbation" and "your child" have never been particularly harmonious to the ears of the American parent. After centuries of vague concern over wasted seed, high anxiety over childhood masturbation seems to have been ignited in 1710 by the appearance of a pamphlet entitled *Onania, or the Heinous Sin of Self-Pollution, and All Its Frightful Consequences, in both Sexes, Consider'd with Spiritual and Physical Advice to Those, who have already injur'd themselves by this abominable practice.* (You get the picture.) By the end of the nineteenth century, the subject of childhood masturbation was an American obsession. We have their fervent allegiance to the antimasturbation crusade to thank for Dr. Kellogg's cornflake and Mr. Graham's cracker. A bland diet, they believed, would curb a child's sexual appetite.

Years later, your grandmother may have had her own method. "Don't touch that," she might say on those special occasions when she supervised your bath. "It'll fall off."

"My, how times change," you muse contentedly.

Then it happens to you.

"I was on the phone with a friend, and I glanced over at Ella," Leann recalls. "At this point she was about two-and-a-half and her favorite stuffed animal was a big Barney. So there's Ella, and she was sort of lying on him. Something seemed a little odd. And then I noticed her hips were moving. She was sort of rocking. 'Oh, my God,' I realized, 'Ella's humping Barney!' "

What is it about seeing your child masturbate that feels so . . . weird?

Well, first of all, it's *masturbation.*

Now, maybe you're so cool that you can turn to a stranger and tell him that you like to masturbate as if you were giving him directions to the IHOP. Or maybe you're like some others among us, and just trying to get the word out tips you into an altered state. (Try it.) Thanks to ten seconds of research on the Web, we have uncovered 974 euphemisms for the word *masturbate,* evidence that you are not the only one who doesn't like to say it. But even snappy phrases like "doing time in the hand slammer" don't entirely disguise the fact that you're talking about giving yourself genital pleasure, an idea that may still trip you up. You've heard it's healthy. You've been told it's normal. But you would rather have a tooth drilled than discuss it with your mother. Why?

Consider this. Do you think that your mother is more or less comfortable discussing masturbation than you are? Now bear in mind that your first lessons about masturbation were under your parents' tutelage. You might not have been subjected to impassioned lectures on the evils of self-abuse, but you may have gotten a negative message from subtler clues. Maybe your lessons took place years before you can remember, like having your hand repeatedly pulled away from your genitals as a toddler. Maybe when you were older the family was resolutely silent on the subject—even when your mother walked in on you in high school—making you feel masturbation was just too dirty to discuss, or that you were the only one in the house who did it. Whatever the specifics, there's a good chance that your parents' management of your childhood masturbation was guided by their own embarrassment (itself instilled in them by their parents, who told them it would fall off, too). And the result is this: Their embarrassment became your embarrassment.

Second, it's your *kid,* and frankly, even if the notion of your child pursuing sexual pleasure doesn't trouble you in the least, you might not necessarily want to watch.

"Recently Ella started to do it in the car seat when I'm driving. Sometimes I'll say, 'Oh, knock it off.' Other times I just sit there and try not to laugh . . . or cry." Leann now knows what her parents were dealing with.

Start with your own uneasiness about masturbation in general, add to it the discomfort of facing your little one's sexuality, and you are perfectly primed to raise your child to panic some day when she finds her own daughter rubbing against the furniture. And the beat goes on.

Or you might choose to finally put a stop to this transgenerational chain letter.

The Invention of Pleasure

"Gee, they find it at six months, and they never forget they have it."

Children discover masturbation in a variety of ways over a range of ages. Some children never masturbate. Some pass through a period in their toddler years when they seem always to have a hand on their genitals and then shed the practice as mysteriously as they picked it up. And some, as Ginny's mother tartly observed while diapering her grandson, find their penis at six months and never forget they have it. But if there were a common pathway kids follow in their development, what would it be?

Well, Ginny's mom is right; masturbation can begin in infancy. Diapers are about as effective as iron chastity belts at preventing genital play, so during diaper changes it is not uncommon for infants, both boys and girls, to make the most of the opportunity by exploring their genitals. A boy will get a pleasurable sensation (we can't say how "sexual" a pleasure it is yet—if it's sexual at all) when he rubs his penis with his hand. A girl, who has the same limited dexterity as a boy but a smaller, less accessible target—the clitoris—may use her hand, but she may also get at that good feeling by stretching or squeezing her vulva using her leg muscles or pressing against a blanket or pillow.

This sort of genital play is more casual, less goal directed than what we usually think of as masturbation. Less commonly, though, an infant will practice a more intense, focused sort of self-stimulation. This has been observed in boys and girls before the end of their first year, and the reasons why some children pursue it and others do not is unknown. A ten-month-old girl may squeeze her legs around her teddy or her bottle, fix her gaze, and flush for a minute or more, until she suddenly relaxes. The episodes may look to a parent like the child is in pain or even having a seizure. However scary it may at first appear, though, this sort of masturbation is considered harmless and subsides on its own.

Later, in the toddler and preschool years, children will practice a range of behaviors from the odd tug of which they seem unaware, to a pleasurable tickling of their genitals in the tub, to a goal-directed rhythmic rubbing in which they seem almost to lose themselves. And now they can talk about it. Take four-year-old Avra, whose mother, Irene, heard grunting from the backseat. When asked what she was up to, Avra gave an unexpected response: " 'I'm doing my tush exercises. Don't look.' So I looked," explained Irene. Avra, with a big smile on her face, was rocking back and forth against her car seat strap, which was wedged firmly between her legs. "It was very clear what was being exercised."

A toddler's genital play can comfort her. She may use it when she is in an especially stressful place to block out what feels like too much outside stimulation, or at quiet times as a normal part of the process of winding down.

But let's not forget that even at times like these, kids also masturbate because it feels really good. Consider Noah, who at four, had a habit of fiddling with his penis while his mother would read to him at bedtime. Most nights Trudy would ask him to please stop (this was becoming *her* habit), and he would. Temporarily. One evening after Trudy made her usual appeal, Noah decided it was time to finally help his mother understand the situation. "Mom," he explained without removing his hand from his pants, "if you had one of these, you would do it, too."

Lords of Their Flies

As your little one marches through his elementary school years, you are less and less likely to see him masturbate. As we explained in Chapter 3, he is learning a thing or two about modesty. But don't be fooled by appearances. He is more and more likely to be masturbating as he grows. The boy who didn't masturbate at four or five may very well start at age six. The girl who didn't masturbate at six may get going at seven. How do they pick it up?

While some kids get the news from a more experienced peer ("Hey, swing on the rope like this. It's fun!"), others make the discovery all on their own. One mother explains, "He was 'cruising' around the edge of the swimming pool when—WOW—he found the warm jet stream. Oh boy, did he like that! He looked like a little frog or crab all clutched to the side of the pool—at four years old. Then at five he realized that sliding down the 'fire pole' on the monkey bars at school made him feel the same way. And so on, and so on."

And so on, and so on. The methods kids find to masturbate seem even to surpass their strategies for avoiding chores in their dizzying inventiveness. Seesaws, hoses, pets, even a nice patch of grass may be pressed into service. There are no rules to follow, because it's *their* game. They invented it. The child who discovers genital pleasure in this private way, especially if her family doesn't openly discuss it, may well believe that she has discovered an uncharted territory that is all her own. And in a way, she has.

Who Masturbates?

The actual figures of how many children masturbate and at what ages are hard to determine. Based on what parents observe, prior to age six, a sizable minority of boys and girls have masturbated. As they grow older, more and more children have masturbated until, by age eighteen or nineteen, the vast majority of boys and just under half of girls will say they have.

Yes, boys are typically more likely than girls to masturbate, and girls who do masturbate appear to do it less often than boys. These differences may represent the effect of differing cultural or social expectations for girls and boys. They may point to biological differences between the sexes. Or they may simply prove that boys are happier than girls to tell researchers that they masturbate.

A seven-year-old will typically take her masturbation more seriously than she did as a preschooler. At her age, masturbating is more likely to be a mindful choice pursued in private than an unconscious act at story time. She has a wider repertoire of other comforting techniques now, so she is more likely to reserve masturbation for the purpose of pleasure. And if she didn't know about orgasms before, she may soon discover them.

Although few parents ever expect it, school-age children sometimes find that if they masturbate long enough, they can reach a sort of junior orgasm. Kip, now a dad, became quite familiar with this phenomenon at age eight when he poured vast sums of energy into climbing the rope in his backyard. He knew that if he rubbed around long enough he would inevitably reach "a breathless, dizzy peak." At that age, he never ejaculated. However early a child starts masturbating, ejaculation waits for puberty. When, after four years of "exercise," Kip had his first ejaculation, the feeling he remembers most is disappointment. Now, he thought, I can't get away with it anymore. His orgasms no longer felt like a secret.

By the time puberty is in full swing, masturbation's functions have evolved again. Teens use it to satisfy those surges in sexual desire that once made it impossible for you to get through two chapters of *Madame Bovary* in one sitting. Masturbation may also provide a sort of sexual education. As adolescents masturbate, they can develop an awareness of their own sexual responses and a familiarity with their bodies that may make sex with others less mysterious and potentially more satisfying when it happens.

Of course, back in toddlerhood, when your daughter first discovers the rewards of a well-placed teddy bear, all of this is about as comprehensible to her as particle physics. Wiggling around on her favorite stuffed animal, she has no notion that what she is doing is sexual. Or that grown-ups love sexual things but don't like other people to know that. Or that your boss, who has never visited your home until today, doesn't have children, which may explain the beads of perspiration that seem to be forming on his brow.

No—infants, toddlers, and preschoolers are oblivious to what society makes of masturbation. All they know is that it feels good. It's up to you to explain the rules of propriety to them. The way you choose to respond to your children's masturbation will teach them what sexual pleasure is; what the world thinks of it; and how, when, and whether that pleasure is okay to pursue.

So What Do You Do?

It wasn't really until he was about two-and-a-half when I was sharing a bedroom with him for about nine months that I noticed that he was waking up about two o'clock in the morning and literally humping the bed . . . the problem was, I was sleeping right beside him and he was doing it for two and three hours in the middle of the night.

—*Kirst, on her son, interviewed on Australia's Radio National*

There are two key objectives to keep in mind every time you respond to your child's genital touching or masturbation.

The first is to help your child to develop an accepting attitude toward himself and toward his enjoyment of his body—to make certain that he doesn't learn to be ashamed of his genitals or of himself for taking pleasure in them. Promoting this goal means making sure not to react negatively to your little one's masturbation.

So I was faced with this real dilemma then, because part of me thought it was really, really funny, and part of me was kind of proud, and part of me was just completely pissed off because I'd fallen to sleep. And there's also this kind of inner struggle about wanting them to stop because you want to sleep and not wanting to make him feel guilty, or make him feel like he was doing something wrong, that was the last thing I wanted to do.

Second, you want to school your child in the ways of the world, and more specifically, the ways of your household. You want him to learn what behaviors are appropriate and under what circumstances and gradually to become more and more responsible about meeting social expectations. To further this goal, you'll have to educate him about the times and places he shouldn't touch his genitals. Sometimes, you'll have to say no.

The hard part is figuring out how to reconcile these two goals.

> **What I ended up doing was just generally saying "Stop moving around" and not letting him know that I knew what he was doing. Like I was this complete dummy that had no idea what he'd discovered.**

This dilemma—call it the "Sex is good, but not now" paradox—is really the central challenge you'll face in responding to all of your child's sexual behavior from birth onward. Master it now, and your solution will serve you for the rest of your parenting career.

Whether it has to do with your toddlers' masturbation or your teenagers' love life, our advice on how to manage this paradox will always be the same: It's best for your child when you respond to his sexual curiosity with respect and acceptance along with rational and consistent limits.

Let's see what constitutes a rational limit—one that makes good sense for your particular child at his particular developmental level—when it comes to masturbation.

Learning to Love It

At twenty months of age, Clara has a word she uses for her genitals: "tunnel." Her Mom, Yuni, doesn't know how Clara came to apply a word she learned on her drive to the airport to her genitals, but proudly observes, "It makes sense!" Clara knows that her vagina goes in. She can only have learned this by being allowed to explore herself.

When Yuni changes her diaper, Clara pronounces "tunnel" with glee and starts to play with her labia and giggle.

"I let her," Yuni says a bit sheepishly. She will wait and watch Clara play for a few minutes and then put a clean diaper on her.

When it comes to genital play, your child has to start with the basics. First, she should learn that she has genitals, and that they are valued, not dirty or bad, and that they can make her feel good. Later she can learn the more difficult lesson about when and where to play with them and when and where to refrain.

In the first two to three years of life, when children are constructing their categories of good and bad, they may have trouble understanding the difference between a behavior that is always bad and one that is bad in some contexts (like at the bank) but good in others (in a private place), or bad at certain times (when he's in the bath with his sister) but good at others (when he's alone there). Tell a young toddler not to masturbate in a particular context and he may understand it always to be wrong. One lesson like this is unlikely to stick, but repeat it over time and you risk teaching your child to feel anxiety or guilt about his body, his genitals, and their pleasures. All of which is to say, these are the years to let your child go.

Of course, there are times when this advice is harder to follow than others. Moira explains: "At about age two, Tim started exploring himself in the bathtub. We didn't say anything until a few months later when he started going after himself sitting in someone's lap.

"He would do it with anybody, my friends, his aunt, anyone. They would get a little tense and look at us like, 'Oh God, what are we supposed to do?' "

At moments like these, Moira would tell Tim to stop. "I'm more informed by what goes on in society," she says. "I don't want to hamper his exploration. But if people are uncomfortable, that's where I want to draw the line."

There's another option to consider. During the first two to three years of your child's life, you can try managing moments like these by helping your friends with their discomfort before trying to stop your child. Acknowledge the situation and many people will relax. A statement like "Oh, there he goes again; he sure knows how to entertain himself" can relieve a lot of pressure.

And when that just seems impossible, what then? What happens when you find yourself, as Kirst did, "sitting at the front of the bus which is facing the whole rest of the bus, and he's sitting there just rubbing away, and you're really embarrassed because everyone else can see; obviously all the other parents are looking at you, grinning, but other people are looking at you in a really horrified way, like, 'How can you let your child do that?' "

In such delicate situations, avoid scolding, saying no, or pulling your child's hand away. The best approach is simply to distract your little one with something else: a toy, a tickle, a song. If you are in a situation the two of you can leave, do so. Remember, he may be seeking the comfort of masturbation because the setting is overstimulating for him. Taking him to a quieter place will help him as well as you, and it won't ascribe feelings of shame to the act of genital touching.

Civilization and Its Discontents

You might also console yourself with the following thought: This won't go on forever. Some day he'll learn to save it for home. Someday soon you will introduce him to the rules of the road.

And when you do, this will be good for him, too. Because the kids who make friends, the ones who are smiled upon by the world, are the ones who know how to behave. There are certain rules that all children need to uphold in the social world of their peers, not to mention the world ruled by schoolteachers. Those who don't will get teased or excluded, and that is most definitely not good for any little child.

So when do you do it?

You can begin to enforce a modesty standard for public masturbation at any time between the ages of roughly two and five, depending upon your particular child and your own views.

Children begin to take in and use information about social rules around the age of two or later. Once this happens, it is technically possible to begin schooling your child not to masturbate publicly, just as you will make use of this new aptitude to toilet train your child. Bear in mind that learning to comply with rules like these can be stressful for your toddler. If you notice that potty training or a new sibling or some other stressor is making things tough for your child, you might consider waiting to establish a rule about genital play until your little one is doing better with the other challenges he's facing.

However long you decide to wait, at a minimum, you should

require that before your child heads to kindergarten, she only mastur-bate at home, not outside the house. This will protect her from the shame of being criticized by peers or adults for masturbating at school or elsewhere. Although schools differ enormously, many will begin to demand a certain degree of sexual modesty of their kindergarten stu-dents. True, the staff at some nursery schools will raise eyebrows about genital touching. In this case, you may find that they will respond if you talk to them and explain that your child's masturbation is acceptable to you and not the sign of any problem. However, by kindergarten, you would do better to encourage your child to comply with these rules.

The range of rules parents set for genital play at home is broad. Some decide that masturbation is only acceptable when their child is entirely alone. Shelly, the mother of six-year-old Abe, is a bit less restrictive. She allows Abe to masturbate in her presence in the privacy of the bathroom, but she feels he shouldn't when his younger sister is in the bath with him.

If you prefer a little more modesty at home, you might decide to allow your child's unconscious touching of his genitals in public areas of the house but ask that more driven, purposeful masturbating be done privately. If all genital touching is unacceptable to family members, you may go a step further with the privacy line. Always make sure, however, to give your child a place where masturbation is entirely acceptable.

The Message: Privacy *and* Pleasure

What do you say?

Almost every parent we speak with knows that when a child mas-turbates at the wrong time or in the wrong place, she should tell him about privacy: "That's private—you should do that in your room." Or "Didn't we say you needed to do that in private?" Statements like these are fine, but with a little extra effort, you can do even better.

First, consider paying some extra attention to your tone of voice. If you feel a little tension about your child's masturbation, your lyrics may say it's healthy, but your music may convey a different message.

Then remember that talking about the importance of privacy only takes care of teaching your child about responsibility and social rules. If you want to help him develop a healthy regard for his sexual feelings, you might say a little more. When laying down the law about masturbation, also point out that the feeling he is having is a good one. It's the location you're limiting, not the act.

Without that assurance, what your child confronts at the moment he has found a nice place to rub is your sober face and an admonition that sounds an awful lot like "Stop it, or go away." Think about it. The difference between "If you are going to do that, I am going to send you to your room" and "Don't do that here, you need to do that in your room" may be subtle enough to elude even your brilliant four-year-old.

So, whenever you set your limit on genital play, simply pair privacy and pleasure in what you say:

> "It's fun to make yourself feel good like that. But I want you to do it
> in private, when you are alone. Special feelings like that are private."

You might let your child know that he's not the only masturbator in the world. It is one way to show that masturbation is a fine thing in the right setting.

> "When grown-ups do that, they make sure to do it in a private place,
> like their bedroom. You should do it in a private place, too."

Explain that her bedroom and the bathroom are private places. And remember that if you walk in on your daughter masturbating in her room, she *was* doing it privately.

When it comes to giving your child the house rules about masturbation, harsher reactions than these, like yelling, or punishment, or pulling a child's hand away, are unwarranted. This is true even when—perhaps especially when—masturbation becomes a problem.

How Much Is Too Much?

There are some times when masturbation does represent a problem. Don't try counting how often your child masturbates, however, to find out if there is cause for concern. More than the frequency of genital play, it's the pattern that matters.

Sheema, a kindergarten teacher, explains: "There is usually a pattern to masturbation. Most of the time it is during a downtime, which I think is fairly acceptable. Even at kindergarten you see a fair share of children touching themselves around rest times. I would never comment about that to a child, nor to a parent.

"But if I saw a child routinely masturbating during playtime when you want him to engage in another activity, then I might get concerned. You worry if a child is masturbating to the extent that he doesn't engage in other interesting things."

If you are concerned about how healthy your child's masturbation is, the first question to ask yourself is, "Does her masturbation interfere with other play activities?"

Next, ask yourself, "Is she masturbating in a setting where she once knew not to?" Some children may be communicating a problem by breaking the rules they once obeyed.

If the answer to either of these questions is yes, then your child's masturbation warrants some thought. Problematic masturbation can be a child's way of trying to manage an excessive degree of tension.

The Secret of Sexual Pleasure

I was putting Alex to bed one night, and he told me that sometimes he gets a "tingly feeling" in his penis. He said to me, "Daddy, do you know, are those feelings really nice feelings? Because I sort of think they are nice." I think he was having an erection, and he was asking me for permission to experience it as pleasurable. I said, "Yes, I think it's a feeling that people enjoy."

—Blair, on his ten-year-old son

I asked my mother, "Why does it feel so good?" Mom explained that it was a gift from God to give ourselves pleasure. She said that it was how my body would feel when I

*would grow up and have sex with my husband. I thought it was
cool that I could have a grown-up feeling when I was still a kid.*
  *—Mary Lou, recalling a conversation with her mother about mas-
turbation when Mary Lou was eight years old*

Your child's masturbation will probably afford you your first
opportunity to teach him about sexual pleasure. It's an opportunity many parents never take.

It may surprise you to learn that when a large sample of
American children were surveyed about the purposes of sex, not
one child below the age of nine listed pleasure. When it comes
to sex ed at home, we seem more inclined to outline the process
of meiosis than to point out one simple fact: Sex feels good.

The lessons of sexual pleasure your child can learn are
pretty simple, though. And the timing is easy, too. Start pre-
senting these ideas when you begin to give your child the
house rules on masturbation: That feeling you are having is a
sexual feeling. People like you and me like having that kind of
feeling, and we follow certain rules about how we get it.

This is the very lesson you will be teaching your child for the
next fifteen years. As he gets older, it will take on more sophisticated layers of meaning for him, but the central message never
changes. Sex is a great pleasure for all of us. To accept that pleasure is also to accept the responsibilities that go with it.

Like no masturbating at the dinner table.

Given this possibility, it's best not to focus on limiting the masturbation itself, an approach that may only increase your child's tension.
Instead, try to search out and eliminate the possible sources of stress in
your little one's life. As pediatrician T. Berry Brazelton advises in
Touchpoints, "Don't emphasize the behavior. Don't show disapproval or
try to inhibit it." Rather, he says, "parents should lighten up on any
pressure such as meal behavior, manners, toilet training, and so on."

Is the house too busy and stimulating for your child? If so, try to give him more quiet time in his room and reduce the overall hubbub at home. Have you been working hard to teach your kindergartner a new skill or responsibility that he can't quite get? Give him a breather. Is he being teased by another child? Ask your child and his teacher to tell you of any new stresses he may be facing, and work out a plan that will bring him some relief.

If the problematic masturbation persists, consider an evaluation with an expert. There may be a stress in your child's life that you are too close to see.

Doing unto Others

Developing a sexual career isn't just a solitary enterprise. Kids network. They collaborate. They take meetings.

"Let's see, first there was strip parlor," Chuck recalls, "which was done in the woods and which I can't really describe because I never had

And If It's Against Your Religious Beliefs

Parents sometimes find themselves caught between their religion's teachings on masturbation and their child's wandering fingers. If you're in this position, and you want to put an end to your child's masturbation because it conflicts with your beliefs, we recommend you try to do it in a way that doesn't make him feel bad about himself. A private explanation that masturbation is not allowed will be less troubling than a public or angry rebuke. An acknowledgment that you know it feels good, but that it's not appropriate, may be more effective than a comment that ignores the reasons he might want to masturbate.

We can't say that your young child will fully understand (or that he'll obey), but we think things will go best if you are frank about the reasons you consider masturbation wrong, tying it to other family beliefs. Your religious adviser may have some useful suggestions.

the guts to go watch. But it seemed very . . . established. Then there was something called 'hot dog in the bun,' which—you can probably guess—involved the oldest boy putting his penis between the buttocks of the oldest girl. I said, 'Why don't you put it in the front?' and they looked at me as if I were a true pervert. At age six."

If you thought kids were creative about masturbation, just wait until they discover sex play—the sexual games and experiments kids invent between toddlerhood and their teens.

Of course, what is confounding to most parents about children's sex games is not how varied the pretexts, the subterfuges, and the excuses to get naked with each other (although they can be astonishingly diverse). No, what is truly confounding is figuring out how in the hell to react when you walk in on it.

Jeffrey had his moment of truth one Sunday morning while his wife was out for a run. After a quick scan of the morning paper, he left the kitchen to find the girls. There in the living room were his two daughters, ages four and five, quietly eating their cereal in front of the television, each one naked and each one with a toe in the other's vagina. Jeff decided the best plan of action was to head right back into the kitchen— at least until his wife came home.

What was he supposed to do?

If you're not sure, you're in good company, because when it comes to sex play, uncertainty rules. You have to wonder, Is sex play healthy and should kids be allowed to pursue it undisturbed? Or is sex play a problem? Is it age-inappropriate behavior that kids should learn is off-limits? Could it be damaging if you let it continue?

Come across your five-year-old giggling in the broom closet with his girlfriend's pants down to her knees and phrases like "Stop! Stop! Stop!" and "No! No! No!" may spring to your feverish mind—not unlike the first time you saw him masturbate. As you did then, you may sense the need to protect his budding sexuality from your anxiety, and so you inhibit the impulse to yelp. But this time, you may think that if you *don't* stop him, you are somehow being irresponsible.

So may your neighbor, the father of the girl whose buttocks your son has initialed with a glitter pen. Life has just gotten a little more complicated. When sex play shows up, it adds a new wrinkle to the already formidable challenge of parenting about sex—a wrinkle that you will not soon be free of. The dilemma of the other kid's parents.

Read on and prepare yourself for one of the least comfortable conversations you may ever have with your neighbor, and for one of the most interesting—and when it comes to his sexual development, most important—conversations you may ever have with your child. The talk about sex play.

Or you can wait for your wife to come home.

Jeff was alphabetizing the spices when his wife finally showed up. He gave a mute nod toward the living room, where she found her girls just as Jeff had left them. As Jeff tells it, she frowned, put a hand on her hip, and asked her girls a single stern question.

"What did I say about eating in front of the television?"

Who Does What with Whom?

Sex play seems to be a normal part of growing up for many children. Just what percentage of kids experiment with their peers is hard to ascertain. But the handful of studies that have tried to answer the question suggests that at least a third of all girls and more than half of all boys have played at sex with a peer before they enter puberty. That's a lot of kids.

Games of a sexual sort may start as soon as your little one begins to interact independently with her playmates, like in preschool. When do the games stop? When they stop feeling like games. We tend to draw a somewhat artificial boundary at puberty. After that sex play becomes sex.

For some children, sex play will be a onetime affair, a single incident never to be repeated. For others, more commonly boys than girls, it will continue with the same or different playmates for years. Most often, sex play is shared among friends, although occasionally children pick siblings or cousins to play with. Friends who play together at sex are usually about the same age.

Unlike the more heated kind of sexual experimentation that begins with puberty and dating, young children don't seem to select sex-play partners based on whom they find attractive. They pick the ones who are willing and convenient.

Which explains why children's choice of sex playmates seems unrelated to their sexual orientation. In fact, children appear roughly as likely to experiment with a child of the same sex as they are with a child of the opposite sex.

Silly Willies

In early childhood, sex play is a famously silly endeavor. Take this parent's experience, reported in London's *Guardian* newspaper:

> My son, who was then four, and the five-year-old girl from next door had been unusually quiet so I went upstairs to find out what they were up to. I opened the door to find them dressed only in wellies [rain boots], a "tail" of pink loo paper tucked between their buttocks, faces flushed with excitement.

> ("What did I say about wearing your wellies indoors?")

> Of course it was by no means the only "doctors and nurses" game that my children ever played; but along with the time my son and his cousin wrapped their willies in yellow industrial tape, panicked and had to have a long soapy bath, it is the occasion I remember best.

Sex play before the age of about five is the delightfully carefree concoction of noodlebrains who love to have their clothes off, like to see their friends naked, and will try just about anything that pops into their little heads. Their play has mostly to do with showing and touching and is unself-conscious enough, especially among the youngest set, that it may happen out in plain view. You could just as easily call a lot of it "naked play"—it's not always clear how sexual it really is.

Only later, as they grow, will modesty imbue sex play with its thrilling cloak-and-dagger quality. Approaching school age, children begin to take their games more seriously. Their own modesty makes undressing for a friend a much more charged experience. And they have a new sense that they need to hide their adventures from adult eyes. Secret places have to be found. Pacts of silence are sealed.

Need we say it? Sex play gets better.

The Golden Years

Almost everything that's known about children's sex play was learned from adults. College students filling out questionnaires, psychotherapy patients recounting tales from their past—these are the key informants. And when you ask grown-ups like them for a story about sex play, you typically hear of an encounter between ages seven and ten. These are the golden years of sex play, and they remain forever enshrined as such in the hearts of many.

In literary equivalents, sex play that was once *Goodnight Moon* has become *Harry Potter and the Goblet of Fire*. All 734 pages. Yet, because children have learned to hide, much of middle childhood's sex play goes on without parents ever finding out.

What are you missing? Well, the most common form of sex play is still based on showing and looking, with or without some touching. Often children will strike a simple "I'll show you mine if you show me yours" deal. At other times, the stripping, looking, and touching are egged on by a game of pretend. Doctor and patient are of course the most famous roles enacted for this purpose, and they still remain popular (despite the new requirement that children obtain prior authorization from their HMO for these encounters). But sex charades run the gamut from tame husband-and-wife scenarios to scenes involving pornography or bondage patched together from shreds of knowledge of the adult world (and you thought they were asleep during your little midnight escapade).

Occasionally, children will actually pretend to have intercourse. This sort of posturing usually involves children touching their genitals together or lying on top of one another. Rarely is there any sort of penetration. Pretending is usually enough for children, and the small penis of prepubertal boys makes any real attempt at intercourse unlikely to succeed.

Encounters like these thrill their little practitioners in part through the excitement of discovery, and in part through the shivery early stirrings of attraction and desire that rustle in the background. Other sorts of sex play trade on different kinds of arousal. Some games focus less on the fun of showing and looking and more on experimenting with genital sensations. A group of girls at a sleepover may take turns climbing into the bath and spraying their genitals with a shower hose. Boys may slip away and masturbate each other in just the way they have learned to enjoy themselves when alone. One mother tells of her ten-year-old son and his best friend: "I saw both of them lying on their backs in the sun in the backyard and masturbating each other. I said nothing at the time, but tactfully asked Byron about it later on. His unashamed reply was to grin and say that they were always doing it in bed and that they both liked doing it because it felt so good!"

In still other cases, sex play seems less about the pursuit of nice feelings than about an edgy, taking-it-to-the-limit kind of thrill. Consider Jenny, now a mother herself, who used to bathe at age seven with her best friend Alison: "We used to compete to see how far we could put our finger in—how far up you could get your finger inside yourself." The main excitement for Jenny was one that plays a role in many of the sex games young children pursue—daring herself to explore the dark reaches of the body and its sensations. Finding the forbidden, and sticking your finger in.

The End of Sex Play

Does sex play ultimately stop, or does it simply morph into something we are less inclined to consider "play"? This is a hard one to answer, in part because we have very little good data about the end of sex play, and in part because there may be no single answer that applies to all children.

It is clear that as elementary school draws to a close, the meaning of sexual exploration changes noticeably for kids. As they move into puberty and understand more about grown-up sex, they begin to view sexual experiences with peers through older lenses. Preteens start to believe that sexual explorations should be reserved for someone they are attracted to, someone they are dating, or someone they might want to date. As a result, sex play relationships that have lasted through middle childhood may begin to break up.

Is Sex Play Okay?

As long as your child is a willing participant, sex play itself appears harmless.

In fact, some leading sex researchers see sex play as a valuable element of a child's sexual education and a key rehearsal for healthy adult sex. But we also know that sex play isn't always a good experience. What might have been a pleasant step on the way to a happy sex life can sometimes end up a stumble on the road to self-acceptance and sexual health.

What determines which sort of experience your child will have?

Two factors seem crucial: the degree of coercion involved in your child's game, and the reaction of those—especially you—who find out about it.

Sex play is undeniably best when it is mutual and accepted by fam-

---

Don't Blame Barbie

Anna, my oldest daughter, came to me one day and said, "I'm going to tell you something, and it's really disgusting." She said Olivia was playing a game she didn't like. It was called "Sexy Barbie." At the time, Olivia was six or seven. She was playing this game where she took Barbie's clothes off and put her on top of Ken and had a big make-out session.

I took Olivia aside. Her first response was to totally deny it. "Oh, no, I wouldn't do that." That's how I knew it was true.

—*Lenore, mother of four*

We know what you're thinking. It's Barbie's fault. That crazy bust. Those tarty outfits. They try to palm her off as a solid citizen—a dentist, an astronaut, an aerobics instructor—but she'll never really pass. Plugging away at her campaign after all of these years, Barbie even makes running for president seem sort of naughty. What do they expect? She may be ambitious, but she's still the girl who was modeled on a German sex toy, herself modeled on a popular prostitute. Poor Barbie. It's in her genes.

But if you find your daughter using your nail polish to paint nipples on that improbable chest, don't blame Barbie. Children's sexual curiosity was probably visited on their dolls long before the mid-century birth of America's favorite compulsive shopper.

Sex play with dolls is not so different from children's sex play with each other. Just as with games between children, doll play varies with a child's level of sexual awareness and interest. Give a toddler a doll and within minutes she will pull its clothes off, looking at the buttocks and genitals. As she gets older, stripping and peeking gradually give way to smooching and flirting.

As with sex play, simulated sexual acts like humping and oral sex between dolls are less common. In the case of dolls, though, you have to wonder, is it just because Ken is such a dud?

ily and peers. A child who enters sex play free of interference or pressure is likely to leave with a feeling of excitement and pleasure that will nourish her view of her body and her sexuality. Happily, much of sex play takes place under just these conditions. As long as this is the case, there is no reason for you to limit it.

Sometimes, however, children are pressured into sex play or humiliated by others for having participated. When that happens, sex play can leave scars of shame or fear.

Let's look first at the issue of pressure. Think of any nonsexual game you've ever watched children play. Typically, one or two kids come up with what they consider a brilliant idea, a few others go along for the ride, and the rest have to be inveigled. The same holds true for sex play. Sometimes it takes a little leverage to get a game of "tweak the wiener" going among your friends. Sometimes it takes a lot.

A little pressure is probably okay, but when there's a lot, we worry.

A child who feels substantial pressure to enter a sexual game against his will may join in, but he may feel bullied, taken over, possibly invaded. When these feelings get linked in his mind with sexual behavior, they can cramp his healthy sexual development. In the most extreme cases of coercion, which include manipulation as well as physical force, sex play becomes sexual abuse (a small percentage of all sexual abuse is perpetrated by other children) and can cause psychological damage similar to that wrought by an abusive experience with an adult. Obviously, this sort of sex play is not okay and should be stopped.

Sometimes problematic coercion results when an older child uses her authority to boss or trick a younger one into joining in. The greater the age difference between two children, the more likely that there is an unhealthy element of coercion involved in their sex play. A large age difference may also leave a child with simple ambitions faced with play too adventurous for him to want or understand.

In assessing age differences, you might follow this simple rule of thumb. If two children are different enough in age that they don't naturally choose one another as playmates for other games, then they probably shouldn't play sex games together, either.

Your Crucial Role

The second key factor determining whether childhood sex play is okay—a variable vastly more important than what exactly gets shown or touched or acted out during the play—is the conversation a child has with his parents after the fact.

When adults recall their childhood sex play, the stories they tell are often lighthearted tales relayed with a smile and a wink, or a sort of sentimental longing for the past. When they are not, when they are stories of shame, there is often the harsh reaction of a parent in the picture. A parent's angry disapproval of sex play can cut to a child's heart, affixing an enduring negative meaning to what might have been a benign event.

Occasionally, it is the negative reactions of peers that turn a sex play experience sour. One child becomes a target of teasing by playmates who may or may not have been involved. (Because homosexuality is typically stigmatized by kids, same-sex sex play may be more likely to draw this reaction.) Still, the importance to your child of his friends' reactions will be mediated by you. Parents who openly accept their child's play can lessen the impact of peer teasing. Parents who seem to agree with a child's hecklers may compound it.

So What Do You Do?

The silly sort of peekaboo play your children enjoy in their first few years really requires no intervention at all. It is usually quite clear that sex play at two and three is lighthearted fun and not emotionally laden for your child (unless it gets undue attention). If you stumble across it, do nothing. Just as with early masturbation, if you feel you have to stop it—because the kids have drawn a crowd in the children's book section—simply divert them into a less eye-popping activity.

There is no real need to have a discussion about their behavior at this tender age.

Starting around the age of four, sex play may still be a casual romp, but you can begin to give a fuller response. From now on, you have two decisions to make: what to do the moment you swing the door open, and what to say about it later.

Some parents will still find it unnecessary to interrupt their kid's sex play. Tara explains: "Much more probably goes on than I know about, and that's fine. When I do find out, like when the girls go upstairs and they take out their dolls, and I open the door and no one has their clothes on, that's fine, too. I'll say, 'Is everything going okay?' 'Yeah, it's fine.' I say, 'Okay,' and close the door."

Bea feels differently. "I don't sponsor my children's sexual activity. What they do on their own is fine, but once they know I know, then the game is over. I will clomp down the hall so they know I am there and then say something like, 'How about a game of volleyball?' "

You decide which approach feels better for you. If you do choose to stop the play, it is best to use Bea's approach and do so without a "What are you doing?" or a "Stop that now" sort of scold. This is not the time to comment on the behavior itself. It is a moment ripe for embarrassing your child and feeling flustered yourself, which makes it a lousy time to try to teach anything.

If you weren't able to hold back the "Stop that!" or the "Oh, my God" that leaped immediately to mind, simply explain your momentary fluster and apologize. Then remember that kids are resilient and forgive yourself.

Time for a Talk

Later, however, whether you decided to stop the sex play you saw or let it continue undisturbed, consider having a little talk. This discussion should happen as soon after the event as you can be alone with your child in a comfortable, calm place. Try not to let it go too long. Your child may be waiting anxiously for a word from you, and she may interpret your silence as anger or disapproval, especially if your facial expression revealed surprise or confusion.

What are your goals for this talk? Certainly, you want to put your child's mind at ease about having been caught. At the same time, you want to check on the health of the sex play and help her avoid harmful situations in the future. And you want to make the conversation itself pleasant enough that your child will be inclined to keep you in the loop when sexual things happen that confuse or concern her. As we explained above, there is no place in this discussion for shaming or scolding.

Start by giving your child a little relief. Tell her that you are not angry, and that she is not in trouble. Then focus on understanding. Try to help your child describe just what the experience was like for her. Lead with easy-to-answer questions that don't seem to be looking for blame:

"Was that a game you and Chris were playing today? Does it have a name? How do you play?"

Then look for signs of coercion. Remember your child may have been coerced, or she may have been the coercer.

"Was is fun for both of you? Sometimes not everyone wants to play. Did everyone want to play this time?"

You don't really need to know all of the details. But try to find out enough to get a clear sense of how willing a participant your child and the others were. Remember, a small degree of persuasion is common and probably acceptable.

Then it's time for your reaction. If you sense the sex play was a fun experience for all with a minimum of coercion, you can support it:

"I'm glad you had fun. That kind of play can be fun with a friend like Chris. I don't want you to do it with someone who isn't your age. And only play like that if you want to. You can say no if you don't want to play. Do you understand that?"

Make sure she does understand, and clarify any uncertainty. Then ask:

"Will you tell me if something like that happens and it isn't fun?"

If your child seems to have strongly coerced her playmate, that will be the focus of your comments, but you can still support sexuality:

"Those feelings are nice—but it isn't nice to make someone do something he doesn't want to do. I only want you to play like that with your friend if he wants to do it also."

Because some children who coerce others may have been coerced themselves in the past, take this opportunity to ask:

"Has anyone ever made you do something like that that you didn't want to do?"

If your child was forced to play against her will, you will have a more involved talk with her, and you should carefully revisit the topic if the event has not been defused. Give her a chance to discuss her feelings about what happened. Is she upset? She may not be. Allow her to be casual if that's her response. Try not to amplify the event by expressing your own anger or fear to her. Don't suggest that she has been physically harmed (if she hasn't) or that something has been done to her that can't be undone (such as asking, "Did he break your hymen?").

Tell your child that her friend was wrong to make her do something she didn't want to do. If you're going to talk with the other child's parents about what happened, let your daughter know. At some point, you can explain that if something like this ever happens again, there are a few things she can do. She can say no. She can say she will tell on him if he does anything. Or she can leave the room without saying anything. Tell her these things don't always work, especially if the person is very strong or mean, but she can always tell you afterward and you will take care of things.

In particularly troubling cases, you may want to seek the consultation of a child psychiatrist, psychologist, or other professional.

When sex play was coercive, you also have to decide whether or not to limit the children's access to each other. Use your judgment. Consider the quality of their relationship and the nature of what happened. If the other child is a close friend, and the experience was not very upsetting, separating the two could cause your child more distress than the sex play did. Instead, provide a little more supervision and reduce their opportunities for sex play. You can end joint baths or sleepovers, or you can make a rule that when the children play together, the door always has to be open.

If, on the other hand, your child expresses real fear of the playmate, or if the playmate's behavior seems either cruel or at a level of sexual development well beyond that of your child, separate them until you feel the situation has changed.

Meet the Joneses

You have one more dilemma to face the day you discover your child's tush-rubbing game with the Joneses' boy.

"Should I tell his friend's parents?" you ask yourself in a voice you usually reserve for questions like, "Should I have my spleen removed?"

Well, yes, usually you should tell them, although no one could blame you for being a teensy bit reluctant. If there is one thing harder than talking to your child about sex, it's talking to your neighbor about talking to *her* child about sex. Sex play turns out to be an especially difficult subject among parents, because they often know little about it and commonly disagree about how to react. Add to this your neighbor's fear that her child will be labeled sexually promiscuous or deviant, and things can really heat up.

In the best cases, all parents involved agree that age-appropriate, consensual sex play is acceptable, and then work out a consistent message to give their children. The children either continue their play or move on from it without having been disturbed by grown-up fireworks.

In the worst cases, families follow the age-old rule of problem solving: "First, assign blame." One child is identified as "the instigator," and his parents get accused of irresponsibility if they fail to punish him. Those parents in turn criticize the others as alarmist, and the children, who were actually playing well together, get separated. More than a few friendships have ended this way.

Why take the risk of telling other parents when they may not understand the situation as well as you do? Think of yourself as on a reconnaissance mission for your child. Any sex play you discover this week could just as easily be stumbled upon by your neighbor next week. If she is going to overreact, you want her to do it on the phone with you, not in front of your half-dressed seven-year-old. Preparing her may spare your child a humiliating experience; so may warning your child.

Call your neighbors soon after you discover the sex play. They are less likely to be alarmed if they feel you aren't holding back any information and that you are taking the matter seriously. Simply explain what you saw and how you have decided to react. Tell them what you know about sex play and why you do or don't consider the children's game to be a problem.

If the parents have a strong negative reaction even after you have done some education, then you should protect your child from the surprise of their opinion by discussing the matter with him. You might try some version of the following:

> "You know we think your tush-rubbing game is fine. We spoke with
> Peter's parents and the Joneses don't like it. We disagree with them,

but we still want to listen to them. So you can play your game with other kids, but don't play it with Peter anymore."

If you feel you really can't talk with the neighbors about the situation, because of how they'll react, consider whether it's a good idea for your child to play at their home. Your priority remains to protect your child from unwarranted blame or criticism.

Something Simple

And what about the Joneses, who flipped when you found their kid playing naked with yours. What's with them? Well, probably they were hoping for something simpler than all this—something simpler than having to sort out when masturbation is okay and when it's a problem, or when sex play can continue and when it should stop. The Joneses want an innocent child, a child untouched by their complicated world—a child who isn't sexual yet.

Ask the Joneses and they'll tell you, adult life can smart. And the more it smarts—the more vexed you feel by the complexity of your daily life—the more irresistible that fantasy of a child's simplicity. It's a dream, of course, but it's a dream so damned appealing, it hurts to wake from.

Does anyone really have an easy time with this? Sure, we've found a few parents who seem so comfortable with their own sexuality, so confirmed in their view that sex *is* innocent that they gracefully support— even enjoy—the first expressions of their child's sexual self. As for the rest of us? Let's just say that we have met the Joneses, and the Joneses are us.

The parents of parentsplace.com flip on their PCs and tap out their distress:

> "The problem is that when the two were in the bath the other night, I caught the oldest one playing with the youngest one in such a way that my stomach caught."
>
> "He is tooooo curious for my liking."
>
> ". . . a huge stuffed teddy bear which I recently caught her lying on top of and 'humping,' for lack of a better word."

". . . that's what they do. They look at their penises and bottoms."

". . . in my backyard in the middle of the day taking their pants off."

"I told my daughter that they need to keep their hands to themselves. . . ."

"I, of course, have told them that it is not appropriate behavior."

"I'm afraid that I got a little upset."

"I tried to stay calm."

"Was I overreacting?"

"I am having a really hard time dealing with this."

Once in a while, a parent will seem so distraught, you would think his little one was being taken away from him. In truth, she is being taken away, although by no one other than the girl she is about to become. Maybe this is the hardest part of facing a child's first sexual explorations. The realization it makes plain: She's growing up.

Let's not pretend that there isn't something quietly cruel about being a parent. Just as you grow more and more in love with your child, you are expected to carry on equipping her with the supplies she needs to leave you, and to cheer on that leaving. Nurturing your child's sexual development is no less bittersweet than any other aspect of her growing up. To help her along, you have to let go a little.

Bea, who goes clomping down the hall when she hears her kids fooling around, is right when she says she doesn't sponsor their sexuality. As a parent, you don't have to teach your child to masturbate. You don't have to set up sex-play dates with his friends. You really don't need to be involved at all.

When it comes right down to it, you don't give your child her sexuality. What you give her is the permission and the privacy to seek it out, and the confidence to claim it as hers when she's found it. Letting your child find her sexuality, in the end, comes down to one challenging act of love: blocking your impulse to take it away from her. The impulse that says stop, wait, I'm not ready to let you go.

Chapter **5**

Think about it

CONSIDERING YOUR CHILD'S SEXUAL ORIENTATION

When he came out to his father and me, it was a complete surprise. I was shocked! There was just no way of knowing. I mean, in all of those years of raising him, I'm honestly telling you it never occurred to me that he might be gay.

—EILEEN, ON HER SEVENTEEN-YEAR-OLD SON

YOU ARE IN THE KITCHEN with your five-year-old, fixing him a snack. The television is on and he is glued to it, chattering back to a cartoon. Then an advertisement cuts in. "I love him," you hear him say. You turn around. He's beaming at Pete Sampras, dark-eyed in whites, holding up a watch.

Ben doesn't like tennis, you think.

The grilled cheese sizzles, and the thought disappears.

You have taken your eleven-year-old daughter to buy bathing suits for the family summer vacation. There, in the fitting room together, she gets oddly quiet. You are undressed, and you catch a glimpse of her, looking at you. Her face is flushed.

For a moment you think, "This is different from what it's like with her older sister. Does she feel odd around naked women?" You turn around to adjust your suit. Your son calls in from outside asking if he can come in, your daughter shrieks, and the thought slips out of your mind.

Your seventeen-year-old son is hanging out in his room with a close girlfriend, a sweet classmate who has almost become a part of your family over the last few years. You trust them alone together, maybe because you have never noticed a strong sexual tension between them. Walking past his open door today you overhear a snippet of their conversation. They are talking about boys. Cute boys.

Standing there with a basket of laundry in your hands, half straining to hear what your son is saying, half trying to ignore it, do you consider the possibility that your son may be gay, or does it still feel too remote? More to the point, does the idea feel too upsetting to really let it percolate through your mind?

It doesn't surprise us when a parent says she had no idea her child was gay until the moment he came out to her. There are some ideas that even the most curious and devoted parent won't give a home to. "Maybe my child is gay" is near the top of the list.

Not long ago a mother asked for advice about her sixteen-year-old son. Charlotte, who had an ongoing struggle with her son over his ceaselessly sloppy room, had taken it upon herself to clean out his closet one weekend when Michael was at his father's. Deep in the back of his closet she unearthed a safe she had given him years ago and somehow found herself opening it. Inside was a small pile of pages from pornographic magazines and photographs downloaded from the Internet. They were all pictures of naked men.

"Do you think Michael is gay?" she asked.

Charlotte said she didn't want to jump to conclusions. Michael was still very young. When told that heterosexual teenage boys don't hide gay porn—that the hallmark of sexual orientation is a child's private attractions and that the direction of those attractions, especially in boys, doesn't appear to change—Charlotte nodded. She understood. "That's great. That's a help," she smiled her warm smile.

Was she at all troubled about her son's attractions? "The pictures? Oh, no. You know, Michael knows I love him no matter what, but I don't think he's ready to consider the possibility that he might be gay. He's still so young."

Perhaps Charlotte was right about Michael. But one thing seemed clear. Charlotte wasn't ready, and that, above all else, was why she was looking in his safe and then trying to make what she found there go away.

He Needs You

If we had to reduce this chapter to three words of advice, the words would be these: Think about it.

Consider the possibility that you may have been charged with the responsibility of a raising a gay son or daughter. Undeniably, this possibility presents a few challenges to most heterosexual parents. Your lesbian daughter will pass through some major life experiences that are almost entirely unfamiliar to you. Your gay son will have needs you simply can't anticipate. What coming out advice will you give? What will you say if he's taunted? How will you handle the prom?

But the greatest challenge posed by a gay child, and the most important one to surmount, is getting yourself to entertain the possibility that you've got one.

If you spot your five-year-old boy cooing unself-consciously over Pete Sampras, or find your eleven-year-old daughter rattled by seeing you naked, or hear your seventeen-year-old son discussing the cute boys in his class (and you may—these examples are all drawn from real experiences of parents whose children did indeed turn out to be gay), you might prefer to just let it go. That would be understandable. Imagining your child to be gay can be unsettling; and yes, it is important not to reach a premature conclusion about your child's sexuality.

But bear in mind, too, that your inclination to wait, to tell yourself it's unnecessary or even wrong to wonder whether your child might be gay, may be your child's single biggest obstacle to getting the support he needs. For as long as you are not dealing with it, it is dealing with him.

Your child needs you to be the parent. You may not be an expert on homosexuality, but neither is he. All that's required is that you allow yourself to consider the possibility that your child is gay, keep that possibility in mind, and act accordingly.

A little effort on your part can spare your child the shame of a child-

hood of teasing, the fear of losing your love, and the loneliness of a closeted adolescence. If ever there was a job for a parent, this is it.

As Charlotte spoke, the more she said about her son Michael, the
clearer it became that he was in trouble. He was spending hours alone
in his room, apparently doing nothing; his grades had dropped; and he
had fallen out of contact with his friends at school for months. It was
too late to prevent some of the losses of his depressive episode, but it
wasn't too late to prevent the suicide attempt or unprotected sex that
might be on the horizon. Which is why, despite the fact that Charlotte
was unconvinced about her son's orientation, it seemed essential that she
speak with him, to help him navigate what was probably one of the
toughest passages of his adult life.

Charlotte listened attentively. She seemed genuinely grateful for the
advice and said she would talk to her son the next weekend.

Do You Have a Vote?

If we are going to talk honestly about your child's orientation, there is one
thing we have to acknowledge. It's probably fair to say that most parents
want their children to be heterosexual. That's understandable. Most parents want their children to have lives free of hardship, and although het-
erosexuality has never been a guarantee of happiness, it is true that gay
youth have to face some difficulties that their straight friends never will.

More than that, as a parent, you probably want your children to be
like yourself (or, better, like an idealized version of yourself). If you are
heterosexual, and you want to share some of the most important experiences of your life—falling in love, marrying, starting a family—with
your children, you may fear that you'll miss those pleasures if your son
or daughter is gay.

Then there are your dreams of your child's success, whatever that
means to you. If you could, you wouldn't mind choosing your child's
SAT scores, picking her particular talents, or selecting a favorite candi-
date for her spouse. If you could, you wouldn't mind determining your
child's sexual orientation. But you can't.

Whether your child will grow up to be heterosexual or homosexual is probably shaped by a host of interacting factors. But your wishes and your opinions are simply not among them.

What does decide your child's future orientation?

The road to unraveling this particular mystery is littered with the remains of countless theories that have never panned out. Research has given us some ideas, though. First and foremost, there is good evidence that genes play a major but not determinative role in shaping your child's sexual orientation. In fact, for all its confusion, the extensive research into the origins of sexual orientation makes one thing clear. The only known vote you have in your child's sexual orientation you cast with an egg or a sperm.

Twins Speak

The best evidence for this view has come in the form of studies that gathered up large groups of gay and lesbian adults and then went looking for their siblings' sexual orientations. What makes this research so powerful is the study of identical twins, nature's own little experiments into what genes do or don't determine.

One study of gay men and their brothers found that if a man has an adoptive brother who is gay, his chance of being gay himself (11 percent) is not too far from that of anyone else in the population (estimates vary, but researchers tend to set that chance at 3 to 5 percent). On the other hand, if he has an identical twin who is gay, that man has a 52 percent chance of being gay himself. That's a very big difference.

You might wonder, could twins' orientation be more alike than adoptive brothers' for reasons other than their genes? Could it be because they were born at the same time to the same parents, or because they were exposed to the same prenatal environment? The study addressed this question, too.

The researchers looked at fraternal twins—twins who from conception onward experience the same environment but who, because they result from two separate eggs and two separate sperm, are not genetically identical. As it turns out, the brother of a gay fraternal twin has a 22 percent chance of being gay himself, significantly lower than the rate for identical twins. Being born at the exact same time and place isn't enough. Genes almost certainly play a role.

The same pattern turned up in a separate study of lesbian women and their sisters. A heritable factor that helps shape a child's sexual orientation seems to be the best way to explain these results.

The Other Half of the Equation

The second key revelation of those valuable twin studies is this: Genes can't be the whole answer. There must be some other factors that affect the expression of those genes, some influence that helps shape a growing child's sexual orientation. What could that other influence be?

You may have heard of the close-binding-mother-distant-hostile-detached-father theory of homosexuality. This idea, popularized in the 1960s, essentially maintained that young men become gay because as children they get too much of their mother, and too little of their father. Unable psychologically to separate from an overwhelming mother and identify with their absent dad, these boys were thought to identify with their mother and seek out love partners like the one she chose. The theory stuck, in part, because it struck a cultural nerve in the American household.

First, it gave parents a rationale for their irrational guilt. Their suspicions were right: They *were* to blame; they *could* have prevented this. Second, the theory legitimized already well-established family resentments. What 1960s mother didn't at some point feel anger at her husband for not being as available to their children as she was? What father didn't experience a twinge of bitterness at being excluded from a private intimacy between his wife and his child? When the child turned out gay, their resentments seemed justified. Never mind that the implicated family constellation described a sizable percentage of all American families at the time, regardless of the sexual orientation of their children.

Numerous investigators have since put this theory to the test, and the results are illuminating. For one thing, the mother finding doesn't hold. Gay men are no more likely to report having had a close-binding mother, however that's defined, than heterosexual men are. The father finding, however, stands up somewhat. Gay men are more likely than their heterosexual peers to tell researchers that their relationship with their father is poor or distant. Importantly, however, that finding has been substantially reinterpreted since the 1960s. The arrow of causality has since been reversed. An example will clarify why.

A psychiatrist specializing in the study of gay men once had an opportunity to study a pair of identical twin bothers, one of them gay, the other heterosexual, who had grown up together with their parents. The psychiatrist interviewed the brothers separately, asking each to describe his father. The gay man's response went something like this: My father had very little to offer our family. When he would come home at night, he would sit through dinner and hardly speak a word. After dinner, he would disappear into the basement where he had some sort of shop. And that was about it.

The heterosexual twin's response: My father was a man of few words. He worked hard all day, but he always made sure to have dinner with us. He didn't talk much, but when he did, you listened. He was a wonderful craftsman. After dinner, he would often go downstairs to do some woodworking. I had great times down there with him.

Same father. Different sons. Different relationship.

It is now generally thought that the poor relationship that can sometimes be found between a gay son and his father is the product, not the cause, of that boy's orientation. We'll say more about this later.

What We Do Know

Despite the failure of the old theory, no other explanation of the non-genetic contributions to sexual orientation has taken its place. If any such environmental factors are discovered, they will probably be found to act in the earliest years of a child's life during a sensitive window period. When that window opens and closes is not known. But it seems that while an environmental factor may operate as early as the prenatal period, it is unlikely to have its effect after a child reaches four or five. By that age a child's future orientation is probably well established. There is no evidence that any later influence can change it.

Although we may never know what these early influences are (one possibility is hormones circulating in the fetal environment), we have a fairly good idea of what they are not. When behavioral scientists talk about "environment," they are not referring to a child's learning about homosexuality, meeting gay or lesbian people, or watching *Will and Grace* reruns. In other words, there is no reason to believe that familiarity with gay people leads to homosexuality, or that lack of familiarity prevents it.

Maybe It's a Phase

Remember how we once learned not to say, "Maybe it's just a phase"? There was a time when it was pretty hard to imagine a kid calling up the courage to tell someone she was gay if she wasn't certain. In fact, it's still hard to imagine for most teens.

But over the last generation or so, we've found that some teenage girls say that they are bisexual or gay in high school or college, and then later go on to consider themselves heterosexual. Sometimes, it turns out, it *is* a phase. Has something changed?

Yes. There are now some environments in which the stigma against homosexuality is low enough that teens can test out the idea of being gay or bisexual without fearing an unfriendly reception. And so, occasionally, a girl may, for a period of time, identify herself to friends and family as lesbian or bisexual. Later, if she finds her attractions to boys really are stronger than those to girls, she either recants, or simply goes back to dating boys without much fanfare.

These girls are doing exactly what adolescents are supposed to do when it comes to crafting an identity. Healthy adolescents test identities out. They try a style on for size, and if it doesn't fit, they slip into another. Look at your own teenager: one day she's a goth-chick with black nail polish and a grudge, the next day she's braiding her hair and baking cookies for the school fund-raiser. There is not always great depth or substance to these little jaunts. Still, we bite our tongues and respect our teenagers' adventures, because they represent a serious and deeply felt search for self-definition. (Which is why it's still insulting to tell your daughter you think she'll grow out of being bisexual, even if you turn out to be right.)

This degree of subtlety is likely to be wholly unnecessary in dealing with your son. These days, when it comes to hetero-sexual teenage boys, trying out being gay seems to have all the allure of a body cast. Apparently, the negative consequences of saying you're gay remain so great among boys as to prohibit any public exploration of that identity. There may also be an inherent difference between male and female sexuality that allows girls to discover and explore their orientations in ways that boys do not. In any case, until things change, if your son comes out, odds are he isn't experimenting. He's gay.

Sissies and Tomboys

Though you can't select your child's orientation, you can certainly influence the route he takes to discovering and accepting it. For many kids, the road to gay adulthood is a rough one, with stress and hardship beginning as early as preschool and increasing in intensity until the moment they finally come out. If your child is on that road, a little well-focused help from you can make his path dramatically easier than it might have been. To get started, you'll need to know what challenges your kid is up against. How, for example, is the life of a kindergartner who will someday be gay different from one who won't?

"Oh, I always felt different," explains Evan, a man who says he's been gay his entire life, "even in kindergarten."

Do you mean you knew you were gay when you were five?

"I didn't know what 'gay' was. But I knew I didn't fit in. I just wasn't like the other boys. First of all, I was much more into the way I dressed. A couple of times, I was actually criticized by my kindergarten teacher for spending too much time in the dress-up corner. I hung out much more with the girls than the boys back then. Do you think the other boys were playing house? They were swinging from the jungle bars.

"Let's face it," Evan says with a rueful smile, "I was a big sissy."
What's this about?

To understand the early childhoods of gay and lesbian people, you need to know a bit about temperament. Understood as a constellation of personality traits that are considered inborn, a child's temperament shapes how eagerly she seeks out new experiences, to what extent caution guides her choices, and how reliant she is on the approval of others. A key element of a child's temperament, and the one we're especially interested in here, is the degree to which a child enjoys or avoids boisterous, knockabout play.

There are some kids who love to take a flying leap into the mud, who will throw themselves into the path of a ball if it threatens to whiz past them, who like to shout and roll around and rough it up. Call them the bold ones. On the other hand, there are children who hang back when a ball is tossed, who are afraid of getting hit, or dirty, who like quiet play. Call them the timid ones.

There is a great degree of diversity among women and among men when it comes to boldness and timidity. But, although some women

Can You Tell?

Some parents ask if they can predict their child's future sexual orientation based on her interest in rough play. The answer is definitely not for girls, possibly for some boys.

The great majority of tomboys grow up to be heterosexual women.

As for boys, the research seems to show that the majority of those who are the most "sissy-ish" in childhood do grow up to be gay. But because some of them don't, and because some of the rough-and-tumble boys grow up to be gay, you can't make a reliable prediction of your boy's sexual orientation based on his play style. What you can do is create an environment where a less-approved style doesn't subject him to ridicule and shame, regardless of what orientation he's headed for.

are very bold, and some men are quite timid, in general, boys are more likely to pursue and enjoy rough-and-tumble play than are girls. From what we now know, the difference seems to be somewhat based in biology and then, importantly, magnified by culture, as girls are discouraged from playing rough and boys are praised for it.

What does this have to do with gay kids? Well, although kids who grow up to be gay or lesbian have a full range of temperaments, from delicate to tough, a number of gay adults, upon looking back, say that they were timid boys who avoided rough play, or bold girls who loved it. Many gay men say they were, to adopt the word so often used against them, "sissies," and many lesbians remember being "tomboys."

And that is where their trouble begins.

The (Hard Knock) Life of a Gay Child

Children whose temperaments differ from what their parents expect (or want) for a boy or girl face some of their earliest challenges right at home in their preschool years. A timid four-year-old who is afraid of loud noises or being flipped upside down may find an afternoon in the backyard with his rough-and-tumble dad an uncomfortable experience. His father, who finds he just can't get his son to enjoy playing with him, who sees his son hurry back into his mother's arms when given the chance, may start to feel a bit rejected by his boy. Without really knowing it's happening, the two of them may withdraw from each other. Remember the twins whose father had a woodworking shop? Of course, this kind of disconnect isn't limited to same-gender parent-child pairings, and it isn't even limited to gay kids. But it probably represents the riskiest household situation for a kid who will eventually discover that he's gay. Before he reaches kindergarten, a boy like this may develop the sense that he can't please his dad.

Then, when elementary school gets under way, peers present the next challenge. The world of school-age boys is highly hierarchical. To picture young boys' society, imagine a totem pole with one boy on the top, one on the bottom, and the others ranked in between. Athletic skill, speed, and strength are the surest routes to the top of the pole. Weakness, timidity, and anything boys associate with being a girl send a boy right to the bottom (whether he's destined to be gay or not). And that's a dangerous place to be.

Timid boys relegated by virtue of their temperaments to the lowest rank on the totem pole are commonly bullied by their peers. The top boys are his leaders, so when they tell him he's inadequate, he believes them. If that message connects with the impression he's gotten through years of mismatched play dates with Dad, it carries even more weight. The result is a child on the cusp of puberty who hasn't an inkling that he might be gay, but who already senses that there is something intrinsically flawed in him, something to be ashamed of.

Tomboys fare a little better in these years. Their mothers are more likely to see their departures from the girly-girl norms as positive, a sign of strength or independence. Their fathers, too, may be taken with a daughter who can throw a punch with the best of them. And these girls can thrive in grade school. Compared to boys, early school-age girls seem to give their peers much less of a hard time for being unfeminine. In fact, tomboys often win the respect of classmates who respond to their boldness.

It can be an awful jolt when puberty rolls around and things start to slip in a lesbian girl's world. If boys' society looks like a totem pole, picture the early adolescent world of girls as a series of concentric circles. While boys struggle to reach the top, girls try to get to the inside of their peer group. The more connections a girl makes, the more she will be seen as a member of the inner circle. Anyone who has spent an hour in a middle school lunchroom knows girls forge these key connections by sharing confidences in intimate conversations. No conversation is more intimate, no confidence more valuable, than who you think is cute.

Tomboy or not, a lesbian girl can have a hard time finding her way into these conversations. She can't match her friends' enthusiasm for the cute boys, she doesn't have boy crushes of her own to share, and if she doesn't learn to change the pronouns when she describes her fantasies, she will begin to avoid true confessions over lunch. As she does, a lesbian girl may find herself slowly drifting to the outer circles of her social network. Instant messages sent online slow down. Invitations stop. The cold shoulder that girls give their lesbian peers may be subtler than the taunting a gay boy endures on the playing field, but it is no less painful.

As a gay teen grows and his sexual attractions strengthen, there's even more for him to worry about. Unless he's prepared to come out, he'll have to make sure to hide any sign of his desires. And yet he'll be placed in situations that make his attractions terribly difficult to disguise. Teenagers not uncommonly find themselves in emotionally intimate friendships and in close physical contact with same-sex peers. They may hang out with each other late into the night and share a room or even a bed at times.

For the gay teen who has come out, this may be no big deal—even if he develops a crush on a friend, he can talk about it, if not with the object of his affection, then at least with another friend or, perhaps, with you. But for the gay teen who hasn't revealed that he's gay, it can all be too stimulating to hide, but it must be hidden. And if concealing their reactions from their peers weren't hard enough, many gay teens, not wanting to know they're gay, also pour their efforts into keeping them a secret from themselves, telling themselves that they're admiring a classmate because they want to be like him rather than admitting to themselves they think he's cute.

As a result, these teenagers may turn away from the healthy group dates and liaisons of the high school years, burying themselves in schoolwork or the tennis team or the band. Many will succeed in stopping the developmental clock, at least temporarily, only to discover years later that a wonderful opportunity for growth has been lost.

Some teenagers will comfortably come out to themselves and to others—too self-possessed and secure for anyone to threaten them, they are a wonder to behold. Other teenagers will be so severely shunned by peers (or will fall so powerfully in love) that they can no longer hide the evidence of their orientation from themselves or their friends. Still others will freeze, fully aware now that they are gay, but afraid to take the leap into openness.

The period between a teen's acknowledgment to himself that he is gay and his admission of that fact to the important people in his life appears to be the most likely time for a suicide attempt. Boys who are gay have been found to be much more likely to make a suicide attempt than boys who aren't: In one study, 28 percent of homosexual or bisexual boys had made an attempt compared with 4 percent of heterosexual boys. Lesbian or bisexual girls don't appear to have a greater risk than other girls, although all girls have a higher rate of suicide attempts than boys.

Making a Home for Your Gay Child

If your child turns out to be gay, you will not be able to protect him from all of the pain we've described, but through a few focused efforts, you can unquestionably guarantee him a substantially happier and healthier childhood, and greater prospects for happiness in the years that come. What can you do?

A good place to start is to make your or your partner's relationship with your child as good as it can be, especially if you sense there's a disconnect. Try to reinvent the ways you play with your child based on her own unusual interests. Your gender nonconformist is bound to benefit from any effort you can make to meet her on her own turf. Mom, you may have been a girly-girl, but if you're raising a tomboy, think of this as an opportunity to brush up on your free throws. Let her teach you.

And if you're an I-don't-even-know-how-to-turn-the-oven-on kind of dad, why not try to schedule some time in the kitchen with your son, if baking is what he loves to do. Entering your son's world, and sharing some of his passions with him, will speak volumes about your affection and respect for him.

Lindsey, the mother of a six-year-old girl, felt uneasy with her daughter's pleasure in cuddling with her mom. "The only person I feel she is attracted to is me," she said. "I worry, if I encourage it and if she grows up to be gay, I'll feel responsible." Should she put a limit on the intimacy, she wondered.

No, family romances don't create homosexuality. Rather, like the more expected father-daughter or mother-son crushes so often seen in early childhood, they are thought to be the results of its early stirrings. A six-year-old on the way to a lesbian adulthood may set up the kind of affair of the heart with her mom that other girls might reserve for their dads. Boys growing up gay may pitch the woo at their fathers. Actually, heterosexual kids can court their same-sex parents, too.

Here is your next challenge as the parent of a possibly gay child: Find a way to accept her amorous attention for the treasure it is. Only this acceptance can instill in your little one's mind the sense that she is lovable.

Fathers, are we right in guessing that you may have a somewhat rougher go of this? You may find it odd to let yourself be courted with a fistful of daisies by another guy, even if he's in kindergarten. Even if all he really craves is a wink and a tickle. Do your best—and try not to reject his little offerings and invitations.

Peer Protection

Then it's on to elementary school and, for boys, those daunting totem poles. What, you might wonder, can you do about that?

"Nathan is an incredibly sweet kid," says Nell, the mother of a ten-year-old boy. "He's really a wonderful boy and he's very interested in gems, in gemology. So he has a lot of rings, with various stones, which he loves to wear. He's been wearing them all summer."

Interest in adornment is one of those attributes that gets a boy called a sissy. This seems to be how Nell sees her son, and not only because of his rings. She and her husband, Reg, have never given Nathan a problem about wearing his rings around the house. At the end of summer, though, he is going to start sixth grade, and Reg has decided to draw the line at Nathan's wearing them to school. He's certain that Nathan will be teased by the other kids for it.

Reg is probably right. Nathan has a fairly good chance of catching some flak from the boys in his class if he shows up with his rings on. But Reg and Nell need to consider how to present this to Nathan. If they just declare that Nathan has to leave the rings at home or convey their own belief that wearing them is sissylike, they will be allying with those boys against their son.

Instead, Reg and Nell can say that "there is really nothing wrong with wearing rings anywhere, and if that's what you want to do, we'll back you all the way." They can warn him that some boys might make fun of him, but they can also make it clear that they feel those boys would be wrong.

They can brainstorm with Nathan some ways he might respond if he gets teased, and even try acting out a confrontation with a peer together.

If Nathan chooses to go ahead with his plan, they can praise his bravery while keeping a watchful eye on just how much negative attention he gets. (There are some schools where it's just too dangerous for Nathan to be so clearly different, and so his parents may have to intervene.) If Nathan decides to leave his rings at home, they can support him in his choice but also make him feel comfortable expressing himself around the house.

Rather than working to divert your sissy from the path he prefers, try smoothing it for him instead. The goal with a sissy or a tomboy is not to change your child's inclinations, but rather to develop his or her talents and enthusiasms, and try to expand the sorts of pleasures available to the child, all the while helping him or her learn how to respond to the negative reactions of others.

The natural choices your child makes in play, and dress, and so on grow out of her emotional responses to the world. Although influenced by those around her, they are also expressions of her authentic self, and importantly, she experiences them as such. Sure, she can hide them or abandon them, and she will if she feels that doing so is the surest route to keeping you close. But then she will have abandoned a part of herself, and with that she'll lose some of her zest for life, some of her spirit.

There are few sadder things than a child who has managed to satisfy her parents by sacrificing her spirit.

What Every Child Should Learn About Homosexuality

Meanwhile, there are a few things you should let your kids know.

Simply discussing homosexuality with (and in the presence of) your child is one of the easiest and most effective ways to improve her chances of a happy childhood and adolescence should she happen to be gay. Learning early on that gay and lesbian people exist and are acceptable to you can spare your child painful confusion about her desires, reduce her fear that you won't love her should she come out, and diminish the effects of other children's bias and teasing on her delicate self-esteem. Whether she is gay or not, your teaching can also help her learn to appreciate the diversity of the people around her and help make her a better friend to the gay and lesbian people she is bound to know.

Now, some parents feel uncomfortable discussing homosexuality with young children because, in their minds, to talk about homosexuality is to talk about sex, and that's not something they are prepared to do with their four-year-old.

You may feel this way because when you hear a reference to homosexuality, you may think about sex. But the chances are that although the term may conjure up a few images in your seven-year-old's mind, sex won't be among them. One researcher surveyed second graders, asking them what a gay person was. "Someone who can't play ball" was the overwhelming response.

Gil, at age eight, is a boy who ought to know about homosexuality. His parents have several close friends who are gay, including one who has been living in their guest room for the past year. In preschool, he was the first kid in the class to notice that one of his classmates had two dads, and that boy quickly became a close friend. Gil's parents had used each of these opportunities to teach him about gay people.

When over dinner Gil presented a fairly screwball explanation of the origin of skim milk (horses, not cows) and attributed it to his friend Ari, his parents encouraged Gil to be a little more skeptical of Ari's view of the world, since he often gets things wrong.

"You're absolutely right," Gil replied with great seriousness. "Do you know what he told me yesterday? He said that gay men have sex with each other!"

Gil's parents were dumbfounded. How could he not have known that? In all of those years of learning about gay people loving each other and having different kinds of families, he hadn't been told the sex part, and so he simply never guessed it.

Thanks to their concrete thinking style, young children learning for the first time about homosexuality take comments about gay people literally and don't abstract to ideas about people having sex. So, you can discuss homosexuality with your children without having to worry that you are talking about sex with them sooner than you want to. In fact, you don't have to wait beyond preschool to tell your children about gay and lesbian people.

Words for Young Children

How do you talk to your five-year-old about homosexuality?

You might wait for your child to ask a question about a gay person he's met, or to use a term he's heard that refers to gay people. If he uses the word *gay*, ask him if he knows what it means. Then give him a simple definition:

> "A gay man is a man who loves another man, just the way your mother
> and I love each other. A lesbian is a woman who loves another woman,
> in the same way. When two lesbian or gay grown-ups meet and fall in
> love, sometimes they start a family just like Mommy and I did."

Ask your child if he understands, and expect that you will have to repeat the lesson over time before he can fully master it.

Since they haven't yet developed their own different ways of loving, young children sometimes have trouble distinguishing between romantic love and the love between friends or family members. Your daughter may say, "I love Emma. Does that make me a lesbian?" Don't expect her to understand this one immediately. It's a hard concept to grasp because it is too abstract until she has fallen in love herself—but you might use a story about romance your daughter already knows:

> "That's friendship love. That doesn't mean you are a lesbian. The kind of
> love a lesbian has for another woman is like the love Cinderella felt for the
> prince. If Cinderella were a lesbian, she would fall in love with a princess."

(And she wouldn't have to wear such ridiculous shoes.)

If your child doesn't bring up the topic of homosexuality, she might at least ask about a family that is different from yours—a family with one parent if she has two, or a family with two parents if she has one.

Use this opportunity to teach about homosexuality by explaining about the different sorts of families people can have:

> ". . . and some people have two mommies, or two daddies. Two women who fall in love and make a family are called lesbians. Two men who fall in love and make a family are called gay."

It needn't be any more complicated than that.

Always bear in mind that when you tell your child about gay people, you aren't just delivering the facts. You are showing her how you feel about gay people and how you want her to feel. Do you respect them? Could you be friends with a gay person? Could you love one? Think of each little discussion as communicating how you would react if she were to make fun of people because they are gay, or if she were to someday tell you she is a lesbian herself.

You'll also be conveying your general beliefs about how to relate to people who are different from yourself. Even if she doesn't turn out to be a lesbian, the openness she sees in you will help her if she ever wants to turn to you with something she fears may disappoint you or diminish her in your eyes.

You can communicate even more directly that you would accept your child if she were gay. "When the idea of dating would come up with Krisianna," Sally explains, "I would always refer to some day when she would be dating a 'boy' or a 'girl.' This started when she was still in elementary school, so dating was a ways off." Sally feels her approach works well. "One time she said, 'Mom, I don't think I'm going to be a lesbian.' She didn't sound annoyed or embarrassed, just factual. That made me realize it was working. I said, that's fine, but you're still rather young, so it can be hard to know for sure. I just think I'll keep it open until you're sure."

So, when your eight-year-old asks on the way back from a wedding if he can have chocolate cake when he gets married, you can say:

> "Some day, if you meet a girl or boy and fall in love and want to have a wedding, you can have whatever type of cake you and your partner want to have."

Remember, acknowledging various options isn't going to make a heterosexual kid gay.

Introduce Them

Teaching your child what the words mean is even more effective when there is a real person attached to them. A flesh-and-blood example puts a face on the concept of homosexuality for your child.

People you care about, and ones who will be a part of your children's lives for a while—best friends, aunts and uncles, and teachers—are all prime candidates. Often it's a matter of just not hiding someone's orientation from your child. If your kids have a lesbian aunt, there is no need to wait until they reach a particular age to tell them; they can certainly know by kindergarten. Not discussing their aunt's orientation risks creating a family secret with the unintended message, "We are ashamed of her." (And it takes a lot less energy than coming up with contrived explanations for their aunt's partner—they're friends who just happen to live, sleep, and travel together.)

When children begin to sketch in the categories of boy and girl, they tend to begin with fairly exaggerated distinctions that they hold to rigidly. As a result, some children in the preschool years who have learned that boys only date girls may find the fact that their uncle dates guys a bit confusing. If they have questions, let them ask him about it.

As children progress through their elementary school years, they will begin to absorb the reigning attitudes toward gay people among their friends. A boy who has learned on the playing field that "fag" is what you call the kid who misses the ball may need some time to square the negative views he's acquired about gay men with your friend who always cracks him up. Ideally, your child will know someone gay before he reaches this point, and his own experience will deflect the stereotype bandied about on the school bus.

Dealing with Bias

Recent years have seen some major changes in the lives of gay kids. They can see gay characters on TV and read about gay people in the newspaper. In some schools, they are now much more likely to know a gay teacher, to hear a guest speaker describe her life as a lesbian, or to know of another gay student. One thing hasn't changed, though. The words *gay, fag,* and *queer* remain three of the most common put-downs among children from elementary school through high school.

Lydia, a high school student, puts it this way: "Hardly a day goes by when I don't hear someone use the word *gay* as an adjective meaning stupid, useless, or worse." Another high school student remembers the discriminatory comments of middle school: "It was the most popular joke-insult to accuse others of homosexuality and to mockingly call one-self a lesbian. . . . I was afraid to get close to any out gay person for fear that someone might think that I was gay."

Gay kids may not be the only ones to suffer from the kind of unchecked antihomosexual bias these girls describe. William Pollack, Ph.D., author of *Real Boys,* has come to see their antigay attitudes as compounding the inhibition heterosexual boys feel about expressing their feelings, treating each other warmly, and pursuing their creative lives for fear of being labeled a fag. And what adolescent doesn't feel vulnerable to someday dropping out of favor, to being the one left out. When one group is shunned or stigmatized with impunity, every child's sense of security is eroded.

As it turns out, many kids use these words without really thinking about what they mean, and without harboring any particularly strong negative feelings against gay people.

"Gay doesn't mean gay," a group of tenth graders recently protested, "it just means, you know, gay."

If your thirteen-year-old complains he doesn't want to watch the DVD his younger sister picked out because "it's so gay," call him on it. Ask him if he means the movie is about homosexual people, and when he tells you it isn't, have him pick a more specific word. Tell him the movie may be a flatulent, tendentious screed served up as a treacly paean to itself, but it isn't gay.

You might also explain that while he may not feel his words are directed at homosexual people, if someone gay were to hear him, she would certainly be hurt (a reminder about the gay friend or aunt is especially helpful at a time like this).

When You Think Your Teen Is Gay

Several weeks after she had resolved to talk with her son Michael about the gay pornography she found in his closet, Charlotte hadn't yet had the conversation with him. But neither had she stopped wondering about her son. One weekend, while Michael was visiting friends out of town, she found herself seated at his desk, looking through his drawers. There was a folded slip of paper on which Michael seemed to have penned a combination of letters and numbers. A password.

Charlotte switched on his computer and made her way into her son's saved e-mail. In between messages from classmates about school assignments were notes from guys, some offering support for the fears and loneliness he described, some asking him for a date, and some confirming where they would meet for sex. There was no question about the kind of sex they were talking about.

Charlotte got into her car and began driving around town, stopping at each of the places where Michael was supposed to find a teenager on the corner, or press the third buzzer. She looked at the apartment buildings, the buzzers, the corners. A few days later, when she picked Michael up from his friend's, she made no mention of her excursion.

What held her back?

"You know, maybe I'm a coward, but I just don't feel I have the right to confront him with something he has chosen to hide from me. To confront him, I think, would be acutely embarrassing to him."

Perhaps you understand what it is to feel like Charlotte—to have some information about something, maybe even just an inkling, but to set it aside with some seemingly logical reason, because you would prefer not to know. If the subject you're struggling with is your teenager's sexual orientation, we suggest that once he reaches high school, the time for waiting should be coming to a close. Remember, boys who think they may be gay but haven't told anyone have an elevated risk of making a suicide attempt. Their risk goes down if they have discussed it. Also, kids who are more satisfied with their relationship with their parents have been shown to practice safer sex—all the more reason to open the lines of communication about his orientation.

Find a quiet time alone with your teenager and introduce the subject of dating and attractions in an uncharged way. Ask if he knows of any gay kids in his class. See how he reacts to a few comments about what it might be like to be gay and to have to keep it a secret. Then ask, without suggesting that you believe the answer is yes, if he has ever had attractions to someone of the same sex. This is an easier question to answer than the self-defining "Are you gay?"

If he says no, you should consider that you may be wrong, or that you're right but he isn't yet ready to own his attractions. Let him rebuff you, affirm that you love him, and move on:

> "That's fine. If you ever find that you are attracted to guys, I'm here
> if you want to talk about it. Since some parents don't react well to that
> sort of thing, I want you to know that I will love and support and
> respect you whether you're gay, straight, or in between."

Having your child come out with a definitive statement about his orientation is not the chief goal of these conversations, although that may be the ultimate outcome. Your goal here is really to open up the subject for discussion and thought. Your fourteen-year-old shouldn't feel pressured to declare his orientation, but you do want to diminish any fears he may have if he's contemplating telling you.

If, on the other hand, your child says yes, he has had attractions like these, you can feel pleased and proud to know that you have, in an instant, relieved him of a burden he's been bearing for a long, long time. Of course, that may not be all you feel.

Now You Know

Sitting in a wide circle on an assortment of mismatched armchairs and plump sofas, thirteen parents gather in the early evening to hear one another's stories. They begin by introducing themselves. One soft-spoken mother gives her name, and says she has known about her lesbian daughter for three and a half years. She has been coming to these church basement meetings of Parents, Families, and Friends of Lesbians and Gays (known as

PFLAG) for almost as long. Beside her, a garrulous couple in their seventies have brought their grown daughter, her partner of fifteen years, and an album of baby pictures. Across the room, a woman with a sniffle looks stricken. She found out that her teenage boy is gay six weeks ago.

How is she doing, the group wants to know.

"I'm on the path, I guess. I don't know. I read that book about the boy who comes out to his parents and then their marriage breaks up. I sort of fell apart. I don't know why I did that. I was being self-destructive." She gets some warm words of encouragement from the room. A father with two gay sons congratulates her: "Remember your first meeting? You cried all the way through. You have come a long, long way!" The others nod and smile.

"I got a phone call from a friend of mine last week," the mother goes on. "She wanted to tell me her son had just gotten engaged. She doesn't know about Alan. I just—I couldn't say anything. I had to get off the phone." One of the more seasoned parents explains that since she told her friends about her daughter they are a little more careful discussing the experiences she's likely to miss.

"Listen," the older man chimes in, leaning over his photo album, "when my beautiful daughter and her beautiful partner had their ceremony ten years ago, Ruth and I didn't miss a thing! There was a chuppah, flowers, the breaking of the glass, even a *rabbi*. You can't imagine how proud I felt, walking her down the aisle that day, before a rabbi. And then afterward, the music and the dancing. Let me tell you, if you want a wedding, we had it all. All the trimmings!"

Parents at PFLAG meetings like this one often talk about being on a "path" or a "road." Some are clearly very far down that road and have drawers full of "I love my GAY SON" buttons to prove it. Others have just taken their first tentative steps. Their paths will probably lead in different directions, but they all seem to start in the same place. They start with one of those intense, hyperreal experiences, a moment that once it's passed will have altered everything: The moment your child says, "I'm gay."

What will you encounter along the way that begins with a bracing moment in the kitchen and ends (if it ever ends) with you passing around baby pictures at a PFLAG meeting? Well, there will certainly be decisions to make, like which relatives to tell and when to let her little sister know. There will be gaffes and recriminations. But mostly there will be a gauntlet of emotions to run. Consider the following a partial list.

Grief. Some parents we know swear they never really imagine the specifics of their children's futures. As for the rest of us, well, we may nobly resist those "Class of 2024" onesies, but it is hard not to dream a little. Maybe you imagine your daughter as a young woman, excelling in one way or another, finding love. You can get pretty attached to dreams like these after fifteen or twenty years.

And then she comes out just as you feel she's on the verge of fulfilling your hopes—just as she's moving out into the world. Suddenly the fantasy upon which you have pinned so much is shaken, maybe briefly shattered. You haven't lost your daughter, but you have lost the future you've imagined for her. And so you feel grief.

Estrangement. Or maybe you feel you *have* lost your daughter. How can she not feel to you like a different person from the one you thought you knew? In fact, she may soon begin to behave differently. You may find her more alive, more communicative, or less compliant. She may begin to talk about a world that seems quite foreign to you.

Shame. Now she's out, and suddenly you're closeted. You may find yourself avoiding conversations that might lead to questions about how your daughter is doing. You may find that when you talk about her, you censor the details about her new relationship, or the organization she's running at school, even though you thought of yourself as genuinely pleased, even proud. Worse, you may catch yourself feeling that in that silent competition that gets waged between parents everywhere, you have fallen embarrassingly behind. Her daughter didn't get into Stanford, but your daughter is gay. It's hard to grow up in America and escape the feeling that there is something shameful about gay people. As the parent of one, you may have to work hard to shake that feeling. Coming out yourself helps.

Fear. After your child comes out, all the news stories you've ever heard about gay bashing, discrimination, and AIDS may begin to swarm around you like the Furies. Yes, there are reasons to worry. Your average gay man is more likely to be exposed to HIV than your average heterosexual man. Scary incidents of harassment and baiting are all too common.

One way of responding to your worries is to take some protective action. Of course you should talk about the details of safer sex with your child (you should do this whether your child is gay or straight, as we'll discuss in later chapters), but you might also consider meeting with the principal to improve the environment at school and, if necessary, get him greater protection there.

Anger. Your anger these days may be an equal opportunity employer. You get angry at your partner, who you feel isn't reacting well. You get angry at your friends for their discomfort or their thoughtlessness. You get angry at the man calling in to the talk radio show, at the state representative, at the woman ahead of you in the checkout line, for their bigotry. And you may even get angry at your daughter for being gay.

Guilt, reliably, arrives when you imagine yourself responsible for your child's sexuality, or when you think of the struggles he went through without feeling he could turn to you.

Then there's the *isolation* of thinking you are the only parent you know dealing with something like this, the *confusion* about how best to talk to your child now, and, finally, the *fatigue* that comes from managing so many conflicting feelings.

And now you know why it never occurred to you that your daughter was gay until the moment she told you driving back from the beach. If you had really thought about it before, you would have had to feel like this.

It really is fascinating the way the mind manages to work these things out. You can have a perception that your daughter has only ever developed crushes on girls and at the very same time a curtain is pulled that effectively exempts you from really having to think about the implications—in fact, from having to draw any conclusions at all from your observation.

Gay kids go through this, too, which is why many cannot answer the question "How long have you known?" Some seem to know in an instant ("I saw a picture of a naked man in a magazine, and I thought,

'Oh my God, I'm a homosexual' "). But others take years to say it to themselves. They have both known and not known for years.

Now that you know, you may go through anger, resentment, and all the rest, but for the first time you will also have a chance of genuinely understanding your child, and through that understanding the two of you may develop a richer, more honest, and ultimately more rewarding relationship than you ever had before, back when things were easier.

Whom to Tell?

Everyone in the immediate family can find out that your child is gay as soon as your child is comfortable with their knowing. Although it may have flashed through your mind in a moment of weakness, we hope you have already rejected the (sometimes tempting) notion of keeping your spouse in the dark. Secrets of this magnitude work wonders on a marriage (see, for example, *Ethan Frome*). If your partner doesn't already know, support your child in coming out. Granted, there are some families in which that simply is not feasible. If your partner would kick your child out on the street or make his life miserable, secrecy may be necessary.

The other kids will need to know, too. Some parents ask their gay children not to tell a younger sibling out of an apprehension that the child will be upset or that discussing homosexuality with a young child is inappropriate. By now, we should have laid the latter concern to rest. As for the former, some siblings *will* be upset. Kids who have learned that gay equals bad may not react well to the revelation of an admired older brother's homosexuality. They will need some time alone with their older sibling to understand that he hasn't really changed, as well as some education from you about sexual orientation and how it works. If your child doesn't want his friends to know about his orientation, you might want to help him consider whether his siblings can keep the secret.

"Somehow He's Let Me Down"

Recently, at a chance encounter, Charlotte provided an update on her son. It had been about a year since she first looked inside Michael's safe. "Michael? Oh, he's fine," she said. "He'll be a senior in the fall, and we're planning our college tour. Soccer's going well, his grades, too. He strikes me as a fairly well-adjusted kid these days."

Had she broached the topic of his sexuality with her son?

"Well, I went out of my way to make it clear that I don't condone discrimination of any sort, but no, no one has said anything directly about it. I decided the risks were too high to confront him. I'm afraid that he would feel that somehow he's let me down or that he would be too uncomfortable to discuss it. I don't want to do that to him."

But there was no cause for concern, she was certain. Michael didn't seem depressed as he once did, and he had friends. "Maybe he's got his own internal demons," Charlotte said, "but they're not to the point that they affect his daily function."

Perhaps she had forgotten about the e-mails, about his loneliness and fear? What about the corners and the buzzers? Charlotte's attention shifted. She was in a hurry.

"Anyway, even to this day I'm not sure what his orientation is. He has as many friendships with girls as he does with boys. He seems to be a pretty well-rounded guy." And she was gone.

What would you say to Charlotte? What advice would you give her? Here's what we might try to say.

Your child is not what you wanted, we would tell her. He is himself.

You *have* been let down. But your son's becoming what you wanted was not part of the deal when you had him. It *is* terribly uncomfortable to discuss. But being a parent means doing hard things to help your kids. It's in the job description.

Make the effort to know your kid. Take the leap and embrace him for who he is, and if it's disturbing or scary, be brave.

Be the parent.

Chapter **6**

Going over the bump

Weathering the physical changes of puberty

You're sitting in the waiting room, wondering how much longer it's going to be. Thankfully the pediatrician squeezed you in, but has he forgotten you? You look at your watch again. Okay, so it's only been twelve minutes.

Rose is reading a book. You're getting worked up over nothing, you tell yourself. She's only ten, and you can't get breast cancer if you don't have breasts. Although, couldn't it be a metastasis? Kids get bone tumors. And leukemia. No, that's the blood one.

Maybe it's some kind of . . . *carbuncle?*

The nurse comes out, mercifully stopping your train of thought, and calls out, "Rose?"

A few minutes later, you're telling the doctor about her bump. Rose thought it was a mosquito bite, but as you explain to the doctor, it doesn't itch, and it's under the skin. "It's like a little marble. I just thought it could be, you know"—you make a gesture you hope will communicate "dreaded disease"—"and so I really appreciate your seeing us right away."

Dr. Rodriguez examines Rose. His facial expression doesn't change. Is that good or bad?

He tells Rose to put her shirt back on, looks up at you, and smiles. "I've got a diagnosis. The technical term is thelarche, but to translate into layman's terms, it's her first sign of puberty."

"Oh . . . She . . . ?"

"It's a breast."

We interrupt this book for a lesson in biology.

Remember puberty? Acne, sex drive, bad photographs you destroyed when you were twenty—it would be impossible to forget this stuff. Do you need a refresher course on all those diagrams they flashed past you in health class? Probably not. But you might benefit from some coming attractions of your children's impending transition to adulthood. And it wouldn't hurt to have a look at the questions your kids might ask you as their bodies start to morph.

Knowing what to expect during puberty can prevent a lot of anxiety—and not just yours. Some girls who don't learn about menstruation before it happens think they are dying when they get their first period. And boys who discover ejaculation without having heard about it can panic. A twelve-year-old patient who had just started to have wet dreams recently asked if he had to worry about using up all of his sperm.

Now there's one you could probably answer without a hormone graph.

Viewed from the sylvan fields of childhood, puberty can seem fairly formidable: the mood swings, the self-consciousness, the infamous irritability. Will your little girl stop letting you hold her on your lap? Will you stop wanting to?

At eight, Jemma has a sense of what's up ahead; her friend's sister is thirteen. She has her period. She's mean to them. Jemma came up with her own name for the shock of puberty: going over the bump. "I was driving with her the other day. I don't remember what provoked this," Jemma's mom remembers, "and she said, 'I don't want to go over the bump.' I said to her, 'You know, Jemma, it may not be so bad.' She said, 'Mom. Everyone goes over the bump, and it's *always* really bad.'"

Read this chapter, and you should know virtually everything you will need to give your children Lesson Three—the puberty primer for eight- to twelve-year-olds—all the facts about what will happen to them before it happens. Perhaps we can also help you tackle some of the challenges that follow puberty's first bumps. Though puberty may feel like it starts with a jolt, once it does, you've still got a long road ahead.

Timing

We know very little about what triggers puberty's first stirrings. We do know it to be the complex product of a host of hormones acting together on various body organs to create the physical changes of adolescence. Biologists credit the early pumping of the adrenal glands, a pair of organs perched atop your child's kidneys, with the start of the hormonal cascades that herald your child's maturation. Adrenarche, the name given to their little coming-out party, seems to start as early as six, and as their chemical signal gradually grows stronger, it may be responsible for your child's first glimmers of sexual attraction (commonly experienced as early as age nine or ten). But the bigwigs behind your child's physical transformation into a curvy, hairy grown-up are those sex glands, the testicles in boys and ovaries in girls, which, under the tutelage of the brain's hypothalamus and pituitary, start pumping the testosterone and estrogen responsible for most of what you see.

Over the past century, there has been a shift in puberty's timetable. Adolescents have been developing earlier and have been growing larger in much of the industrialized world and in other places as well. (Curiously, most of the extra height has come from longer legs, not from taller torsos. Go figure.) The reasons for this change are unknown, although there is a general consensus that the improvement in children's nutrition has something to do with it. At any rate, the changing age of puberty's onset has been leveling off for the past few decades, leaving boys' and girls' maturation happening about two years earlier than at the end of the nineteenth century.

As for the more immediate matter of timing your own child's development, you can expect to spot the first signs of puberty in your daughter between ages seven and thirteen (or as young as six if she is African American) and in your son between ages nine and fourteen. It is hard to give a better prediction than that for any one child, but there is a genetic component to the timing of puberty, so if your child's relatives developed on the early or late side, there's a good chance he will, too. Nutrition and other environmental factors play a role as well. Indeed, malnourished girls, such as those with anorexia, tend to develop later, and girls who are heavier tend to develop earlier. One theory holds that a girl will start menstruating when she reaches one hundred pounds, regardless of her age, because that weight guarantees her enough stored calories to support a pregnancy.

There is a general sequence of events to puberty's various innovations, but the events seem to get out of order in some children. Most girls, for example, begin to develop breasts before they get pubic hair, but some go in the reverse order. And there is a lot of variability in how much time adolescents take to go from one milestone to the next. Still, knowing the general sequence of events may help you prepare your child and yourself for what's coming. As a rough guide to the changes in their usual order of appearance, girls tend to start with breast budding, followed by pubic hair, the fastest phase of their growth spurt, and then menstruation. Boys start with growth of their testicles, followed by pubic hair, penis enlargement, ejaculation and wet dreams, and then the peak of their growth spurt.

Beanstalks

Let us take you through the changes you can expect as puberty has its way with your little one. First a few words about growth spurts and skin, and then we will take on the particular changes girls and boys experience separately.

Julie's son Chuck lived with his father across the country, and she hadn't seen him since Christmas vacation, although they talked every week. She was looking forward to spending his fourteenth birthday and the rest of the summer with him. She got to the airport early and waited for Chuck as everyone came off the plane. The steady stream of people petered out. No Chuck. Did he miss the plane? She would've gotten a call if he had, she thought. Then there was a booming shout in her ear: "Yo, Mom!" She turned to see her son standing behind her, laughing. "He had walked right by me, and I hadn't recognized him. He was a baby just six months before. Now he was an adult—well, not an adult, but he was so much taller."

Ah, the growth spurt. One minute you're looking down on your son, and the next he's looking down on you. This is every clothing manufacturer's dream—adolescents outgrow their clothes even faster than the styles change. Once the growth spurt begins, it typically lasts about two or three years.

Now, children often go through a transient acceleration of growth sometime after age six, attributed to adrenarche, which might give you the mistaken impression that puberty has begun. But their major growth spurt will come a bit later, and you will know it when you see it. Your daughter will probably start her growth spurt shortly after her breasts begin to bud. Her hips will also widen around the same time, and a little later, she should be getting more fat and muscle. You may not have noticed, but she probably started building additional fat reserves before budding began. By the time she reaches menarche (the beginning of menstruation—the showstopper of every girl's pubescence), she will be approaching her adult height. Girls tend to grow another two to four inches after menarche. Boys will start their spurts about two years later than girls and will grow more than girls during their spurts. Even after it seems like puberty's over, your son may still grow another inch or so.

You're not imagining it. Growth really does start at the bottom and work its way up. Your son's feet started stretching before the rest of him. His legs are next, and it may be another half a year before his upper body starts its burst. One bone can grow before another, and muscles don't always adjust right away, which is why kids can go through a clumsy phase, wreaking havoc on their confidence and your nerves.

Other bones are growing, too. Your son's jaw may become more prominent. As we said, your daughter's hips will widen; but actually, hips grow for both boys and girls—in part this may be harder to notice in boys because they're also getting broader shoulders.

Both boys and girls grow larger muscles, although they become more prominent in boys, courtesy of testosterone. Muscles increase in size about a year before they increase in strength, so you've been duly warned—when you see those muscles growing, it's your last chance to beat him in arm wrestling. Girls generally add more fat than boys do. On average, about a quarter of a girl's body weight will come from fat, compared with about an eighth for boys. Some fat is important. If a girl's fat drops to less than 17 percent of her body weight, her menarche may be delayed. Nevertheless, girls are often bothered by the new shapeliness of their bodies, which they can view as too heavy.

Your son's voice box (the larynx) undergoes its own mini growth spurt, which causes his vocal cords to lengthen and consequently leads to a deeper voice (in the way a cello is deeper than a shorter-stringed viola), but not without an occasional crack along the way. Voice changes are quite variable, but, on average, they begin around age fourteen, and the voice reaches its adult quality within a year. (This doesn't mean that he won't still sound like a child when he whines about having to take out the trash.) He'll also develop an Adam's apple, which is formed by cartilage in his neck that grows at more of a protruding angle in boys than girls.

The First Heartbreak

He mopes. He snarls. He snaps back. Did he fail his test? Did his team lose the big game? Did he get turned down for his first date? No, far worse; far, far worse. Your son's first pimple has arrived.

The bane of adolescence and the boon of an entire industry of special soaps, creams, and cover-ups, acne cannot be ignored.

Eighty-five percent of kids get acne. It generally begins after your child has started getting some hair under his arms, and it can last long after he's moved out of the house.

You've seen the diagrams. Little skin glands secrete some oily goo, the glands get stopped up, bacteria get trapped, and then the bad stuff happens—blackheads, whiteheads, papules, pustules, cysts, nodules. Why now? You can thank the same chemical that's been toying with your kid's sex drive and temper, the Eddie Haskell of hormones, good ol' testosterone.

Advise your child to avoid using oily cosmetics or moisturizers. Tell her to look for ones that say "oil-free," "nonacnegenic," or "noncomedogenic." Washing repeatedly throughout the day just makes things worse, and picking can cause more scarring. The good news is that the medicines are better than when you were a kid, and if your child is worried about scars down the road, there are treatments that might reduce their visibility.

If you notice your child developing bad acne around the same time he's also putting on the muscles, don't ignore the possibility that he's using anabolic steroids (aka 'roids), a practice that builds muscles but can also cause liver damage, testicular atrophy, and stunted growth. Girls on 'roids can have menstrual problems.

Now for the Girls
Budding Geniuses

I couldn't believe it. Hannah came home and told me that her friend Maddy came back from camp with breasts. I have to say I saw them, and they are not much to write home about. But Hannah started worrying, "I'm going to be the only one in the fifth grade who's flat." Here we go.

—*Jessica, on her ten-year-old daughter*

Breasts have to start somewhere. When your daughter first feels a nascent breast, it may be no bigger than a pea. There might be several tiny peas, and there might be some on both sides. Your daughter might not even notice them; and if she does, she might have no idea what they are and come to you to find out. Even if you've been through your own breast development, it's easy to forget about the pea phase.

If you have any doubts, you can take your daughter to her clinician, who can double-check. Believe us when we say you won't be the first or last family to leave with a diagnosis of "normal breast development," and you'll feel a lot better.

Esther remembers that she had just turned eleven and was away at camp for the summer. She felt some "knots under my skin. They were near my nipple, and I was convinced I had cancer." She didn't tell anyone, though, because she was scared, but once the lumps got bigger, and there were more of them, she realized this was the beginning of getting breasts. "About half my friends already had breasts, so I knew it was going to happen. I guess it just didn't feel anything like what I thought breasts would feel like."

For most girls, breast development is the first sign of puberty. The ovaries and uterus have already begun to grow by then, but these are not visible, of course. The little peas soon grow big enough to push the skin out a little; this is called breast budding. About a year later, her breasts may be rounder and fuller, and her nipples and the areola (the darker area surrounding the nipple) get larger and darker. In still another year, the areola will protrude from the breast as a distinct mound, although some girls skip this stage. Finally, after about two more years—but sometimes as many as nine, and sometimes never—the areola will stop protruding, as the breast reaches its adult shape.

Puberty is not synchronized swimming. Your daughter's breasts may develop at different rates, with one noticeably larger than the other for some time. You can reassure her that within two years or so, her breasts should be much closer in size. If she's self-conscious about the difference, you may find her putting tissues in her bra to make the two look more even. This may not fit the ideal of loving her body for what it is, but it may also be something that helps her get through this phase. When her breasts are fully grown, it's not uncommon for one to still be a little larger than the other.

Once you notice that your daughter's breasts are beginning to bud, a trip to pick out a bra usually follows. When is the right time to start wearing a bra? There really is no right time. The fact is that most girls don't actually *need* a bra for any physical reason, unless they are uncomfortable during exercise or have very large breasts that are affecting their posture (in which case a bra can add support). Wearing a bra more typically serves a social function.

The biggest influence on the bra decision is what other girls are doing. If your daughter's best friend gets a bra, she may want one, too, and just as there is no practical reason to give her one, there is no strong reason not to.

Sometimes the bra decision is made by a parent, perhaps a parent who feels uncomfortable with the sudden visibility of his little child's budding sexuality.

"I wasn't ready to get her a bra, and she wasn't ready to get a bra, but she was going to a family function with her father—my ex—who called and asked me to get her one," Janice says of her nine-year-old, Savvy. "I knew where he was coming from. When Savvy and I showed up at my parents' house a few months ago, everyone got a bit quiet, a bit sheepish. My parents and my brothers said vague things like 'She's really grown' or 'She put on a little weight' out of her earshot in serious tones. I actually believe they were all a little embarrassed."

Girls themselves may ask for a bra for similar reasons, hoping it will conceal these new body parts, knowing it will keep them from bouncing visibly. On the other hand, some don't like to wear a bra because it feels uncomfortable or hot.

Janice talked with Savvy about getting a bra. "She got excited about the idea. It was a grown-up thing to do. I coupled it with a shopping trip. She tried on all three models of kids' bras and picked the kind she liked, and we bought two. At home, after she had one on for twenty minutes, she said she didn't like it. Now she wears it occasionally at home, but not outside the house. None of her classmates has a bra that she knows of."

Some girls may not be as eager to get a bra. They may not want anyone to notice that they are changing and may hide within baggy clothes. Sonia had started to develop breasts, but she didn't tell anyone. "My sister's old training bras were in her drawer, so I just took one. Some days I would wear it, if I didn't think it could be seen through my clothes, and some days I wouldn't. I remember one day when my father gave me a pat on the back for something I'd done, and I was petrified he would feel my bra strap. He never said anything."

If your daughter is one of the later girls to develop, she may be eager to get a bra even before she starts budding. Should her self-esteem be wrapped up in her breast size? Of course not. Are you feeding into that notion by allowing her to wear a bra before she's really developing? Maybe, but it probably depends on how you handle the situation. If she's embarrassed that everyone else has a bra, she may not be in the most receptive state for learning about the objectification of women and why she shouldn't care what others think. On the other hand, if she's unconcerned about her lack of breast development, insisting that she wear a training bra or a padded bra may make her needlessly self-conscious.

Tanya's twins barely looked like sisters, so it was no surprise when Alfreda began developing breasts and Katrina didn't. But Tanya wasn't going to let this turn into a chance for Katrina to feel inferior. So on their eleventh birthday, she told them they would soon begin changing into young women. She said they shouldn't expect for both of them to go through every change at the same time. She then surprised them with a trip to the department store to get their first training bras. "Bras turned out to be easy," Tanya observed. "Now if I can only figure out how to get them both asked out on their first date at the same time . . ."

Hair and Shaving

What flipped her out was the underarm hair. She felt funny at the swim club and began to ask about shaving it. I suggested she wait, because once she starts, she really has to continue. I heard her talking to one of her friends about it. It went like this. "Molly, have you started getting hair under your arms yet?" Molly: "Ooh, no." Sarah: "I have." Molly: "I'm sorry for you." Sarah: "It's okay."

—*Vanessa, on her nine-year-old daughter*

She begged me to shave her legs. I wanted her to wait, but it really bothered her, so she got in the bathtub, and I was shaving her legs, and all of her sisters were there asking when they could shave their legs. She was very proud of it. She was thrilled.

—*Tess, on her twelve-year-old daughter*

If your daughter is growing breasts, pubic hair is probably not far behind. It'll probably start within six months of her getting breast buds, although she could get hair before breasts or not until much later. Other hair, such as armpit and leg hair, probably won't grow in until her pubic hair is fairly full, although again the timetable varies.

With body hair comes the question of shaving, waxing, and so on.

The Menstrual Cycle: A Refresher

The full story of the menstrual cycle involves multiple glands and organs pumping their hormones together with the precision of a finely choreographed ballet. The details could fill a few lectures in a biology course, but here are the basics. (For a diagram see the books we recommend on page 184.)

The cycle lasts anywhere from twenty-one to thirty-five days. It's usually described as running from the first day of bleeding of one menses (the "period" itself) up to but not including the first day of bleeding of the next menses. However, we start our description here several days into the cycle, just after menses is complete.

Follicular Phase

A girl is born with all the eggs that she will ever have. Each immature egg rests in its own cocoonlike follicle, and the follicle is stored in one of the two ovaries. At the beginning of the follicular phase, two hormones stimulate the development of several follicles in one of the ovaries. Gradually, one of these developing follicles becomes dominant while the others regress. As the dominant follicle matures, it secretes increasing amounts of the hormone estrogen, which stimulates the lining of the uterus (called the endometrium) to grow. This phase lasts about ten to seventeen days. The variability in the length of the menstrual cycle generally comes from the variable length of the follicular phase.

Ovulation

A hormonal burst from the pituitary gland causes the follicle to rupture. The egg is released and is swept up by the eager fingers of the adjacent fallopian tube, down which it travels to the uterus. Some women feel a cramping or a twinge when they ovulate (called mittelschmerz), but most feel nothing.

Luteal Phase

The remains of the follicle turn into an organ called the corpus luteum, which secretes the hormone progesterone as well as some estrogen. Together, these two hormones urge the endometrium to become even thicker and richer in blood so that it can support and nurture an embryo. The progesterone causes an increase in the body's temperature, which can be measured if you need to know whether ovulation has occurred.

This is the time when pregnancy can occur, the fertile period. During intercourse, as many as 300 million sperm enter the vagina. They pass through the cervical mucus within minutes, and within half an hour, there may be several hundred thousand sperm in the cervical canal. Some sperm travel up the fallopian tubes right away, while others take a rest stop for up to several days before making the journey. Sperm remain functional for seventy-two hours and possibly up to five days. The egg can be fertilized for up to twelve to twenty-four hours after ovulation, so the odds a woman will become pregnant are highest if sperm are already present in her fallopian tubes when she ovulates. Fertilization usually occurs toward the top of the fallopian tube, and the embryo moves down the tube to the uterus within two to three days. Implantation in the wall of the uterus occurs six to seven days after fertilization.

If an embryo implants in the newly enriched wall of the uterus, the corpus luteum will live on through gestation. If there is no pregnancy, it regresses in about fourteen days.

Menstrual Phase (Also Called Menses)

When no pregnancy occurs and the corpus luteum deteriorates, it stops producing estrogen and progesterone, so the endometrium loses all stimulation. It shrinks and sloughs off as blood, tissue, and mucus, which together make up the menstrual flow. On average, the menstrual phase lasts four to six days—four to six very meaningful days for your teenager, especially the first time.

This again is a matter of style and custom. There's no medical reason for her to shave, and women all over the world live perfectly happy lives with underarm hair and leg hair. But, obviously, many American women shave. You may find that by the time you get around to discussing shaving, she's already learned from a friend, or she's already taught herself, having watched you or someone else.

Menarche and Menstruation

I'll never forget when I got my first period. I had been bitten by a dog earlier that same day, and I thought it was some kind of internal bleeding from the bite. I wasn't supposed to be at the house where that dog was. So I didn't tell my mother about the period. Eventually, I figured out what it was.

—*Julia, mother of two*

Drum roll, please.

About two years after your daughter begins to develop breasts (about three years if they develop on the early side), she will typically reach menarche, her very first menstrual period. "When people talk of the indelibility of a strong memory," Natalie Angier writes in *Woman: An Intimate Geography,* "they speak of recalling exactly where they were when Kennedy was shot or the *Challenger* space shuttle exploded. But what a woman really remembers is her first period; now there's a memory seared into the brain with the blowtorch of high emotion."

Twelve is the average age of menarche, with most girls starting between ten and fifteen years old. In the several months before menarche, girls may have a small amount of vaginal discharge that is thin, clear or milky, and odorless. This fluid comes from the uterus and is normal. Think of it as the final warning before her period. If you haven't talked to her about menstruation yet, the time has come.

The lining of the cervix is maturing now but may not be fully grown until late in adolescence. The less mature lining is not as resistant to STDs, which makes it easier for adolescents to become infected when they are exposed to certain diseases. (More about this in Chapter 11.)

Sanitary Pads, Tampons, and Sponges: Notes for the Uninitiated (i.e., Dads)

Sanitary pads (also called sanitary napkins) have rectangular layers of cotton or some other absorbent material and a protective plastic lining on one side. They are about the size and shape of one of those old blackboard erasers, only much flatter. Most come with adhesive strips that help the plastic side adhere to a girl's underwear so the cotton side is against her labia. Pads come in different sizes and thicknesses (e.g., maxi), and your daughter may need to vary the thickness with how heavy the flow is on any particular day. Many girls start with pads, which are easier to use than a tampon when they're not yet very familiar with their own anatomy.

Tampons are made of an absorbent material shaped into a cylinder that fits directly into your daughter's vagina to absorb menstrual flow. She can insert the tampon with her fingers, but most come with an applicator. It should be inserted far enough that she doesn't feel it. If it's not comfortable, it isn't in right. To remove it, she pulls on a string that hangs out of her vagina.

Like pads, tampons come in different sizes, with size chosen based on comfort and the amount of flow. Most girls should start with the small size. If it's difficult to get the tampon to slide in because her vagina is dry, she can use a lubricant. Many girls ultimately find that the tampon is more comfortable and practical than the pad.

You may need to disabuse your daughter of some tampon myths.

Myth #1: Some girls worry that a tampon will "get lost up there." It won't. There's nowhere for it to go. The only opening is the cervical os, which is tiny (except when it expands to deliver a baby). Likewise, the tampon won't fall out—except perhaps when she is straining on the toilet—because her vaginal muscles keep it inside. Your daughter might forget she has a tampon in, especially if the string disappears into her vagina. It's not hard to remove a tampon without the string; she can just reach inside her vagina to get it.

Myth #2: Some girls think that if they use a tampon they are no longer a virgin. Tampons can tear or stretch an intact hymen, but not usually. Many girls won't care, but if your daughter doesn't want to do anything that might affect her hymen, she should use a pad. If it's hard to get the tampon through, she might be able to stretch her hymen with her fingers. Otherwise, she'll probably find it easiest to use pads until her hymen becomes more flexible or until she's had intercourse.

Menstrual sponges are similar to tampons in that they are inserted into the vagina, but they are reusable. It is very important to wash them carefully before reuse. They are not widely available.

Whatever your daughter uses, she should change it every few hours, especially with heavy flow, in part to prevent toxic shock syndrome.

Toxic shock syndrome is caused by bacteria that release a toxic chemical that spreads throughout the body. Symptoms include fever, muscle aches, vomiting, and diarrhea, so at first it may seem like a virus. But within two days, she may become light-headed and dizzy; develop a rash that looks like a sunburn; get red, irritated eyes; have less urine; and get swollen joints. If these symptoms occur, your daughter should go to a clinician immediately.

You can get toxic shock if you're not menstruating, if you've never worn a tampon, and even if you're male, but it's thought that tampons increase the chances because bacteria can grow in a tampon that stays in too long. This syndrome is very, very rare, but the best way to prevent it is to change tampons regularly. Some people also recommend using lower absorbency, unperfumed tampons. It's also a good idea to use pads when sleeping so the tampon isn't in all night.

At menarche, although the menstrual flow begins, the eggs are usually not quite ready to be released; but about a year after the first period, they will start their monthly routine of growth and eruption, a process destined to last for the next several decades. This doesn't mean your daughter can't get pregnant in her first year after menarche. We're talking averages here, and some girls will begin releasing eggs earlier.

Menstrual cycles can be a bit quirky in the beginning. The blood flow might be light or heavy, it can last for a short or long time, and there may be a particularly long time in between periods. Stress, travel, and changes in your daughter's life can cause her to skip a period. (Although missing periods is not unusual, if she could be pregnant, she should get a pregnancy test.) Most girls will have more regular periods by a year or two after menarche.

Flow will generally range from a few teaspoons to about half a cup. If your daughter's flow is heavier than usual, she should see a clinician.

Now, there has long been a lot of nonsense about girls needing to restrain their activities during menstruation. It's not true. Your daughter can do just about anything she's comfortable with. If she finds that she feels light-headed or a little weak when she menstruates, she may choose to take it easier on those days, but in general that won't be necessary.

So one day, you may hear a little voice calling out from behind a closed bathroom door, "Mom?" and you will probably know exactly what it means. Hopefully, before this day arrives, your daughter will have had a chance to learn the basics of menstruation.

When Kathy was eleven, she found a box of pads on the top shelf in her closet. Her mother had put them there. She hadn't started menstruating yet, but she knew from friends what they were for. "My mother was never comfortable talking about anything related to bodies or sex. I asked her what the pads were for, and she told me I'd need them some day."

When Kathy finally got her period, she called her best friend, Wanda, who came over and showed her how to use a pad. "It wasn't hard, but you need someone to show you the first time. You've got to rip the thing off, stick it there, do this and that. It's confusing at first."

The two girls eventually decided it was time to try tampons. "We both had our periods, and we wanted to go swimming."

They picked the smallest box at the drugstore because they thought small would be easier. Those turned out to be ones without applicators. "Applicator-free was definitely not the way to start." They flipped a coin to see who would go first. "Wanda was in the bathroom trying to put it in, but she couldn't. So then I tried. They're not easy to use. My muscles were tightening up. It was hurting. I didn't know what I was doing." Kathy got hers in most of the way, which spurred Wanda to try again, and she succeeded.

"Then we went swimming. The little bit of tampon that was sticking out of my vagina expanded with the water. You could completely see this weird bulge in my bathing suit. It's funny now, but it wasn't funny then. I was horrified. Later we found out about applicators. I'm definitely going to tell my daughter everything she needs to know."

Carl, a single dad, learned from friends what to say to his daughter. "I told her all about her period before she got it, and I told her how to use pads. I was an instant expert, having just learned myself. I also got some tidbits that you'd only know from experience—like she should keep some pads and an extra pair of underwear in her backpack." Carl doesn't plan to teach her everything, though. "When she's ready to use a tampon, my sister's gonna come over and help. I think that's one where she really needs to talk with someone with firsthand experience."

Boys' Life

Not only will your son begin puberty later than your daughter, but when he does begin, you and he will be less likely to notice. Boys' bodies begin developing with a lot less fanfare than girls' bodies. Probably some time between the ages of nine and fourteen, your son's testicles will begin to enlarge. That will be the first sign.

Your son is a bit more likely to notice his penis growing, but many kids don't really catch that at first, either. His penis will typically start to grow after he reaches ten and before he hits fourteen. At first it will grow longer, and then thicker and maybe darker. It takes about three years to reach its full adult size. What boys *will* notice is what they can do with their penis—or rather, what it can do for them—but more about that in a moment.

Carol found out Carter's puberty had begun when he shouted with glee from the bathtub, "Mom, I have a pubic hair!" This is the first sign your son probably won't miss. On average, pubic hair starts growing when boys reach twelve (typically, about a year after their testicles begin growing), but, as usual, there's a wide range. Your son's first hairs will be around the base of his penis, and they'll usually be rather straight. At first, he may be able to tell you exactly how many he has, but soon they'll become too dense to count. His hair will get curlier and thicker and spread up toward his belly button, down onto his scrotum, and partway down his thighs.

Peekaboo

Vanita had developed something of a morning ritual with her son. She'd wake him for school, he'd beg for five more minutes, she'd let him sleep some more, and then she'd stand over him and demand he get up. It worked. "I'm a professional snooze alarm, except I have only one station in the morning, and it's set on cranky," she says with a sinister smile.

"One day he wouldn't get out of bed after he'd already had his five minutes, so I pulled back the covers to yank him out, and there it was, peeking out of the top of his underwear. It never occurred to me. I threw the covers back down, and said something stupid like 'Okay, five more minutes.' As he headed off for school, he told me he was going to need a few extra minutes some mornings, and then he gave me a grin that told me things were okay."

As we explained in Chapter 1, boys start having erections before they're born. But as your son reaches the end of elementary school, his erections will more and more be triggered by sexual attraction. And as his penis grows, they will become more obvious, both to him and to anyone else who cares to notice. Some boys can be very private about their erections, and very concerned that someone might know they have one.

Spermarche!

I was dreaming about a pop-up book. There was a man with a pop-up penis, and it was popping in and out of the book. I turned the pages, and there were more pop-up penises. And then I woke up as I was coming. At first I thought I was peeing in my bed, but it felt good, and I realized what it was. My dad had told me this might happen. I mean, he'd told me about wet dreams, not about the pop-up penis part of it.

—*Sam, remembering when he was thirteen*

The wash has been piling up, and you know it's your wife's turn to do the laundry. But what are you going to do? It's either wash it yourself or go to work tomorrow with no socks. So you separate the whites from the dark clothes, and pull the dry cleaning out into its own pile. White, green, white, white, jeans, white, white, whi—stiff. Your son's underpants have a stiff spot on them. You recognize it in an instant. An old friend from long ago, the wet dream.

Should you say something? Does he know what it is? Has your wife already told him?

Should you wash them in cold or hot?

The first ejaculation (spermarche) can occur anytime during puberty. If there is a single recognizable event that announces to your son that he's hit puberty, this is it. Now, not all boys get wet dreams. For the average boy, the first ejaculation will happen while he is very much awake and masturbating, often between ages thirteen and fourteen. Boys will typically not have mature sperm in their first ejaculation, but as with girls and ovulation during the first year after menarche, this is not a form of birth control to count on.

Eric, at twelve, came running into the den where his father, Sheldon, was reading the paper. Sheldon looked up to see his son naked, holding his penis with one hand, and cupping the product of his exuberance in the other. Sheldon was startled by Eric's lack of modesty, but then realized his son was really scared. Eric thought he was bleeding. Sheldon wondered later, "How could he think blood would be white?" But he also felt bad that his son had to experience such fear.

Sheldon thought he had told his son about ejaculating, but when they talked about it later, he realized his words hadn't made much sense to Eric. He had explained how to make babies. He had felt pretty good about adding that sperm can come out while sleeping and that Eric could make his sperm come out if he wanted to, but Eric couldn't imagine why anyone would want to do that, so he hadn't given it much thought. "I explained and made sure to be clear this time, that it can feel good to rub your penis with your hand or against the sheet, and that if it feels really good, you can ejaculate. It didn't occur to me to use a lot of detail the first time. It's not the sort of thing I was used to talking about."

Telling boys in advance about ejaculation can save some anxious moments later. Boys come up with all sorts of worries, and because they often sense that this is something to keep secret, they may not ask you about it. By talking to your son before his first ejaculation, you can plant the seed (sorry) that ejaculation is normal, a sign of his growing manhood.

If your son isn't as open with you as Eric was with his father, you can educate him about ejaculation while leaving him his privacy. There's no need to press the issue of whether he's had one or not, as long as he knows you're open to such topics if he has questions.

Mowing the Lawn

Learning to shave is the other notable milestone for boys—another chance to officially acknowledge that puberty has arrived.

Regis hadn't really noticed that his son was maturing until the day his daughter volunteered to "mow the lawn" on Jim's face. It was hardly a lawn, more like a weed or two peeking up through the parched desert sand, but Regis swung into action.

As his wife describes it, "He was thrilled to teach Jim to shave. This was one of those days he'd been waiting for. He went to the store and came back with a razor and shaving cream. I wrapped it in gift wrap for

The Locked Door

> *I used to play with myself in the shower, and then one day I couldn't stop stroking myself. I was about thirteen. I just kept stroking and stroking as if I was possessed. And then I burst out, and it was the most amazing feeling. And it suddenly all made sense, and I realized that this was what an ejaculation was. I swore I'd never do it again. I made it through the next day okay . . .*
>
> *—Jamie, recalling his own youth*

Charlie is rather matter-of-fact about his son's need for privacy. "At a certain point, he started going into his room and locking his door. He'll stay in there for hours with that door locked. I don't really listen in, but I've walked by very slowly, and I can't hear anything. My friends find the same thing. What do they do behind those doors?"

Using privacy productively is one more product of puberty. Adolescents are more likely to choose to go off alone than elementary schoolers. As early as middle school, they may benefit from privacy in a way that younger kids don't—as a constructive way of managing strong emotions. You may not feel as welcome in your daughter's private world as you once did, because she's practicing new abilities to take care of herself that weren't available to her before.

Sometimes your newly pubescent kid is lying on his bed daydreaming or going over the conversations of the day. Sometimes he's listening to songs that capture how he feels about life and love and school and you. And sometimes he's masturbating.

Kids this age hole up in their rooms to explore their bodies and see what feels good. They look at themselves in the mirror, or look at pictures of naked boys, naked girls, or both.

They read the sex scenes someone carefully highlighted in a dog-eared copy of the potboiler that's being passed around the seventh grade. But they're also doing their homework, surfing the Web, and doodling.

We had a good bit to say about masturbation in Chapter 4. When puberty hits, more kids are masturbating than at any prior age. Thanks to their maturing genitals, the increased juice in their sex drive, and the development of their sexual fantasy life, teens may find masturbation feels better than ever. With all of these changes, they may also begin to think of their masturbation differently from the way they did back when you first told them it was fine.

"My mother made it very clear to me when I asked her about it in grade school that masturbation was a really good thing," Susanna says, "but when I got into high school and I started doing it a lot, I just felt incredibly guilty. It became the big, dark secret of my youth."

The new intensity to her pleasure and the fantasies she was now having while masturbating may have played a role in Susanna's newfound shame. "Maybe," Susanna says, "it was also because except for my mother, no one ever mentioned it. It was like there was this great conspiracy of silence. It didn't even come up in sex ed. I began to think my mother had just been trying to make me feel better as a kid by telling me it was normal."

After a few years of silence, at the age of seventeen, "I finally admitted to my best friend that I masturbated. It was this huge revelation. I was shaking. It was the scariest thing I had ever told anyone." To Susanna's great relief, "She said she did it, too."

Is there anything more Susanna's mother could have done to lessen her daughter's teen angst?

"I know she told me all about it when I was little, but I guess I could have used a reminder."

After puberty begins, you can remind your kids, without commenting directly on their solo flights, that sexual feelings and masturbation are healthy and normal:

"Some kids masturbate, and some don't. Some people will tell you it's bad or dangerous, and because no one ever talks about it, I just wanted to make sure you know that I think it's perfectly fine."

him. He wanted to make it a big deal. I think he never really felt he had much of a chance to connect with Jim. Jim wasn't into sports, and I was the one who helped him with his homework. Now here was something they could do together."

Your son's first shave is in some ways a little like your daughter's first bra. Facial hair begins to grow about two years after pubic hair starts coming in. The first several times your son shaves, there will probably be no compelling need for it. But taking your son through this ritual can be a way of helping him feel your support of his growing up.

In families in which religion prohibits shaving, boys still need to learn to take care of their beards. Of course, boys don't need religion to inspire them to grow mustaches and beards, which can become a source of conflict at home, if you take the bait.

Babe's son, for example, has a beard about four inches long and about an inch wide that comes out of the center of his chin with muttonchop sideburns. Now if every boy has this beard by the time you are reading this book, keep in mind that when Babe's son had it, he was surely the only one. "Do I like the way he looks? Absolutely not. Do I say anything about it? Absolutely not. He does his homework, he meets his curfew, he's polite. I'd have to say everything is perfect, if it wasn't that he looks like a member of ZZ Top. So, if this is as far as his rebellion goes, then I consider myself lucky." She adds with a chuckle, "And you *know* he's going to be mortified a few years from now when I show some future girlfriend these pictures."

Breasts?

As if a cracking voice and pimples were not enough, between one-half and two-thirds of boys also develop breast tissue (often just a tiny pea-sized lump, but sometimes a good deal more) on one or both sides, usually because of estrogens circulating in their body. Minor breast development usually goes away within a year or two, but it may be the subject of teasing and the source of self-doubt.

Your son should know that a little breast growth is normal. If some of the men in his life also went through a phase in which they developed breasts, he may find it reassuring to be told. If he is heavy, his breast development may be more noticeable and last longer (he will have slightly higher estrogen levels because testosterone is converted to estrogen in fat cells). His clinician can discuss treatments if his breast tissue is particularly disturbing to him.

How Do I Look?

Your thirteen-year-old daughter is locked in the bathroom. For the past two hours she has absorbed herself in the critical process of dressing for a night at the mall. As her father, and tonight's driver, you sense that there is a script for this moment. It involves jangling the car keys and yelling up the stairs some half-mocking, half-irritated comment about girls and mirrors and leaving without her.

Instead, you sit and flip though the paper, proud to resist the path down which so many generations of dads have stumbled. Your daughter is your pal, and for now you are happy to support her decision to cloister herself with a copy of her favorite teen magazine and enough eyeliner to satisfy the court of Nefertiti.

What's this? The door is opening. Footsteps sound on the stairs.

You pick up your coat and amble over to the stairs, ready to make an encouraging comment about whatever it is she has found to put on.

She appears. Her hair is brushed back and gleaming. Her lips are red. She is wearing a tiny black dress with bare shoulders and a silver bracelet hanging around her left wrist. She looks at you. She is your daughter. She looks . . . sexy.

A Visit to the Clinician

Around the start of your child's puberty, her doctor, nurse practitioner, or other primary clinician should tell you that the time has come for them to have a private, confidential talk at each visit.

Private meetings give your child an opportunity to take responsibility for her health—for describing her own symptoms, for asking her own questions, and for acting on the clinician's advice about prevention or treatment. They send a signal that she is growing up and will need to make decisions and look after herself. Most important, they give your child and her clinician a chance to discuss health matters that may be too awkward to discuss with you around. Sexual health is high on the list of such matters.

If your son's clinician doesn't ask you to step out, discuss with her what you think is the right time for this change. You can also encourage privacy by excusing yourself after you've asked your questions.

Laws vary from state to state, but your teen's clinician will generally be able to give completely confidential care when counseling about sexual matters, treating STDs, and providing contraception. In the rare circumstances in which the clinician feels that she has to break confidentiality—such as when someone's life is in danger—she will usually warn your child in advance and explain why, and then give him a chance to tell you himself.

Because the clinician's bill often undoes confidentiality by specifying the type of care that was provided, you can tell the clinician you're willing to have all bills sent to you without the service specified. It takes a certain amount of confidence in your adolescent and his clinician to facilitate such independence, and it also takes some fortitude to resist investigating what the care was for.

Some parents find being excluded from the exam room a bit trying. If you are one of them, bear in mind that the issues you feel most curious about may be the very ones your daughter most needs privacy to discuss. When faced with a choice, for example, between telling their parents about an STD symptom and not getting treatment for it, many teens choose the latter. The result can be a worsening of their infection and complications like infertility.

Some adolescent girls give another reason for delaying treatment when they have an STD: fear of the *pelvic exam*.

At some point after puberty begins, your daughter will have her first pelvic exam. The exam allows the clinician to assess whether there are any abnormalities of her reproductive system, to screen for STDs, and to check for cancer by performing a Pap smear.

Adolescent girls are generally advised to have a pelvic exam and a Pap smear within the year after their first vaginal intercourse and annually for two more years. If these initial Pap smears have been normal, some recommend a repeat every two to three years, while others recommend continuing annually throughout adolescence because of high STD rates. If your daughter has not had vaginal intercourse, the traditional recommendation is for her to start having pelvic exams with Pap smears when she's eighteen, although nowadays some clinicians feel it's okay to wait until she is older.

Parents usually step out during the pelvic exam, although your daughter may want you to stay with her to hold her hand, at least the first time. Even with a warm and gentle clinician, the exam can be disturbing. Your daughter may be afraid, so it helps to discuss the process in advance. Don't be surprised afterward if she wonders if the pelvic exam is what sex feels like. Tell her that the two are nothing alike and that not liking the pelvic exam does not mean she will not like intercourse.

Finally, bear in mind that while many clinicians who are

wonderful with babies are just as good with adolescents, some are not. Sex is still an awkward subject for some clinicians—and if your child's clinician can't talk about it without stumbling over his words or changing the subject prematurely, you might want to make a switch. Your kid, in particular, needs to feel comfortable talking about sexual matters with her clinician.

You gasp.

And as the wave of recognition of what you have inadvertently done slowly breaks over you, your daughter bursts into tears and runs to her room.

You sit down at the foot of the stairs, your coat on your lap and your head hanging low, and think, "Shit. Fatherhood is destiny."

Don't despair. However doomed you may feel to meet the fate of your forebears, fatherhood is not destiny—it's an entry-level position with tremendous growth potential. There is, though, one nearly inevitable fact of parenting a teen that you will have to fumble through, whatever your particular skills may be. Teenagers are a teensy bit sensitive about how they look.

Why wouldn't they be? The sudden physical unpredictability of puberty worries teens terribly that their bodies will betray them. Pick up any teen magazine and flip to the perennially popular and gruesomely riveting column, "My Most Embarrassing Moment." You will find countless horrific tales of the abominations of the body. My fly was down! My skirt flew up! My legs weren't shaved! I had a blood spot! I sneezed on him! I threw up! I farted! Everyone saw/knew/heard/laughed! I thought I would die!

At an age of such physical upheaval, clothes are the one aspect of their appearance teens can control, and the one necessary disguise to hide the ever-threatening leak, or bump, or smell. Which means that now would be a fairly good time to cut your child some slack when it comes to choosing what he wants to wear, either by avoiding comment altogether or finding ways to make blandly informational remarks when some sort of comment seems necessary:

> "Are you okay with that shirt? We're going to a place that might be pretty cold."

> "I know you love those pants, but let me know if I can get you a new pair. They've got holes in some pretty odd places."

Sometimes it can be a bit of a challenge to project the sort of neutrality needed to pull these comments off:

> "Say, that's a great color you dyed your hair. What would you call it, chartreuse?"

> "Oh, by the way, the shower is working this week, if that matters."

You aren't always neutral, and in fact, one of your least neutral experiences may be seeing your daughter ready to pop out the door in a top that in some countries could pass for postage.

A child's first passes at sexiness can be disturbing, angering, even frightening. Your brave battle with those feelings may unpredictably erupt into the awkward jokes and cracks that send kids running to their rooms. Did you know that when ten- and eleven-year-old girls are asked who teases them most about their breast development, parents are first on their list? These parents aren't trying to be insensitive. They are probably contending with a reaction to their daughter's body they don't know how to handle.

With these tensions simmering in the background, how do you respond when your child is wearing something you find too revealing?

"At dances, the girls dress really provocatively. They wear these strappy, low-cut things," Jean, the mother of fifteen-year-old Deena, says with some obvious reservations. "They all started dressing like that around three years ago."

(Notice by the way that we are talking about girls here. When boys come of age, they seem to adopt aggressively concealing baggy pants and shirts that if they provoke, do so because they fall off. This, however, is a matter of teenage fashion and may have changed completely by the time we put the period at the end of this sentence.)

"At first it really bothered me."

Jean recalled seeing the halters Deena, then twelve years old, was dragging into the fitting room as so many jaunty little scarlet letters she was threatening to affix to her chest. But, as Jean soon discovered, for better or worse, the halters were unlikely to make her daughter stand out as the loose kid at school.

"I found out it was how all the girls were dressing. Which meant that she wasn't going to grab all the attention if she dressed that way, too. I wasn't about to make her feel weird and different. So we bought her the clothes she needed."

As Jean and her husband saw things, "in middle school, if you don't dress according to code, you're toast." Which brings us to the paradoxical fact that in seventh grade, showing off your belly button can actually be a way of concealing your body. If you were worried about your looks, and you needed to hide out in the open, what would you wear? Camouflage.

Of course, your kid's dress may go well beyond blending with her peers. If her choices stray from standard peer mimicry, it's worth wondering what your child is trying to say, and to whom. Some kids dress to tell their classmates that they are not one of the gang. Sometimes if you feel provoked by your daughter's get-up, it's because she meant to provoke you.

Ask about these potential messages if the opportunity arises. Try a time when your child isn't wearing the article of interest and will therefore feel less exposed. With a little tact, you can honestly convey your thoughts on the outfit without expressing a criticism of the kid who wore it:

"When you decided to put that on last night, were you hoping people would react in a certain way?"

"Would you be surprised if I told you I was a little taken aback?"

"I think some people would see that other dress as kind of revealing/aggressive/quirky. Is that the look you're shooting for?"

Still, you may ask, what happens if while you carefully walk the tightrope of a tactfully honest, empathic, and cool dad, you instinctively let out an audible gasp the night you first see your daughter dressed up like an attractive young woman and send her sobbing to her room?

Something like this happened to the husband of psychologist Jodi Messler Davies, who in a recent article described the frightening moment in which her husband knew he had to go to their daughter's room, but had no idea what he could possibly say.

He bravely knocked, disappeared into the room, and, as Davies tells it, a few minutes later father and daughter were chatting and laughing together.

What had he done?

" 'I told her the truth,' he said, 'that I had never seen her looking so beautiful before—in such a grown-up way—that it had taken my breath away. . . . [I told her] that I liked it, but that it was something I was going to have to get used to.' "

What did she say?

Nothing, he told his wife. She didn't say anything. " 'But she smiled the most beautiful smile.' "

My, How You've Grown!

The other side to the scary physical changes of puberty is the power it can give some kids.

There's something magical, and frightening, about being a teenager and discovering you have power over people because of some new contour that wasn't there yesterday. One day you're a prepubescent waif able to slip in and out of a room unnoticed. The next day you're turning heads. This can be a little bracing for parents, too.

You may discover that your daughter has learned how to flirt her way into a bar when she's still sixteen, or get the guy at the amusement park to let her in for free. The secretary at school provides hall passes a little more freely now when your son rolls up the sleeves of his T-shirt. Over the next few years, your kids will be learning how to use their sex appeal, but for now, they may not know their own strength. And it's possible they can get in over their heads.

Obviously, not all kids develop this kind of clout. Those who don't may be envious and feel unfairly left out of the game. Some boys try to work this out through time in the school weight room, which can, of course, be either productive and esteem building or a Sisyphean effort to feel good enough. Some may look for a boost from steroids. Likewise for girls and dieting.

These pubertal years can be a cruel collision between children with fragile self-images and the judgmental and competitive peer society they make. Telling your teen she looks great as she heads out to a party won't change her world, but it can make it a bit easier to live in.

A Different Drummer: Early and Late Bloomers

Someone's always got to be first, and someone's always last. Here are some thoughts if your child's development falls out of line with his peers.

Early Puberty

Starting early can be a challenge, especially for girls. If your daughter is one of the first at school to develop breasts, she may get teased. Boys may snap her bra. Older boys may pay attention in ways she doesn't understand or like. Girls may make derisive comments. If none of her friends is older, she may not have peers with whom to compare notes and share feelings.

And her development can affect how adults treat her. Family, teachers, and strangers may all treat early maturers differently. They may assume a level of sexual precocity that is not there or expect her emotional and intellectual development to be keeping up with her physical development. Her social skills may be those of a child, even though her body is looking more and more like an adult's. You may even catch yourself expecting her to act older than she is.

All of this may have something to do with the findings that girls who go through puberty very early enter adulthood somewhat less well adjusted than their peers. These girls tend to be more likely to get involved with various risk behaviors, including unprotected sex and drug use.

Of course, the research on these kids averages the effects of early puberty over many children. You've only got your daughter to take care of, and your reaction to her experience might mitigate any challenges she's facing. Adjusting your own timetable of expectations may help her feel that what's happening to her is fine.

"I was not happy when I realized she was already developing," Evelyn says of her daughter, who got breast buds at eight. "It really caught me off-guard. We adopted her, and I had some medical information, but they don't give you this sort of stuff. I'd been rather average on the development front, but one of my friends was the first in our class to get breasts, and I saw what she went through. I told my daughter everyone gets her turn to start on the road to womanhood and her turn had come up. I talked all about menstruation and all the body changes, but what really helped was that I invited her older cousins over more often, so there would be opportunities for her to talk with other kids about the changes. I think it made a difference."

Boys who mature early are more commonly the objects of envy than ridicule. Their deep voices and muscles can give them a kind of authority in their peer group, and they rarely feel a need to hide the evidence of their development. They may be treated as more capable, even though they may be no more socially advanced than their peers. Some studies have found that the social benefits these boys gain in junior high and high school dwindle as they get older.

Late Puberty

Boys and girls whose puberty arrives late can struggle, too.

Patty got her first period when she was about seventeen. "I thought

Early and Late Puberty: When to Go to the Clinician

"Look at this!" Pesha was pointing at pubic hair, which I had never noticed. I said "Oh, that is natural. Your body is growing." Inside I was thinking "What the hell is this? She is only seven!" Pesha had been clumsy for the preceding weeks, and was having headaches, so I got worried about a brain tumor. I took her to the doctor, who said lots of times kids develop at different rates, that he wanted to make sure she was healthy, so he ordered a CT scan. Pesha also got a bone-age X ray. She was anxious, but everything turned out to be normal. Pesha feels pretty okay about it now. We've read some books about puberty, and everything's fine.

   —Arlene, talking about her now eight-year-old daughter

We recommend that adolescents have an annual medical visit so the clinician can detect any abnormalities with puberty, but if you are concerned about something, there's no reason to wait a full year between visits. Go ahead and make an appointment.

There's some scientific debate over exact cutoffs, but basically, when African American girls start developing breasts or pubic hair before six or seven and when white girls start before age seven or eight, they are said to have "precocious puberty." Most girls who start early don't have a medical problem — they're just very early bloomers — but they could also have hormone problems or other diseases, so it's best to take your daughter to the clinician if the timing of her development seems abnormal. If she gets some pubic hair but no breast development before these cutoffs, that's usually fine; but if she starts growing faster, or her clitoris starts enlarging, or she develops acne, she should go to her clinician.

Unlike girls, when boys develop early, they are much more likely to have a medical problem that warrants immediate attention, such as a tumor, so check out any concerns with a clinician. If your son's penis or testicles are growing early (you might not notice) or he's growing faster than other boys, that warrants a visit. It's probably easier to detect if he's got acne before age nine or pubic hair before age ten—both are reasons to go to the clinician.

Puberty is considered delayed for girls whose breasts don't begin to develop by about thirteen or who haven't reached menarche four or five years after breast development begins (or by age fifteen, whichever comes first). Puberty is late for boys whose testicles don't grow by fourteen or whose testicles and penis don't look adult five years after starting to develop.

What's not big enough for a testicle? If it's not at least 2.5 centimeters long (a little over an inch) by age fourteen, he needs to get checked by a clinician. Of course, while you may catch your son measuring his penis, he probably hasn't taken a ruler to much else, and we'll guess you haven't clocked a lot of hours measuring testicles, either. Again, an easier marker to follow is pubic hair. If your son hasn't started growing pubic hair by fourteen or seems otherwise less mature than his peers, you can ask his clinician.

Most of the boys and girls who are late will turn out to just be late, nothing more, and they'll catch up eventually. We call this *constitutional delay.* Many children with constitutional delay in puberty are also on the small side for height even before reaching adolescence.

Medical problems, some of them treatable, can cause the delay. A chronic illness can delay puberty, possibly because it drains energy needed to go through puberty. Among girls, ballet dancers and other athletes may have delayed puberty because of diversion of energy to their exercise and a reduction in body fat, although it's probably more complicated than we currently understand. Medicines and environmental toxins can delay puberty; so can malnutrition, as with anorexia.

something was wrong with my body. All my friends had had their period. First I'm a year late. Then I'm two years late. I'm like, what's up with this? But I didn't have anyone to ask. There's no way I could have talked to my parents about it. I read that ballet dancers get their periods late, and I had taken ballet lessons as a little girl, so I thought that was the reason." Patty's parents didn't say anything, and Patty didn't make it to the doctor very often. When she got her period, she was elated. " 'Finally,' I thought, 'I guess I'm normal.' Later I found out that all the women on my father's side don't get their periods until they are seventeen, eighteen, or nineteen, but no one ever told me."

Boys can have as much trouble with late puberty as girls. They can see their small stature and high voices as a kind of "wimpiness," and so may the other boys in the locker room. But as far as we know, in the end, once puberty arrives, most boys will adapt fine.

"I don't think I noticed that I was developing later," Marshall, who took his delay in stride, says. "I'm not sure I ever saw another boy's penis. I knew I was smaller and not as strong. I could tell that other boys were developed. But I didn't realize that I would become like them. I didn't think I was late, just different. I just thought it was part of being a wimp."

Some studies have found that boys and girls who develop late may be treated as less responsible and dependable than more physically mature peers. That's a mistake that you'll want to watch out for. Your late bloomer may be miles ahead of others in less visible categories.

Time for Lesson Three: Expect Puberty
Who Does the Talking?
Many parents in two-parent homes wonder if mothers should talk to daughters and fathers to sons about puberty. The answer is yes, but you should mix and match as well. You may know more than your partner about the pubertal changes of both genders, so why shouldn't you be the one to talk about them? Better yet, you and your partner can talk together with your child, although you might not want to sit him across the table with the two of you facing him, bright light shining in his eyes, FBI-style.

The point here is to get these conversations going, and if there is a pairing that for whatever reason feels relatively comfortable, go with it. Then try to work on the other relationship, because the more points of view your child gets, the better.

You never know when the topic is going to come up. One day when your partner's out shopping and you're home with the kids, your son may ask why girls get a period and boys don't. (Maybe next time, when he wants to know what a blow job is, you'll be the one at the store.)

Make sure your child knows that he can ask questions of either of you (if, in fact, that's true), but respect his choice to gravitate toward one of you in particular, or to someone else in or outside the family. What he needs most is guaranteed access to a sensible, informed adult.

Other Resources

Clinicians, sex education teachers, religious advisors, grandma, and favorite uncles can all help out here. A few minutes online should also help you find some of the excellent books and informative websites available for preteens and teens. There's enough diversity in these resources to help you identify at least a few that present information from a perspective that fits with your values and cultural background.

Two of our favorites are *It's Perfectly Normal,* by Robie Harris and Michael Emberley, a great puberty picture book we mentioned earlier, ideal for school-age kids just learning about puberty, but sophisticated enough for teens already going through puberty, and *Changing Bodies, Changing Lives,* by Ruth Bell and colleagues, a comprehensive guide for middle and high school students.

And What Should You Say?

So how much should you tell your child about puberty, and when should you start? Do you give a lecture and ask him to take notes, or do you just wait for him to ask questions? Well, probably both. We recommend that you give your child an overview before puberty starts—most parents will be safe starting at age eight—and then repeat those lessons in greater detail as puberty marches on and they become more pertinent.

Some children will want to know all about puberty, how it feels, and when everything will happen. Others will be less curious, or at least seem less curious. Still others will balk if you mention tampons or threaten to sit them down with a puberty primer. You know your child best, of course, so you are in the best position to choose which material to share with him from this chapter. There are a few key points that we think virtually all preteens should know.

Girls should definitely know about menstruation. If there is a menstruating woman in the house (you?), this shouldn't be too hard to bring up. Your kids can just learn as a matter of course about your monthly cycle. Some children pick up more than you realize, but others don't, so when you notice your daughter developing breasts, it's time to make sure she understands menstruation. She needs to know the practical aspects, such as how to wear a sanitary napkin or tampon. She will probably also want to understand why she menstruates. Details about the menstrual cycle will help her understand pregnancy and contraception. You can let her know about the clear or milky discharge she may notice from her vagina, which is perfectly normal.

Tell her about the little bumps she might feel in her breast just as it is beginning to bud. She'll probably also want to find out about bras at some point.

Boys will have been getting erections since they were infants, but now they will probably become more aware of them and more self-conscious about them. You can let them know that erections are a normal part of a boy's life.

Ejaculation is probably the big surprise for boys. Let your son know in advance that this will start happening when he is in the midst of puberty, so it won't scare him. Be specific about wet dreams and masturbating to orgasm.

Depending on your cultural perspective, someone needs to teach both boys and girls about shaving and deodorant, but if you forget, both visual and olfactory stimuli may remind you.

If you have a daughter, perhaps you skipped the sections on boys, and vice versa if you have a son. But it would be good for each to understand what the other sex is going through.

How to Talk

There's no need to try to squeeze everything into a single conversation. As we discussed before, education about sex and puberty should not be provided as a onetime lesson. Seize any opportunity fortune provides you to get in a little teaching. Small doses are fine. A question about what your tampons are for. A question about when he'll grow a beard. An uninhibited display of affection between two dogs in the park.

Try to depict puberty as a natural process and a good thing. You may have some ambivalence based on what your friends have said about piercings, mood swings, and the kid who sold his dog to buy a bong, but try to put all that out of your mind. It's got to be hard to be ten and thinking that you need to survive rather than enjoy the next period of your life, especially when that period is about as long as the number of years you've already been alive.

You can be frank, acknowledging that some of what's coming up will feel strange, but remain upbeat. This is going to be a time of discovery, of increasing intellectual and physical strengths, of learning the mysteries of adulthood. Okay, that might not impress them much. Try another tack. Let them know that puberty provides the transition to being old enough to drive, to go to an R-rated movie, and, for the civic-minded among your kids, to vote.

Cracks in the Wall

One final thought on talking. No matter how hard you try, no matter how much you care, talking with your child about puberty won't always be easy, or even, necessarily, possible.

Ellie was looking forward to sharing in her daughter's transition to womanhood. She had envisioned doing all the things that her own mother had never done: showing her daughter how to use a tampon, teaching her how to shave, enjoying long talks. From the time Jill was old enough to ask questions, Ellie had given honest answers and sought to convey that Jill could ask her anything. Jill knew where babies come from, that sex feels good. Ellie had told her about menstruation when

Jill wandered in on her in the bathroom and again when it came up on TV. But when Jill began puberty, "the puberty wall went up."

Jill was about nine years old when Ellie noticed that she had the very beginning of breast budding. Ellie arranged a special walk through an arboretum to explain how Jill's body worked and what Jill could expect. They went and sat by a little pond where they could have some privacy. But Jill would have none of it. "She stomped off. With all that attempt at modern openness, I couldn't get her to talk at all. She didn't want to deal with it. None of her friends was going through it yet. She thought she was weird."

Ellie later learned that Jill had begun menstruating when she smelled something in the bathroom and found a used sanitary napkin wrapped in tissue in a drawer. Ellie knew that she had taught Jill enough over the years for Jill to have a basic understanding of menstruation and how it fits into a woman's life. But she had wanted to be a part of it. "Well, I didn't get to live my mother-daughter fantasy. But I had to respect her privacy. I had to accept that this was about her, not about me. So, I let her know that I was available to discuss whatever she wanted, and I made sure she knew that the proper place to put a used napkin was in the trashcan and not in a drawer."

Ellie finally found a way to tell her daughter the things she wanted to say. Jill had a friend whose mother had died. The friend would ask Ellie a string of questions when she would visit. Ellie was especially generous in answering the questions because it allowed Jill to hear a lot of information without having to ask about it. From Ellie's perspective, it was also nice to show Jill that she could be valued by her own best friend. A few years later, "the puberty wall came down," and they were able to talk about everything again. "My friends and I have decided that no matter what you do, all adolescents have a two-year rough period. There's no way around it."

Yes, all the details behind the physical changes of puberty can be a bit complicated, but what may be the most complex of all is the fact that when puberty happens, when your kid goes over the bump, she's not the child she used to be. She's an adolescent girl, with an adolescent mind. And that, friends, that is an organ that can really behave in some startling new ways—ways capable of altering the landscape of your relationship at home.

No doubt, a young teen's new body can pull off some amazing feats, but it's his or her mind that is responsible for the next great leap forward of adolescence: the reinvention of love.

Chapter **7**

Then comes love

FLIRTING, DATING, AND OTHER

HEARTBREAKS OF ADOLESCENCE

Speak low
When you speak, love,
Our moment is swift,
Like ships adrift,
We're swept apart too soon.
　　—"SPEAK LOW," LYRICS BY OGDEN NASH,
　　　MUSIC BY KURT WEILL, 1943

Oh no! I don't want to be the only one who doesn't have a
boyfriend!
　　—SARAH, AGE NINE

"YOU REALLY DON'T HAVE TO go to this party if you don't want to,
honey."

Perched on the edge of his bed, your twelve-year-old son—who has
just resolved the bitter dilemma of which shoes look more grown up—
may be a brave kid, but you still know when he's freaked, even if he is
too old to grab the back of your thigh and weep at the sight of a room
full of screaming kids and a clown.

"I think I should try it," he says, sweetly reaffirming his place at the
top of your list of all-time favorite males.

So you drive the fifteen minutes together largely in silence, get out of the car at the end of a long driveway, and walk your only son to the barn where, in honor of the seventh grade's spring party—the very first dance of your little boy's life—his school has re-created Studio 54.

The music throbs, a mirrored ball rakes the crowd with little flecks of light, smoke spurts out of a machine in the corner, and the girls . . . the *girls,* who look like they just walked out of a music video, flock together, shimmying in backless outfits and strawberry lipstick. Your son is the shortest kid there.

"You know my cell phone number, right?" you shout over the pumping disco beat.

"Yeah." There is a glazed look in his eyes.

"I'm just going to be doing some shopping, so if you decide you want to come home early, just give me a call."

"Okay."

Minutes later, at the grocery store, the cell goes off. The little voice at the other end is succinct:

"SOS!"

"I'm on my way."

You make it through the checkout and head back to the party, where you find your son hurrying to meet you at the car. Mom to the rescue.

He's smiling. "Mom, I think it's going to be okay,"

"What do you mean?"

He gestures for you to lean down and, when he's got your ear, carefully whispers, "I asked a girl to dance, and she said yes."

He stays.

As you stand there at the bottom of the driveway watching your only son race back to the dance with the sound of kids' laughter and the music spilling across the lawn, an odd feeling creeps into your chest. What is that sensation, hovering somewhere between anxiety and grief?

Could it be you feel . . . jilted?

You get into the car, fasten your seat belt, and take a long hard drag on an imaginary cigarette. "So what you're saying is," you address to no one in particular, "this is what's next?"

That's What We're Saying

Now that your child has entered adolescence—that period of develop-ment that begins when he starts puberty and ends when he remodels his kitchen (or endures some similarly harrowing event that strips him of his last scraps of innocence)—he will start to do adolescent things.

Around about now, if all goes well, he will begin to explore the world of romance.

As you might expect, your child's forays into dating and love may pre-sent certain emotional and tactical challenges for you and your mate. Young lovers are provocative creatures. They have been known to stir a complex whirl of feelings, not all of them benign, in the hearts of many an adult, par-ticularly their parents (see, for example, Adam, Eve, and God).

Consider this chapter a heads up. We will detail the path you and your child are about to travel as he makes his imperfect way to becom-ing someone's love. How will things change? What does he need from you? Why do you keep dreaming that you're planning a middle school graduation party on Temptation Island? We will explore some of the reactions you may have to your child's amorous innovations. And because they will all take place in the midst of the emotional and cog-nitive leaps forward that characterize adolescence, we will look at how, in shepherding your child through the mysteries of love, you may want to adapt your parenting practices to suit his new needs, talents, and urges.

A new world of hurts and happiness, passionate declarations, betrayals, and bliss awaits you and your child, ready to spring to life that afternoon your son first finds it in himself to ask someone to dance. Before we get to that moment, though, let's skip back to where it all began, to a time before the complications of barn discos and sparkly eye shadow, a time when the courtship of boys and girls was in its adorable infancy.

Love in the Time of Coloring

I had a boyfriend, but then he sort of forgot.

I liked him, but then my life went on and his life went on. And

now he's like, he's dumb. Like I got a ring from someone else.
Things happen to me. And he's just still, you know . . . he spits
when he talks.

—*Gillian, age nine*

"In the third grade," Hugh, now in his thirties, recalls, "my friends and
I were aware of one girl in the world, Carol Anne." A little blonde classmate who wore her hair in two braids pinned up on top of her head,
Carol was sweet and cute and looked like the lady on the Swiss Miss
Instant Cocoa box. This made her the ideal object of fascination for an
eight-year-old boy. Carol's signature outfit was an orange crocheted pon-
cho, on the front of which her mother had knit the letter C, "and probably because we all found Carol so irresistibly pretty, we decided the C
stood for Corrosion. 'Danger, danger!' we would shout ecstatically
whenever she came into view. 'Carol Corrosion is coming! Don't let her
touch you! Aaaaaaaaaargh!!!' "

Did you do stuff like this?

If you did, it was probably because you knew, as any third grader
does today, that a shivery, invisible wall separates boys and girls in middle childhood, and that to breach that wall is alternately titillating and
repellent.

From about the age of three, toddlers all over the world erect this
wall by choosing—when given a choice and for reasons not entirely
understood—to play with children of their own sex. As they grow older
and are freer to pick their friends, kids segregate all the more, until
between the ages of eight and eleven, gender segregation reaches its
peculiar peak—especially in public where other kids can see. Lunch
tables and swing sets turn into no-fly zones for one sex or the other. Boys
become convinced of their intrinsic superiority to girls. Girls swear boys
are icky. And when the two groups have to interact, usually because a
teacher or a parent has mandated it, kids approach the venture as if
entering a foreign country with odd customs and suspicious drinking
water.

Which is not to say that boys and girls have no use for each other.

In fact, the very taboo against fraternizing with the other side lends thoughts of touching, kissing, or (and this is really the ultimate) *liking* the other sex an unbeatable shiver of excitement—a thrill they will chase when it suits them.

"In my grade, there is one person who two people like," Greg, a fidgety seven-year-old, explains. "Gordon and David both like Arianna. It got passed around. Everybody found out. So like there was this *huge group* of people all looking for David and Arianna. It was really, really funny! Oh, by the way, don't write down names."

Don't tell. Don't say who likes whom. It's too exciting/embarrassing/weird/icky/fun. Only, let me tell you everything. The earliest stage of social romance, if you even want to call it that, has this tension running through it. Run-catch-kiss is compelling, because to be kissed by the other sex is as desirable as it is disgusting. Liking and hating are hard to distinguish, because they blend into one cross-eyed reaction. She's cute. Corrosion!

Girls may be a little more willing than boys to risk a liaison with the other sex. But they have their limits. Take nine-year-old Gillian, who, after explaining her need to move on from her latest crush (at the start of this section), took a peek at what her father was doing. He was reading a novel. She scanned the page. Suddenly she was seized with a catastrophic gastrointestinal ailment that caused her to collapse on the sofa, clutching her stomach and retching loudly.

"What?! What's wrong?!"

She paused mid-puke to point out the offending phrase on the page. It hideously read: "He grabbed her and kissed her deeply on the mouth."

Designating a boy as your "boyfriend" may briefly be tolerable at the tender age of nine, but kissing one is far too appalling even to consider.

This yes-no-ishness of grade school girl-boy play makes it a thrilling but, ultimately, baffling activity for kids who can't easily reconcile their contradictory feelings for each other. And so it remains an elaborate game of keep-away. Until everything changes.

Gender Blender

"Last year boys and girls were separate," explains Collin, a serious-minded twelve-year-old considering the changes in his life from sixth to seventh grade. "This year, boys and girls can talk to each other without someone calling you boyfriend and girlfriend. Last year, if a boy and a girl were friends, it meant that they *liked* each other. This year it doesn't."

Perestroika!

It happens this way all the time. At some particular point between the beginning of fifth grade and the end of seventh grade, in schools all over the country, the segregation that boys and girls have so scrupulously maintained breaks down. The revving engine of puberty, a step forward in cognitive development, a greater emotional maturity, and in some cases the move from an elementary school to a middle school probably all play a role in fomenting this revolution. And when the new order finally arrives, it opens up a door for boys and girls to get just a little bit closer.

Freed to mix outside of class without risking social annihilation, kids start to test their courage with the opposite sex. Understandably, after years of segregation, most fifth-grade girls and boys feel utterly perplexed about how to approach each other. First forays almost invariably take place amid the safety of numbers. Clusters of boys and girls may hang out together on the playground, almost talking to each other, or they will run into one another at the mall for a few charged minutes before they go their separate ways. Soon they will invite each other to their parties. Which will turn into dances.

How do kids navigate the transition to coed life?

"Someone asked me to dance," Collin says. "I didn't know how, but I think I figured it out. I didn't know the way it was supposed to work, that she put her hands on my shoulders and I put my hands on her waist. But now I can ask girls to dance. I'm getting a lot of occasions to learn exactly how I feel about it, because a lot of kids in my class are having mixers."

And so it begins. A boy and a girl touch each other out in the open where everyone can see. They bop around a little to the music. A few tentative words are exchanged, and, gradually, it's fun. Of course, not every child will be ready to take advantage of a chance at a slow dance the moment it appears.

Collin continues, "There are some kids—I was one of them at the beginning of the year—who are not quite used to the way things work in seventh grade. I've managed to learn how to enjoy it, but my friend, poor him, he hasn't. He tends to sit on the sidelines at dances."

Collin's friend will have his turn, and if it's any consolation to him, from the girls' perspective, both of them are probably desperately behind.

As Alexandra, also twelve years old but a head taller than Collin, explains, "You can't talk to boys in our grade. They're sooooooo immature. They act ridiculous around girls and they won't dance. They think they're too cool for that."

Actually, Alexandra, they're too flipped out for that.

This famous middle school schism, of course, has everything to do with puberty. The girls are simply further along, and that matters because the strong attractions of puberty are a major incentive to brave the fearsome prospect of talking to the opposite sex. Yes, a girl asked Collin. But he *wanted* to be asked.

"It's quite fun for me these days because I'm really starting to *get it* about what attraction really is," Collin says. "I start to *notice* how the girls in my class look, and I start to *like* it."

And let's not forget how important puberty is to the pleasure of a little spin around the dance floor. When Collin had his first dance, "I was happy! I also—I don't know if this is too—often when I dance with a girl, I feel a . . . tingling feeling . . . in my crotch. Is that too private?"

Ah, yes, as love makes her careful play for the heart of a child, sex is with her every step of the way.

A final question for Collin, a mere two months after his first dance. When does he think he might start "going out" with someone he likes?

"I'm pretty sure about one thing," he says. "I'm not ready for that right now. I don't know when I will be. I guess I'll let time decide that."

And so it will. Quite possibly sooner than Collin thinks.

Going Out on a Limb

Having a boyfriend is O.K. when you're 13 and it's considered a normal thing. Adam, my boyfriend, was angry last night because some guys had said that they liked me, and he got really jealous of that, and some girls were saying that I was flirting back with them. And then Adam got mad at those girls because he thought that they were trying to break Adam and I up. Then one of his friends came up to me to tell me that he wanted to talk to me just to make sure I wasn't mad at Adam. But I thought that he was coming to tell me that Adam was going to dump me!

— *Monica, age thirteen,* New York Times Magazine

Fairly shortly after the gender divide tumbles, some middle schoolers will take a stab at going out. Now don't let us confuse you. There were "boyfriends" and "girlfriends" a few years ago. But as nine-year-old Coretta explains, "We just call it boyfriend and girlfriend. You don't go out. You just like them better." In middle school, however, boyfriends and girlfriends do "go out," although at this age the kids who are going out may seem to the unassisted adult eye to be going exactly nowhere. When it comes right down to it, there may be little more to going out in middle school than simply saying you are.

Most middle school kids just aren't up to sustaining romantic intimacy. And so all of the excitement about the opposite sex gets poured into thinking about going out, talking about going out, asking someone out, telling your friends you're going out, breaking up, and being jealous. The courtship can go on forever, but call yourself a couple and the thing evaporates. Fast.

Monica continues:

So I just like walked away from him, and then Adam thought I was mad at him. And then we finally got together and were dancing, and he just said he was never going to dump me and that he never thought of that, and that it was great going out with me, and I like agreed. And everything was great then.

Well, sometimes these connections do last a bit, say for a few months. When they do, such pairings become group property. They stir endless, heated discussions at school, and everyone gets into the mix. A few years from now, when two teens get romantically involved, they will pull away from their friends into a secret intimacy, but for now these liaisons are conducted out in the open and rarely stray far from the central theme, "We're going out, aren't we?"

When a seventh grader talks about going out, the talk *is* the going out. But, oh, that talk.

"When I was thirteen and I was into this guy, Henry," Karenna, now fifteen, explains, "we had the deepest conversations on AOL, but the thought of talking to him in person made me nauseous. I practically only knew him by his screen name."

"The real relationship is online because everyone is scared of what the person is going to say," Karenna's friend Loren adds.

"And then you meet him," Karenna gasps, "and you think, God!"

What Karenna and Loren can tell you is that behind their elaborate flirting lies a deep fear about how the other sex will see them. When you're thirteen, there isn't much in the way of a self-image stockpile to fall back on. These teens' reactions feel like the answer to your daughter's insistent query, "Am I attractive?" And so getting a response from the first guy you have the nerve to ask out is something like being pulled from a cave in the forest where you have survived on tree bark and birds for forty-two years and having a mirror thrust up to your face for the very first time.

No wonder your teenager conducts her every interaction with boys solely through the medium of instant messages (IMs), where every reply can be carefully edited and where friends, opining from other corners of the screen, can secretly back her up. And no wonder your son strikes the elaborate pose of a "player" crowing about "one girl on the front burner and one girl on the back" to his older sister. Desperate times call for desperate measures.

Then somehow, amid this sea of self-conscious fakery and fear, someone gets up the guts to say something.

Karenna: "I knew Henry from school, but I only talked to him online. The phone takes more effort. It took me four months to call this guy. After four months of being in love with him, I thought I should finally tell him. So I called him, and I told him. And then I made an excuse to hang up as quick as I could."

How did it go?

"He didn't say anything the whole time on the phone. Then when I hung up, I found him online and we talked for five hours."

What happened then?

"Um, we sort of got interested in different people."

That, as they say, was that.

And if you think strolling through the streets of Paris with your love, dodging into Café Lipp for a *tarte tatin* as the clouds suddenly burst, and then walking hand in hand out into the cool night air is more exciting than this . . . then it's been too long since you were thirteen. This, gentle readers, is heady stuff.

The Real Thing

It depends on how you define it. If you mean I'm completely . . . I don't know. I've felt like I really, really . . . I don't know how I feel. I really, really like this person both in the way they—how do you put it? Mentally? How they act, their internal qualities, and their external qualities. I've felt that, definitely. I still haven't felt the kind of love that I hear makes people want to marry. You never know.

—*Jared, age twelve*

Amid all of the glitter makeup and the freaked-out e-mails, the panic about what to wear, and who likes whom, lies one revelation destined to make the whole horrible soap opera worth it: love.

Life Online

While your teenagers are making their first forays into the world of love online, you may find yourself wondering if the Internet is a safe place for them to be spending their time. When it comes to the Internet, parents tend to raise two main concerns. The first worry is that a child will be solicited by an adult online. The second is that a child will find his way to an explicit sexual site that they don't want him to see. Let's look at those two possibilities.

Online Solicitation and Abuse

Actually being seduced online to meet an adult for a sexual encounter happens, but it happens very rarely; more rarely, for example, than sexual abuse by a family member or date rape. A 1999–2000 survey of 1,501 Internet-using youth found that none had ever been sexually assaulted by someone who made contact with them over the Internet.

Being asked to have sex by a stranger, however, is common. Twenty percent of ten- to seventeen-year-olds in the study reported being solicited at least once. Kids who were older, who spent more time in chatrooms, and who talked to strangers online were all more likely to be solicited than others. Some of the kids felt quite disturbed by the event, especially the younger ones and those who received offline follow-ups, like phone calls from the solicitors.

Disappointingly, in this study none of the monitoring efforts that parents are often advised to use made a difference in a child's risk of being propositioned online. Keeping the computer in the open, using filters, checking the screen while teens are online, checking web histories when they are off, and asking kids what they do online all failed to reduce the likelihood of these solicitations. There isn't any information as to whether parents' monitoring and rules make those very rare offline meetings between a child and an offender who met online less likely.

But if you cannot prevent your child from being solicited, you can prepare your child for the experience. We don't suggest you discourage your child from entering chatrooms. They can be a great source of fun, support, and information. But make sure your child understands that a person who tells her he's fifteen may actually be a fifty-year-old who says what kids like to hear in order to entice them. Warn your children that at some point they may get an IM from a stranger asking them to meet for sex or even just to talk. Tell them they will be safe as long as they don't respond and don't give out any identifying information, like their address or phone number. Tell them to block the IMs from that sender, and then always to tell you what happened.

Encouraging your child to confine his chatting to one of the few kids-only sites (such as KidFu) monitored by chat jockeys may also help protect him.

Soliciting a minor online is illegal. You can report the incident to the police or online at www.cybertipline.com, a service of the National Center for Missing and Exploited Children, which forwards reports of solicitation to law enforcement agencies.

Explicit Sites and Filters

If your child has access to the Internet and a shred of curiosity about sex, sooner or later he will find his way to a porn site.

As you probably know, if you want to prevent this, you can get a filter. Filters come built in to the most popular Internet service providers and need only to be switched on to start screening out sex-related material. They can also be purchased separately and installed. Most work by denying access to websites that contain certain key words, like *sex*.

The problem with filters is that they are notoriously over-inclusive. A filter will largely block your child's ability to access porn, but it will also prevent him from getting into some valuable sites as well. The Declaration of Independence and *The Adventures of Sherlock Holmes* were both blocked by a filter used by some public schools. And even the cleverest filters will make it impossible for your teenager to get genuinely helpful information about sex on the Web (let alone about breast cancer).

Importantly, the children most likely to lie about their age to view a porn site—boys ages fifteen to seventeen (about one in four of whom do this)—are the very kids most likely to also use the Web to learn about sex and other sensitive topics that they feel uncomfortable discussing with parents (about one in four of them do this, too). So if you block pornography, you will block their online learning about abstinence, safer sex, and a lot of other health issues—not an optimal trade-off.

One way or another, many kids seem to happen upon the occasional porn site—if not at your home, then at the neighbor's. Rather than trying to protect your child from material and ideas he is bound to come across, consider pouring your energy into helping make him a critical consumer of such material. This means keeping an eye on his surfing (and TV watching, and moviegoing, and music listening) and inviting him to discuss with you what it all means. Ask him how realistic he finds the depiction of women on a particular site. Tell him what you think and why. If you are opposed to these sites, explain why, and make an argument for his avoiding them if you feel he should. If you feel it's fine for him to go to them, you might want to make sure he understands the difference between fantasy and reality. (We'll say more about pornography in Chapter 10.)

Will you know if he is following your advice? You may be aware that you can enter the history of your child's browser and find the names of the most recent sites he has viewed (unless he's deleted them). Checking the browser history has a lot in common with reading your child's diary: both are seductive shortcuts around building a functional connection with your kid, and both can render the privacy of the medium, one of its main assets for encouraging discovery, moot. If you decide to check the browser history, tell him when you first get the computer so that he's been duly warned. But why not fulfill your curiosity about your child's online habits the hard but direct way—ask him what he's doing.

Finally, consider eleven-year-old Barry's instructive story about browser histories.

"Last year my friend Julian and I were on the Web on his dad's computer. We accidentally went to—on Internet Explorer, you know the dance sites, where the hamster is dancing? We were looking for one of those sites. It turned out we got a porn site. We got scared his dad would find out, so we went into the history to try to delete it. It turned out there were tons more. Tons and tons of porn sites! We weren't sure how they had got there. We ran away really fast."

As the saying goes, oh history checkers, live by the sword, die by the sword.

All kids feel love. It may not have escaped your attention, for example, that your kids loved you long before they were capable of typing a comprehensible IM. But sooner or later a new kind of love—romantic love—is going to arrive on the scene, and as it does your family life will take another turn.

When will this be?

Well, romantic love is a little like middle age. It's impossible to say precisely when it starts, but at some point you know you're in it.

An odd thing happens if you ask kids when they first fell in love. Eighth graders will tell you they were about ten when love struck, tenth graders say they were twelve, and twelfth graders say they were fourteen. What's going on? Have these kids simply forgotten how they felt when they were younger? The likely answer is that children experience a junior version of grown-up romantic love at very young ages. As they get older, their feelings grow progressively more powerful and complex, making the love they felt a few years before look to them like child's play.

"I went out with Alyssa for three months in the eighth grade. Then she broke up with me," Josh, now sixteen, recalls. "I was upset, but it wasn't a tragedy. I wasn't really ready for it. I thought having a girlfriend looked cool, and it sounded good. I never really thought about the possibilities."

From his perspective as a teenager who now considers himself truly in love (with Alyssa, it turns out), Josh feels certain that what happened between them a few years earlier was merely a pale imitation of the real thing.

"I knew that she liked me, and I never had a girlfriend before, so I thought I'd try it. A few of my friends had just started getting into girls. They thought it was pretty cool. We didn't have such strong feelings. No sexual feelings yet. We kissed a couple of times maybe. It was like we were just bragging for our friends."

A year after their breakup, Josh and Alyssa, who had met at camp, found themselves in the same high school. They started hanging out together, usually with other friends. Alyssa was dating other boys, and gradually Josh became her confidant.

"The whole time we were getting closer and closer as friends. I started to get feelings for her. I was more mature. Now I knew I was feeling for girls. I grew up. There was a lot of talk now about girls. I just felt—I don't know—I just started changing mentally and physically. I just became interested in girls."

And so, eight months ago, they started going out.

How is it?

"Unbelievable, amazing. It just seems like it's never going to end.

It's been a long time, but we just keep feeling more and more for each other. Now we've gotten to the point where we're just best friends. I don't hang out with my other guy friends very much anymore. I spend most of my time with her.

"It's just great in every aspect."

Sounds Like Love

As you may recall, falling in love in the teenage years is sort of like being shot out of a cannon and landing in Oompa-Loompa Land. The intense emotional states that are unleashed upon the tender adolescent mind are so powerful as to temporarily bend his perceptions of the world ("Oh, my God, that song is about *us!*") and melt the structure of his reasoning ("She's *perfect* for me!"). Don't ask this kid to baby-sit.

His chief preoccupation now will be the stadium show his limbic system is putting on. It's the struggle to simply withstand this whirlwind of emotion that drives teenagers to close themselves in their room listening to dreamy or raucous music that matches their mood states, to write the name of their loved one all over the cover of their calculus notebook, and to talk-talk-talk about their feelings, although not necessarily to you.

Tanisha recently got to watch her teenage nephew fall in love for the first time. The whole thing lasted only a month, but oh, what a month it was! "He would come by, wearing one of those unmistakable goofy grins and actually say things like 'My heart feels so big!' and 'It's almost like I'm floating!' "

Ah, the glow of young love. It really is breathtaking to watch someone go through this. "But even as I was moved by his bliss, I had the distinct impression that he wasn't quite aware I was there in the room with him, even while he was talking to me."

Which brings up a funny thing about love. Unlike the wildly inclusive dating life of the thirteen-year-old, true romantic love admits two. Love might seem to be all about building attachments—and from his and his new girlfriend's perspective, of course, it is—but love also separates. Every time your kid falls in love with someone, he falls a little out of love with someone else. Just as—you may have noticed—starting a new relationship is sometimes the best way to get over your ex.

But if this is your kid's very first girlfriend, who exactly is he leaving behind to love her?

Dare we say it?

Midlife on the Rue de Rivoli

Julie worried for a few years that her daughter, Beth, wasn't finding her way into the dating world of her friends. "I really wanted her to start to have love in her life," Julie explains, but Beth showed no signs of interest. What was wrong? Had she been too intrusive and spooked her daughter about intimacy? Was Beth gay but unable to deal with it? Julie toured all the popular penitential sites visited by guilt-ridden parents, until in Beth's freshman year of college, she got a boyfriend.

"And a pretty good one!"

Delighted, Julie and her husband Patrick drove up to visit their daughter and meet Lars, the new boy. They spent a happy afternoon together. Everything went perfectly, and as Patrick drove the two of them back home, a contented Julie fell asleep and dreamed the following dream:

"The entire world has been destroyed by a nuclear holocaust. There is no longer any rule of law. The men are all going to rape the women. At first, I'm afraid that I'm going to be raped, and then I realize the men are going to rape my daughters. I decide that the only way I can protect my two girls is to kill both of them."

Okay, so maybe the visit wasn't *perfect*.

Julie's dream, a vivid example of the standard-issue blood-and-guts images that percolate through the healthy human unconscious, is a lot less unusual than her ability to talk about it openly. "It is clear that I felt enraged at the idea that she had a boyfriend," Julie says, "and I wanted to kill her."

Julie is not alone. Many parents find their child's fresh discovery of love surprisingly disquieting. Surprising, because you're supposed to want your child to be happy; and if there are roads to happiness, surely one of the major ones passes through love. And disquieting, because however wonderful it may be for your child, this step she is taking can throw a glaring spotlight on what life has been doing to you.

You're used to watching your child grow through the loving eyes of a parent, but let her run to grab the phone and turn away, cooing a soft hello into the receiver, and you may find yourself seeing her through your old adolescent lenses. Your past flies back, bringing with it a sweet nostalgia for what was beautiful then and, perhaps, an ache of regret over what pleasures you may have missed.

"The thing about kids is that they are so powerfully evocative," sighs Morgan, who brought his seventh-grade son, Max, to a party much like the one that started this chapter. "I had had a very negative reaction to the dance. 'You don't have to stay here,' I kept saying. 'Just call if you want to come home.' Knowing Max, I thought he would be terribly uncomfortable there."

But he wasn't. In fact, he triumphed.

"I realized then," Morgan says, "that what I took to be my attempt to protect Max had everything to do with the anxiety I had as a kid, feeling that I didn't fit in—that I was a nerd. Without realizing it, I was dealing with my own adolescent shame and the very confused sense I had then of my sexuality. Once I figured that out, I was able to get out of Max's way."

But not, it should be said, without a pang.

"You see, seventh grade was a memorable time for me because we lived in Paris that year. And as I look at the girls at these dances, the girls in Max's class, I suddenly remember the seventh-grade girls in Paris in 1959. As if it were yesterday! I remember the sense of their bodies. These kids have these budding bodies. It's just extremely evocative for me."

Ah, Paris. The city of (longed-for) love. Remember that Doisneau photograph of the two young lovers, absorbed in each other, kissing in the midst of a black-and-white sea of Parisians? You see this photo in your teens and you wonder, "Will that ever be me?" See it in your twenties, and you think, "That's us!" But see it as your thirties turn into your forties and you notice, as the writer Adam Gopnik does in *Paris to the*

Moon, a memoir of his years in Paris, that the couple is standing outside the BHV, the frenetic French department store. "Anyone who has spent time at the BHV," Gopnick observes, "knows that they are kissing not from an onset of passion but in gratitude from having gotten out again."

This, dear friends, is what middle age can do to you. You see two ecstatic lovers, and you think they're excited because they got a good toaster.

Thank goodness irony doesn't shrink with age, for a wry observation about young love may provide the only safe distance from which to watch it. Let yourself get a little closer, and you risk the tug of recollecting the joys of youth and the pointed recognition of how life has changed.

But what if the Doisneau lovers are giggling in your very own living room—nightly? Will your powers of irony be overwhelmed? Will the sharp recognition that you may never again experience the heady infatuations that once filled your youthful days pierce your toughened hide? What then?

You have heard the cliché that adolescence is hell for parents. You may have thought that this was because children, once they hit puberty, morph into monstrous beings. This is only partly true.

There exists a secret reason for the stress of raising an adolescent, one far more stealthy and invidious than the teen-as-tormentor explanation, one that may nibble away at your psyche for years or may sandbag you one evening with a sudden thudding realization as you peer into the bathroom mirror. Your child's adolescence may gall you, because through a cruel trick of nature, it has happened to arrive at the precise moment you stumble into midlife.

Now, your midlife may be a boon. Your love—and your sex—with your mate may be getting richer with each passing year. Or, if you're divorced, you may fall in love again, only deeper and better this time. Your home life may be great. Or your career may take off, and with it so may your sense of optimism about the future. If so, your fulfillment in life may make your adolescent's blossoming feel like a gorgeous gift, or an opportunity to share in a new adventure together.

But if entering these years feels, as author Helen Simpson puts it in *Getting a Life,* as though middle age has come and "sat down on you with its enormous bum," then you may have a harder time.

Oh, look! Your child's body is becoming beautifully mature. Her mind is sharper (sharp enough to judge your shortcomings). Her future seems bursting with promise, and love and romance are suddenly, brilliantly, there for her.

Then you catch your reflection in a shop window and are startled by the difference between the way you actually look and the way you think of yourself. You're not seventeen anymore. Neither is your husband.

And there's your teenager again, nervous and uncertain but suddenly, irresistibly entitled to everything in life, everything she wants.

"What makes you think you can go out again tonight?"

"I don't think you're listening to me, miss!"

"Yes, I know it's unfair, but guess what, life is unfair!"

No wonder parents fight with their teenagers. Just as your children discover the wonderful possibilities of life, you may be coming up against its limits. Of course, it's also one of the great satisfactions of having children to know that life goes on, youth goes on, even as you age. And that satisfaction may well win out. But the collision of adolescence and middle age is the painful moment when the rubber hits the road— the moment in which you are asked to surrender some of your own hopes and place them now in your children.

And Then They Dump You

**Speak low
When you speak, love,
Our summer day
Withers away too soon, too soon.**

—*Ogden Nash and Kurt Weill*

"It started a year ago with my fourteen-year-old," Gerry says of her oldest daughter. "First she picked on a few little things. The way I wear my hair. The fact that I don't wear makeup. Recently, I've noticed if we're out together and I laugh, she cringes. Her dad is dumb. Our jeans are wrong. We talk with our mouths full. 'You two are so gross!'

"It hurt," Gerry says, "because she was once so adoring."

Losing the adoration you once enjoyed is one more poke in the ribs for you to feel as your adolescent reaches for her first romance—that is, her first romance outside the family. It can't be helped.

Children build their selves and their loves out of idealizations. In their first several years of life they idealize you, their parent, endowing you with unparalleled talents. The more wonderful you are, the more secure they feel in their own worth. After all, they belong to you. Being the object of this idealization is one of the great perks of parenthood, but if your children are going to be able to leave you for another love, you'll have to come down off that pedestal. And so the picking begins. As one mother responding to a parenting survey put it, postidealization life with adolescents can feel something like "being bitten to death by ducks."

Of course, your child still needs to maintain her self-esteem by connecting to the greats, but now her friends, or her favorite celebrities, become the stars in her life. She dresses and talks like them. She wants to be seen with them, not with you. And then she finds a person to idealize and not simply to imitate but rather to join forces with fully. She finds her first love.

As we said before, when your child falls in love with one person, she falls out of love with someone else. The first time, that someone else is you. (At least, that's how it may feel.) Like any breakup, this takes some getting over. Especially if you never anticipated having to contend with being dumped by your kid for a college freshman.

"After that weekend with Beth and Lars, I went through a period of feeling depressed that she loved someone more than me, and I thought, this is really weird and sick," Julie says. "I really felt like I was losing her. Then I talked to a number of other mothers, and they said the same thing. They said, 'Oh, this is my big secret I never told anyone.' "

Julie adapted. "I figured out with the new boyfriend you need to shift into mother-in-law mode, which is to extend the attachment you have to your daughter to include him. Lars was very solicitous of my comfort on a hike we all took recently. I thought, okay, just go with this now. This is new."

And so it goes. A few years ago you were starring in a Disney cartoon of your little one's invention. You were Snow White, singing gaily as you hung the laundry, surrounded by your band of devoted dwarfs.

Now you're humming a different tune. The chirpy little birds and bunnies are gone. The enchanted forest has been replaced by an ordinary living room, and you're no longer a dewy cartoon princess. You're a middle-aged woman, sitting on the couch, reading the paper, and waiting for her daughter to come home from a night out with her friends. Suddenly she bounds in the front door, gives a distracted "Hi," and disappears into her room.

So your daughter thinks you chew like a moron, you muse. So what! That's what teenagers are supposed to think. So she doesn't want to climb into your lap anymore. You've been through worse breakups before. You toss the paper aside, grab a CD, and skip to a song in a minor key. You start to sing along, full voice.

Love is a spark
Lost in the dark
Too soon, too soon . . .

Speak Low

Or you might try talking to your kid.

Now, talking with your teenager about her new love is a delicate business, something like tiptoeing through a spring garden of seedlings in a pair of army boots: every step an opportunity to screw up. Your child is embarrassed by the tender feelings she has invested in her new love, and so she may avoid discussing them with you. She may shut you down if you try, and she may react with anger or irritation if she's cornered. It's all too sensitive.

But despite their touchiness, adolescents often describe these conversations with their parents as helpful and important. Fifteen-year-old

Leslie, for example, has advice for parents everywhere: "Keep communication lines open no matter what." She explains, "As a kid, you want
to know that you can talk to your parents whatever happens. If you don't
have your parents there, you'll feel really alone."

Gerry holds on to this notion, despite her daughter's picking. "I was
telling her the other day what I think she should look for in a guy. That
attractiveness isn't the main thing."

Does it mean something to her when you say that?

"It means a lot to her. I can tell she's listening, although at fourteen,
you have to pretend everything your mother says is stupid. I just ignore the
looks and the rolling eyes and blab away. I can tell when it's registering."

It can be a struggle for your teenager to make use of your advice. On
the one hand, as Leslie says, she needs your support. On the other hand,
she needs to differentiate from you, which means deciding that you don't
have all the answers, that she and her friends can reason these things out
better than you can. So while you present your point of view, she may try
to appear like she isn't listening, and sometimes she won't be.

As a parent of an adolescent, you will have your wisdom sneered at.
You may even have the value of your love challenged by a teenager struggling to grow into someone separate from you. It is your job quietly to
hold in mind the fact that your child needs you and that you will always
be important to her. You are the guardian of this relationship, and if she
needs to give it a kick, she also needs you to hold onto it and protect it,
so that next week, when she wants to be your little girl again, it will be
there for her.

The Rules of Love

Even if your teenager decides never to open up about his secret loves,
you may feel the need to discuss at least a few things. Some decisions
have to be made, like what time does he have to come home at night? Is
it okay if he and his girlfriend hang out alone at her house? What if his
grades slip, or his new love takes time away from family responsibilities?
And what if you think the girl he's seeing isn't good for him?

These are the parameters of adolescent love, and sooner or later you'll

Keeping an Eye Out for Sexual Harassment

> *You get dressed up in the morning. Then, a lot of times, you will walk down the hallway and some guy will say rude things that make you feel bad. They're trying to make their friends think you might get together with them, or something. It's upsetting, because you don't want that kind of attention.*
>
> —*Danielle, age sixteen*

Sexual harassment by kids these days ranges from writing pornographic claims about a student on the bathroom wall (or on the twenty-first-century equivalent of the bathroom wall—a website) to aggressive ogling and name-calling, to following, grabbing, and pinching. It's not as uncommon as you would wish. Most teenagers—boys and girls alike—have had some experience of sexual harassment. Girls seem to get it more than boys, and they seem to be more negatively affected by it.

Your child's school is legally bound to take complaints of sexual harassment seriously and to offer protection to your child if she needs it. But you probably don't want to wait for your school to figure out something is wrong.

Once puberty begins (or even earlier), you can ask your child every now and then if anyone is teasing her at school. Only a tiny minority of kids who are harassed at school spontaneously tell their parents, so ask if kids comment on her body or what she wears. If she's too embarrassed to answer honestly, then at least she'll get a signal from you that it's not acceptable behavior. If she answers yes, talk to her about it. If the flak she is getting is relatively mild or infrequent, help her decide what she wants to do. She can choose to ignore it and hope that, unreinforced, the harassment will stop. She might want to confront the kids, or let you give the school that responsibility.

If the abuse is persistent, especially if it is physical or frightening (your child should not have to put up with being afraid to walk to her locker), meet with the school principal. Ask for a plan of action to stop the harassment. At the least, the school should investigate your daughter's complaint, discipline the boys if it's true, inform their parents, and separate the children where possible.

have to decide how to set them. Now, by the time your oldest gets to middle school, you've been making rules for your kids for over a decade. You know what it takes to get them to do their homework, eat like a person, or stop torturing the dog—in short, to live up to the reasonable expectations of a civilized child. You have probably become so accomplished at this over the last few years that you may be tempted to rely on your time-tested strategies to resolve the dilemmas of early adolescence.

Don't do it.

Consider Claire, who discovered that her fourteen-year-old son wanted to go out with a high school senior and decided to forbid it. Outrageous shouting matches ensued in which Daniel would cry that Claire had no right to interfere, and Claire would insist that she was the mother, this was her house, and he would do as she said. By this time, Daniel, who was quite obviously no longer a boy, had grown a head taller than his mother. Claire, accordingly, required that during their arguments, they both sit down because "I don't like him being taller than me." The whole thing went, very directly, to hell.

Claire and Daniel's struggle is typical of the battles that commonly spring up at the threshold to adolescence. These skirmishes share a single, easily understood but not always easily avoided cause. Simply put, children enter their teen years filled with expectations for greater control over their lives before their parents are ready to agree that childhood is over. While young teens are hungering for the freedom they believe they deserve, their parents are typically still oriented toward protecting their kids and organizing their lives.

Angry spats and near-daily struggles for control can result, peaking early in middle school before parents have accepted the need to change, simmering down somewhat in high school, and then subsiding after graduation when mothers and fathers finally hand over the reins—or find them yanked from their desperately clutching fingers. The timetable may vary for your child, but you can spare yourself a good deal of tension by repeatedly adapting your parenting strategies to suit his (and your) needs as adolescence unfolds.

The Authoritative Style

You may recall that in Chapter 2 we introduced the notion of authoritative parenting, a style of relating to your children that combines high demands for good behavior with a warm responsiveness to your children's needs. Compared to other kids, the children of authoritative parents, we explained then, have higher self-esteem, less depression and anxiety, and safer habits; they are more mature and self-reliant; and they even get better grades.

The authoritative style appears to be a useful tool for raising children of all ages, but we're reminding you of it here because when your kids reach adolescence, two of its tenets may prove particularly useful if you want to negotiate the rules of love with your teenager.

Firstly, authoritative parents are known for nourishing their child's development of an independent point of view. True, they lay down the law, but they do it in a particular way. They share the reasons behind their decisions, explaining their logic and appealing to their child's rational side. The technical term for this practice is *induction*.

Secondly, authoritative parents also infuse household discussions with a spirit of *democracy*. When a decision has to be made, they ask their kids' opinion. If the children disagree and have a good point, authoritative parents may modify their rules. But if they don't, they make it clear that they respect their kids' perspective and then explain why they're taking a different approach.

Induction and democracy promote your children's moral development and general mental health. And they strengthen your influence over them when the teen years arrive.

When your kids are little and they see you as their guru, endowed with limitless knowledge, you can say a second dessert is bad for them and they will believe you (okay, they might sneak one anyway, but they'll still believe you). But adolescents are different. They've figured out that you're fallible, and so they want proof that your point of view is right. Because he can now reason abstractly, your sixteen-year-old will wonder whether it is fair that you have any power over his personal choices, like what to wear or how to keep his room. From his new perspective, if you explain a rule with "Because I say so," he'll assume you can't justify your opinion, and he'll oppose you.

Parents who rely on power plays to keep an upper hand at home have been found to reduce their teenager's belief in the legitimacy of their authority. Alternatively, parents who loosen control over their children's decisions in adolescence actually appear to influence their choices more than parents who clamp down. When it comes to adolescents, you have to give power to get it.

With these principles in mind, let's consider how to manage some of the dilemmas your teenager's dating life may pose.

When Love Is Blind

Let's say you don't like the boy your daughter has chosen as her new love. Unfortunately, should you find yourself in this position, there is very little for you to do. Although it can be hard on you and on her, romance is an area where (within certain limits) you should let your child make her own mistakes.

Pitting your child's loyalty to you against her attachment to a new love is a famously losing proposition. The forbidden boyfriend becomes more alluring. She clings to him and withdraws from you, isolating herself with the boy you don't like and making a bad situation worse. Should you succeed in keeping her from her new love, the price may be the loss of her sense of autonomy and of an opportunity to develop her understanding of how to find what she really wants in a relationship.

The risks of forbidding a relationship are serious enough that you should reserve this approach for those occasions when you believe the boy is putting your child in danger—say if he is known to be violent, or to drink and drive.

In less-risky situations, where the boyfriend is not actually dangerous but still more than an annoyance, you might consider telling your child about your objections while giving her the right to stay with him if she likes.

For all other unfortunate boyfriend choices, we recommend supporting your child and quietly praying it will end. This strategy needn't be entirely passive. Stay closely connected to your kid, resisting the impulse to withdraw in frustration. Keep tabs on her schedule, and involve yourself when possible, inviting the two of them to join in family activities. Make sure that she has at least one warm, nurturing, and creative relationship in her life—the one she has with you.

Then wait. And console yourself with this thought: The relationship probably won't last long. The average life span of a fifteen-year-old's love affair is three to four months.

When Love Trumps Homework

Kyle's been with his girlfriend for about three months. I think she's fine, but he worries me. He is not the kid he used to be. Before he started seeing Nora he lived for the track team. He was incredibly diligent about practices. Now he's skipping them. All he seems to want to do is talk to his girlfriend, which he does all day and all night. It worries me that he doesn't care about the things that used to matter to him.

—*Karen, on her seventeen-year-old son*

You may find that you like the kid your son is dating, but that you don't like what the dating is doing to him. It's troubling when your child sheds some of the duties he has so responsibly fulfilled for years in the pursuit of love. Yet, important as it is to maintain high standards for his behavior, even at his most infatuated, now is also a time for you to modify your expectations. Washing the car is great, but learning to love is important, too.

If your son is neglecting important activities and relationships, ask him to talk with you about what matters most to him these days. How does he see his new relationship fitting in with his male friends, the soccer team, and so on? Go over the responsibilities that he has neglected, and try to decide together which ones can't be missed.

Then make a plan together to address them. He should not be getting a D in math, for example, so ask him to decide how he might pull up his grade, perhaps by going out less often. You can also look for ways to lessen his burdens and make room for the new relationship, say by getting someone else to rake the leaves, or letting him out of Friday night family dinners. These days, love and math may be better uses of his time.

When They Want to Stay Out Late

Once your children start spending their evenings out with friends, you should give them a curfew. Remember monitoring, the practice of keeping track of your kids? As we explained in Chapter 2, children whose parents make a habit of knowing where they are, whom they are with, and when they are coming home drink less alcohol, are less likely to smoke, get better grades, and have fewer disciplinary problems at school. They also wait until they are older to have sex than kids who are less carefully tracked. For the fifteen to eighteen set, curfews are the indispensable handmaidens of monitoring.

How you maintain and negotiate your curfew matters a good deal more than the specific time you choose. Curfew times range widely, from before 9 P.M. to after 2 A.M., and tend to vary not only with a child's age but also with the norms of the community. Setting your teens' curfew time is a good opportunity for democratic collaboration at home. Invite your kids to help work out a reasonable deadline for school nights out, and perhaps a later one for weekends. Then decide together how the curfew will be enforced (avoid excessively punitive responses to a missed curfew).

The nightly enforcement of curfews calls for some flexibility. Renegotiating times for special nights, and making a provision for your teen to phone you should he run late, make for harmony at home.

When They Want to Be Alone

"Becca asked us the other day if the boy she likes could come by the house after school. We're not home then," Lynn says. Lynn and Orlando, who both get home late from work, wondered what it was that Becca, at fifteen, wanted from a few hours of privacy with her boyfriend.

Would she feel safer spending time with him on her home turf?

Did she want to play house to try to see if he's the kind of boy she wants?

Was she asking permission to fool around?

"We said, 'No, it's fine if he's here when we are. But he shouldn't be alone with you in the house.' "

"Becca raised an eyebrow. 'What do you think I'm going to do? Have sex?'

"I said, 'I don't think so. But it's a matter of what's appropriate for your age.' "

When your child starts asking to spend time alone with her love, you may wonder what *is* appropriate for her age. Should a teenager be given unchaperoned time during which he or she will have not only an opportunity but also, perhaps, tacit permission (she knows you know what it means to be alone together) to fool around?

As you ponder how much privacy to offer your child, remember that monitoring sometimes bites back. While sensible monitoring is associated with delayed first intercourse, excessive monitoring may spark some rebellion. Rebelling against your parents is probably not the best reason to have sex.

So, what's excessive?

As we explained in Chapter 2, this will have to be an area of experimentation for you. The best you can do is to give your child a voice in negotiating the degree of her privacy, stay attuned to her reactions to your supervision, and pull back when you find your watchfulness becomes too intrusive.

"I think Becca is entitled to a zone of privacy and experimentation," Lynn says. "I don't know how I've communicated that I think it's okay for her to make out with her boyfriend but not to have sexual intercourse with him, but I'm sure she knows."

How does she know?

"Hmm. She knows I wouldn't let him come over when I'm not around. Isn't that code for you're not supposed to have intercourse? Maybe I don't know what she's thinking about this stuff."

Maybe She Doesn't, Either

Behind the raised eyebrow, the cool stare, and the weary retort, your child is no less perplexed by this forest of fears and temptations than you are. Invite a few teens to talk about love and they'll start asking questions. Or not asking, really, but revealing, as if they have just turned up the volume on the track that's playing in their heads.

Listen as they muse: "Do I like him?" "Is it love?" "What should we do?" The deeper their explorations of the world of love, the more their wondering circles back to one specific destination, the next big question facing your teenager.

José, age twelve: "You don't know what's 'right' and what's 'wrong.' Like, for example, when is it appropriate to start doing things? What are sexually appropriate things to do or even think? Especially involving intercourse. Like, I'll often think of the question, am I allowed to want to have intercourse?"

Bennie, age thirteen: "I don't think I feel ready definitely. But I'm starting to think about it. Do I want it? It does click in me that animal feeling, but when I think of what it would involve—what it really means and what I'd actually be *doing*—I feel like I'm definitely not ready for such stuff and I don't think I will be for about five years."

Wendy, age fifteen: "I hate the feeling of having to blow-dry your hair and dress up. It's like who can be more skinny or pretty. No one can win that competition. I'm like, don't look at me like I'm supposed to be that person. But then I end up doing that anyway. It's disappointing, because you want to have the real, caring relationship. But I think the guys might only see you if you're wearing the tight jeans and blow-dried hair. If I put myself out in the blow-dried way, how can I get anything that's more than a hookup?"

Nell, age fifteen: "There was a guy I thought was really hot, but he had a girlfriend. They were in the middle of a fight and me and my boyfriend were in the middle of a fight, so my friends decided to fix me up with him. On New Year's Eve, we invited him to the party, and when the ball dropped, we kissed. I wasn't sure if I was doing it because I wanted to make my boyfriend jealous. Or was it because he was really hot? His girlfriend was giving me dirty looks. We didn't know a lot about each other. So I didn't know what his motivations were. I don't know why I was into it. I know. Because he was really hot."

Giorgio, age fifteen: "My main worry was, am I going to be upset afterward? Will I regret it? Then, am I doing the right thing? Will I hurt her?"

Lily, age fifteen: "You're only in tenth grade. If he likes you and you like him, it's okay. You're not having sex. It's just kissing. So as long as it's fun, it's okay."

Marlon, age sixteen: "I don't think I'll have sex until I'm married. I can't say anything for sure, but that's my plan."

Alyssa, age sixteen: "I'm probably the most honest with Josh of anyone ever. We went to camp together. We were practically living together that summer. We learned so much about each other. If we could do that together, we can do anything."

Josh, age sixteen: "At first it seemed as if sex was going to be a very big step. Now I don't know. We just feel that we're so close that there's nothing left that we have to prove to each other. We are totally open with each other. I've only kissed one other girl before."

What does sex mean, and how does it relate to love? Should we do it?

These are the questions that begin to stir just under the surface as soon as love and dating start. Most teenagers will answer them before they graduate from high school. Hopefully, your wisdom and your warmth will inform your child's answer. The chapter that follows will help you plan an approach to this next challenge. But at least now you understand—as best it can be understood—the heart that is beating beneath it.

There is your child's heart, bravely straying from you and attaching itself to a kid he's fashioned as ideal, because ideal is what he needs in order to leave the best love he's ever had and find a new one of his own.

And there is your heart, startled and sore. How did he get so tall? it's asking. Why don't we play together like we used to? Has he forgotten?

Where has the time gone?

One Touch of Venus

I feel
Wherever I go
That tomorrow is near,
Tomorrow is here,
And always too soon.

—*Ogden Nash and Kurt Weill*

Such is the state of the union between parent and child at adolescence.

There your child is, discovering love for the first time, and here you are, considering where love has led you. You have some wisdom about relationships, while your daughter is a complete novice. Yet here you stand, uncertain how to tell her what she needs to know; and there she goes, determined to act as if she knows it already, and convinced she'll never make the same mistakes and compromises you've made.

Nash and Weill wrote "Speak Low," the song that has been playing in the background of this chapter, for the musical *One Touch of Venus*. The comedy concerns a marble statue of Venus that comes to life one day to experience true love for the very first time. After some exciting flirtation, the story goes, Venus gets a glimpse of suburban married life in all its seeming ordinariness, is appalled, and flies back to Mount Olympus decidedly unattached.

When we hear this story, we can't help but think of all of the teenagers peering with embarrassment at their middle-aged parents, convinced that when they experience love for the first time, it will be a different relationship altogether. One that doesn't involve the imperfections of old dishwashers, bald spots, and chewing. A pristine love.

How can a parent with an ordinary human relationship not feel a little oafish around such sparkling promise?

Lynn recalls one evening when, having resolved Becca's challenge for private time with her latest crush, she and her husband were in the kitchen cleaning up. Lynn was finishing up the dishes while Orlando stood in the door begging the dog to poop. Becca sat at the kitchen table finishing her homework while the radio played, a little loud for that time of night, tuned by Becca to one of her stations. An old disco song came on.

"Orlando headed for the radio dial, and Becca said, 'Dad, wait!' She didn't want him to turn it off.

"Orlando cranked the volume. I looked up as he took a stack of plates from my hands.

" 'C'mon, babe. Let's dance,' " he said. And the two of us hit the floor.

"Becca gave us a look. 'Ew, Mom. Dad is such a jerk. How can you stand it?'

"We kept dancing. 'He's not a jerk,' I said. 'I bet if your boyfriend was doing this you wouldn't think it was jerky. In fact, you'd probably think it was pretty cool.'

" 'Mo-om!' "

Lynn and Orlando spun around the kitchen a little more, chuckling, until Orlando sent Lynn into a final dip, and then lifted her back for one gentle kiss. Becca blushed.

Becca's not there yet, we might have told Lynn. But she will be. With her parents' love, guidance, and a little patience, she'll be back down from Mount Olympus some day soon.

In the meantime, what's an everyday, fallible, middle-aged parent to do but dance?

Chapter **8**

Ready or not

You're helping your daughter pack as she heads off for a summer at drama camp. You hated her being away last summer, and you already anticipate missing her. Why is it that all your friends seem to love sending their kids away?

"Do you think I should take my red sweater?" She reminds you she's still here. "I'm afraid it will get dirty, but I really like it. You know, I've decided, I'm going to take it."

"Sounds good."

"I'm planning to try out for the big musical rather than do the costumes this year. What do you think?"

"Sounds good."

"I'm also going to work on my long-distance running."

"Sounds good."

"Oh, and I think Danny and I are going to have sex this summer."

Why is it that at this particular moment, "Sounds good" seems a little . . . thin?

This Is It

If there was one overriding anxiety that got you to pick this book up in the first place, we're going to guess it was probably this one: What do you do when your kid starts heading toward sex?

Should you try to stop her? Can you? Is there an age after which you should just let her make her own decision?

Of course, as you have no doubt gathered from reading the chapters before this one, managing your kid's decision to have sex or not doesn't simply come down to one moment in front of an open suitcase as she's packing for the summer. Years of discussions, experiences, admonishments, examples, and negotiations have paved the way to this one decision.

And who knows if this is really the first decision your kid has made about having sex? As we will explain in a moment, there is sex and then there is Sex. In your child's lexicon, the words *virginity* or *abstinence* may turn out to be rather fluid terms.

But for now, let's think about your daughter's situation, on the cusp of having sex or of declining it, the way most parents genuinely experience it—as a major life event, the details of which you may or may not hear but about which you definitely have an opinion.

And what might that opinion be?

What Do You Want?

As we mentioned at the beginning of this book, one of the quintessential expressions of the quandary so many parents face came to us from a father who asked, "How can I teach my daughter to have a healthy attitude toward sex, but prevent her from having any?"

Maybe you have a sense of where this guy was coming from.

Adele feels pretty strongly about the issue. "I wouldn't want my daughter to be a virgin when she gets married. I think bad things happen; people get married because of intense sexual pressure without really understanding each other and knowing whether they're right for each other. She should know that she's compatible with the guy she marries. The very thought of her marrying a man she hasn't slept with . . . it's inconceivable. It upsets me."

Garth, whose daughter is sixteen, has a similar attitude. "I don't think we should make so much of a big deal out of virginity. It puts too much pressure on it. It's part of development, and it'll happen when it happens."

Others are ambivalent. Carl and Betty, when faced with the advance warning that their fifteen-year-old might soon have sex with her boyfriend, wanted to support sex as a wonderful experience but just couldn't believe she was ready.

"Why did we not want her to have sex?" Betty asks. "Because it's a big move. It's a big change. I wanted her to be free from that kind of emotional challenge until she had more experience under her belt."

Which raises the question, how do you know when your daughter is ready for intercourse?

"Next year," Carl answers with a grin. "That's the permanent answer. No matter when she asks, she'll be ready next year."

For many, the answer is even more straightforward: no sex until marriage.

Shauna knows what she wants for her daughter. "I don't want her to have sex until she's married, period." When did Shauna first have sex? "On my prom night in high school, but I don't want her to make the same mistake I made. I want her to wait."

So does Helga. "Yes, I want her to wait until her wedding night. I want her to experience sex for the first time with the Pacific beating against the shores of a Hawaiian island. Will I get that? Maybe not. But I at least want her to wait as long as possible."

Why might you hesitate to endorse your kid's first sexual adventure? Well, at the simplest level, you worry about pregnancy and STDs. You don't know if your child can handle the emotional fallout you remember so well from your early relationships. And you're not sure you like the guy.

Moral and religious issues may be very important to you.

Then there's the shadow that's been stalking you throughout the previous chapters: It's just uncomfortable to imagine your child as a sexual person. Or to accept that she's growing into adulthood.

And although you may have balked at them then, you may still have in mind the reasons that got pitched to you by your parents when you were first thinking of having sex. Ann explains: "When I was a kid in the early sixties, you would lose your reputation and become a fallen woman. My mother beat that into my head. I think once Cary moves into a sexual relationship with her boyfriend, she takes risks. You risk the friendship, and you have to deal with the reactions of others."

But Ann continues: "Raising my daughter has helped me become more realistic. I see myself having concerns that my parents had. But these worries really don't mean anything to her. Some of her friends have sex. Some don't. Reputations aren't an issue for them. It's a different world for her than it was for me."

Ah, yes, it's true.

It's a Very Different World

Some parents don't know quite how different.

A few studies have looked at parents' awareness of their own children's sexual activities, and the results are startling. When it comes to knowing that their kids have had intercourse, parents are not entirely clued in. In one study, when parents were asked if their fourteen- to seventeen-year-olds had had sexual intercourse, 34 percent said yes. When the adolescents themselves were asked, 58 percent had. Whoops.

Using 1999 numbers for the United States, 50 percent of high schoolers have had intercourse. Boys are a tad more likely to have sexual intercourse than girls—52 percent of boys and 48 percent of girls do. As you'd expect, these numbers vary by grade—from 39 percent of ninth graders to 65 percent of twelfth graders—so by the time they graduate from high school, nearly two-thirds of kids have had intercourse.

Some kids start especially young. Eight percent (12 percent of boys and 4 percent of girls) have intercourse for the first time before they reach the age of thirteen.

After high school, the percentages jump up even more. In a study of nineteen-year-old men who had never been married, 84 percent had had vaginal intercourse; in another study, 83 percent of twenty- to twenty-four-year-old never-married women had had intercourse.

In case you're thinking that the kids who have sex must all live in some other part of the country, the data show that kids are having sex everywhere. Among the states for which there are representative data, the one with the lowest percentage of high school students who have had intercourse was Hawaii at 41 percent. The highest was Mississippi, at 60 percent.

So, do things seem different from when you were a kid? If so, it's not surprising.

During the mid to late 1950s, 8 percent of girls had had intercourse by age sixteen. Twenty-eight percent of boys and girls in the 1950s had had sex by age eighteen, and 61 percent by age twenty (keep in mind that they married younger back then, so this wasn't all premarital sex). In the 1970s, fewer than 5 percent of fifteen-year-old girls and 20 percent of fifteen-year-old boys had had sexual intercourse. The percentage for high school students rose through the 1980s but started dropping during the 1990s.

We present these numbers as a reality check. Kids *are* having sex. And even those who wait until after high school are generally not waiting much longer. What's going on?

The Widening Gap

For one thing, the gap between sexual maturity and marriage has been growing.

There was a time when marriage followed fairly soon after sexual maturity. However, two trends have changed that. Historians tell us that the average age at which adolescents go through puberty has dropped about two years from a century ago, while the age of first marriage has increased by quite a few years since then. The result is that the wait between sexual maturation and marriage is much longer—longer than many seem to be willing to wait.

Why are people marrying later? Partly because industrialized societies require more formal education and thus a prolonged adolescence. And now that premarital sex has become the norm, there may be less pressure to marry younger, so it's circular. People delay marriage, so society becomes more accepting of premarital sex, and the availability of premarital sex reduces one of the driving forces for early marriage. This cycle, of course, got a bit of a kick from a little thing called the sexual revolution.

Except in certain communities, it can no longer be taken for granted that most people will wait until marriage—or even pretend that they do. The vast majority of men and women in the United States are not virgins when they get married, especially if they don't marry until after their teens.

If you no longer believe it's necessary or even advisable to wait until marriage, what becomes the new standard?

No sex until love? That could work, but how do you know when you're in love? Does intense attraction and arousal constitute love? We venture to guess that the definition of love changes rapidly as the night wears on and the temperature rises (and the third drink kicks in).

No sex until college? Okay, but what is the logic for that cutoff? How would you explain it to your child? Is she different in her last week of high school from her first week of college? And what if she isn't going to college? The marriage cutoff has history, religion, tradition, and an argument about out-of-wedlock children behind it, but almost any new cutoff you devise risks seeming arbitrary to your teenager.

Why Kids Abstain

Now, some kids do, of course, abstain until marriage or at least until they are in their twenties. Why do these teenagers wait?

Some think it's the moral thing to do. Others wait out of fear of pregnancy or AIDS or the unknown. Some think it's important in terms of social reputation. And still others just don't feel interested or ready.

To some kids, virginity can mean purity. To others, it can mean freedom from anxiety. It can mean high self-esteem, obedience to religious teachings, saving oneself for someone special, or eligibility to marry the prince of Japan.

Girls carry the full weight of the historical, religious, and cultural traditions of many societies that made virginity a precious commodity. But boys can feel righteous about it, too. They may feel a duty to respect the wishes of their girlfriend. And just because some of them don't seem to fear pregnancy ("it's not my problem"; "no way the kid is mine") doesn't mean none of them do. It's easy to forget the impact that having sex for the first time can have on a boy, but behind all the bravado, you'll often find a frightened child. He may be insecure about how he'll perform. He may fear that he'll do something wrong when he's in bed, or that he'll be laughed at. He may hear every pimple on his face shout, "Undesirable!"

And then, of course, there are the kids who have held onto their virginity because they just haven't had the chance to lose it. This kind of virginity, although you may value it, may be a source of shame or worry for your teenager.

And Why They Don't Abstain

Teenagers, truth be told, have a seemingly inexhaustible supply of reasons why they wouldn't want to wait for sex. Say your son feels uncertain about his standing as a guy, as a man. He wants to have sex with a girl to prove to himself, and his friends, that he's for real. Or say your daughter is seeing a boy she really likes, but she's worried he won't stick around unless they have sex. These are reasons you'd certainly like to have a crack at before things go too far.

But these are not the only reasons that may be on your teenager's mind.

Teenagers also have sex drives. Opportunities for sex abound, and the consequences—the negative consequences—may seem remote, at least to the body parts that appear to be making all the decisions.

And they are curious. There is so much hype built up around sex, and yet until they try it, they can't really understand what it is that everybody is so taken with.

"Someone I heard of got hit by a bus and was going to be in a wheelchair for the rest of his life," Biff, recalling his youth, says by way of explaining his decision to stop waiting. "He was never going to be able to feel real sex. There was this girl who had been flirting with me. I hadn't really thought I was ready. I'd wanted to wait for someone special, but then I got scared that I might never get to have sex, and I wanted to know what it was like. So we did it."

Why don't kids abstain? There are scores of reasons, and not all have to do with the act itself:

They want to see what all the fuss is about.

They want intimacy.

They are in love.

They want to please their partner.

They feel obliged because they got a nice gift.

They want to prove that they can get someone to have sex with them.

They want to feel more like an adult.

They are afraid to say no.

They want to prove that you can't stop them.

They don't know why they shouldn't.

Ask a group of ninth-grade boys about sex, and their responses are illustrative. The question: "You've been on a few dates with a girl, and she asks you to have sex, and you don't want to. How likely would you be to have sex anyway?"

Their responses? "Why wouldn't I want to?" "Is she a dog?" "I don't understand the question." "Oh, do you want us to assume we're gay?"

The question seems to be "When will I have sex?" not "Should I have sex?"

You may remember Alyssa and Josh, the sixteen-year-old lovers from Chapter 7.

Josh felt so exhilarated by his closeness with Alyssa, his first real girlfriend and only the second girl he had ever kissed, that he wanted to explore the possibilities of being even closer. Sex was the only limit he and Alyssa saw to their intimacy, and so they wanted to breach it.

And there was also the matter of an itch. As Alyssa explains, when puberty started, she began to develop a yen for sex. "When I first got into guys, it wasn't to make friendships. I was, like, horny, horny, horny! There was an itch I wanted to scratch."

Alyssa didn't have intercourse with any of those guys, though. It wasn't until she felt that she was in love with Josh that she decided it was something she wanted to pursue. Why? Well, there was still that itch, but there was more. Alyssa felt that sex would represent the fulfillment of her love and trust for Josh. She sensed that it would feel good in a way she couldn't have imagined back in her "horny" days.

And so Alyssa decided to approach her parents, Dave and Marisol, to tell them what she and Josh had planned. Or maybe to ask them.

Before we get to that moment, let's take a few steps back to acknowledge that things are even more complex than they are about to seem to Dave and Marisol. Before we explore how to handle your child's interest in sex, we ought to point out that intercourse isn't the only issue you may have to contend with.

Parsing Sex

MONICA LEWINSKY: *We didn't have sex, Linda. . . .*

LINDA TRIPP: *Well, what do you call it?*

LEWINSKY: *We fooled around.*

TRIPP: *Oh.*

LEWINSKY: *Not sex.*

TRIPP: *Oh, I don't know. I think if you go to—if you go to orgasm, that's having sex.*

LEWINSKY: *No, it's not.*

TRIPP: *Yes, it is.*

LEWINSKY: *No, it's not. It's—*

TRIPP: *It's not having—*

LEWINSKY: *Having sex is having intercourse.*

TRIPP: *Oh, you've been around him too long. . . .*

—*The* Daily News, *October 3, 1998*

Sex isn't always so easy to define.

If your son said he had *not* had "sexual relations" with a girl he'd only kissed, we doubt you would accuse him of perjury. On the other end of the spectrum, if he had had vaginal intercourse with her, we bet you would indeed expect him to say he'd had sex.

But as far as the various acts that fall in the middle of that spectrum, teenagers are uncertain about what counts as sex. In a 1998 survey at a large university in the West, over half of the students in a human sexuality class thought that men would not consider fellatio to be sex and women would not consider cunnilingus to be sex. When told that there was no orgasm with the fellatio or cunnilingus, even more of the students thought that oral sex wasn't sex. So, no orgasm, no sex? Is that the rule? (Sounds like a lot of women have had babies without ever having had sex.)

Ask the students if a male-female couple would consider themselves "sexual partners" if they had had vaginal intercourse, and over 80 percent say they would. Ask the same question about a couple that has only had oral sex; half think the male would consider the female a sexual partner, and 64 percent think the female would consider him a sexual partner.

If your teenager is not sure what sex is (and neither are we, entirely), what about abstinence?

The next time a friend says she wants her kids to be abstinent, ask her what she means. More often than not, she'll start to answer and stop herself, realizing she's not sure, or she'll say something like:

"You know. No sex."

"But what type of sex?"

"No intercourse."

"So is oral sex okay?"

"No, of course not."

"How about mutual masturbation?"

"Um, I don't know."

For their part, school abstinence programs don't always define what abstinence means. Some don't mention any specific sex acts, which can make it hard to figure out what you're supposed to abstain from. As for the people responsible for teaching sex ed, even they can't agree on what counts as abstinence. Some health educators think mutual masturbation counts, and some don't. Some (three out of ten in one study) say oral sex counts as abstinence.

It isn't any clearer at home. What parents mean when they tell their kids to be abstinent depends on what they care about. If your main concern is preserving virginity or preventing pregnancy, you may care most about abstinence from vaginal intercourse. If you are worried about

STDs, you may be hoping that your teen will refrain from a broader array of sexual activities. If your focus is on emotional readiness for physical intimacy, what doesn't count?

Maybe it all just seems like semantics, but semantics matter.

They matter when you're advising your daughter not to have sex until she gets married.

They matter when your son hears in school that he should use a condom every time he has sex. If anal intercourse isn't sex, then he's not getting the right message.

We encouraged you in Chapter 3 to use precise language when teaching your toddler about body parts. We encourage you to do the same here.

Sex has too many meanings. *Abstinence* hasn't been defined. Even *virgin* may be outdated. A virgin was traditionally someone who had never had sex, which was defined as vaginal intercourse. But it doesn't occur to a lot of people that a woman can have oral or anal sex on a regular basis and still consider herself a virgin.

What Do Virgins Do with All That Free Time?
[I've been] touched, kissed, poked, prodded, rubbed, caressed, sucked, licked, bitten—you name it.

—*Tara McCarthy on her virginity in* Been There, Haven't Done That

They find ways to keep busy. In a nationally representative 1995 study of fifteen- to nineteen-year-old males who had never been married, 45 percent were classified as virgins (no vaginal intercourse yet), but they weren't all just sitting home twiddling their thumbs: 22 percent had been masturbated by a female, 15 percent had had a female perform fellatio on them, 12 percent had performed cunnilingus, and 1 percent had performed anal intercourse with a female.

We don't have national data on the sexual practices of female virgins, but we do have local data. A study of a school district in Los Angeles County found that about a third of ninth- to twelfth-grade female virgins in 1992 had engaged in some type of genital sexual activity with a male during the prior year. About three in ten had masturbated a partner, three in ten had been masturbated by a partner, one in ten had performed fellatio (where the boy ejaculated), and one in ten had received cunnilingus. Hardly any virgins reported anal sex or sexual activity with a partner of the same sex. The findings for the boys in this study were fairly similar. A contemporaneous study of suburban New York high school students also found virgins engaging in oral sex. Lest you think this is just an isolated phenomenon of Big City, USA, a similar picture was found in a study in Salt Lake City.

Bar Mitzvah Blow Jobs: On Becoming a Man?

Remember how at bar mitzvahs we used to put flowers and souvenirs in a glass of water and drip candle wax on top to make a memory cup? Now they give blow jobs.

—*Amy, mother of 10- and 13-year-old boys*

Just in time for the new millennium, with predictions that the sky would fall, came the news that made many a parent think it had: middle school kids were having oral sex. The *New York Times, USA Today,* and the *Washington Post,* among others, ran stories discussing the popularity of oral sex not only among high school students but also among seventh and eighth graders. The stories talked about casual oral sex at parties and quoted adolescents who made it sound no more intimate than a kiss on the cheek. One version of the story is that bar mitzvah boys receive blow jobs as gifts from some of the girls they invite. (We're not sure whether their mothers make them send thank-you notes.)

The reports all seem to be about fellatio. Cunnilingus doesn't appear to be as much of a hit on the party circuit. And from what we can tell, it hasn't crossed anyone's mind to use a condom. The whole idea is that fellatio is the risk-free way to have sex, or nonsex. No pregnancies. No STDs (or so they think). They don't even have to take their clothes off. Just step into the bathroom or behind the garage, give a blow job, and back to the party. Sounds like what making out used to be.

Is this all true? Is there really an oral sex explosion?

We don't know. There is a dearth of data on middle schoolers' sex lives. But we do have data on high school students, and they are engaging in oral sex, so it's very possible they begin in middle school.

And we do know that it's happening in at least some communities. In Georgia, a screening program for meningitis in middle school students serendipitously turned up some kids with gonorrhea in their throats. There's only one way you get gonorrhea in your throat, and it's not from a toilet seat.

Parents are not just concerned that young teens may be having oral sex; it's also the circumstances in which they are having it. As the stories go, girls seem to be having oral sex with boys they barely know. Vaginal intercourse may be preserved for someone special, but oral sex is "no big deal."

"I'm baffled," says Carmen, who is forty-three and has a fourteen-year-old son. "I'm not a prude. I had plenty of oral sex in my day, but it came later, after intercourse. I didn't even know what it was until college. For me, it's still something that seems more intimate than sex."

Parents of boys tend to describe sexually precocious girls as aggressors, going after young boys who haven't a clue what a blow job is. The parents of girls talk of a social network in which girls have found the only way to establish their power is through pleasureless random sex acts. No one is happy.

Now listen to Winston, a fairly nonchalant ninth grader. "Some groups do it, and some don't." Groups? "The slackers and jocks have oral sex. The girls just give it to them." At parties? "In school. In the bathrooms. And I guess at parties, too, but I don't go to their parties." The blades—the kids who go rollerblading—don't seem to get oral sex as readily, at least not this particular blade.

Why the apparent rise in popularity now? No one knows, but we'll take a stab at it. Adolescents are being taught in school and at home that oral sex is much less risky for HIV transmission than vaginal intercourse. It's been presented as an alternative to vaginal intercourse that doesn't risk pregnancy or disease.

And it's true—sort of. It *is* less risky; your daughter won't get pregnant if she performs fellatio on her boyfriend. But she could contract gonorrhea or herpes or some other disease. She could even be infected with HIV, although it's much harder to get it through oral sex. So oral sex is less likely than vaginal intercourse to transmit an STD, but it's not risk free.

Peer Power

What influences your child's choices about sex?

To answer this question, let's return to conventional notions of sex and abstinence. The vaginal-intercourse definition of sex is the one used in most of the research into teens' sexual habits, and we want to take you through some of those studies' more useful findings here. Specifically, we want to look at which factors influence your child's decision to have intercourse for the first time or to wait a little longer. Let's start with peers.

Friends and classmates have a large influence over your child's decision, and probably more and more as your child grows older. Youth with sexually active friends and siblings start earlier. But more important, what they think their peers approve of and are doing themselves makes a difference. If they believe the tall tales their classmates tell about sexual adventures, they will be more likely to try to keep up. "She climbed through my window and begged me to make her a woman" may not sound convincing to you when it escapes from the mouth of a thirteen-year-old boy whose voice cracks every other sentence, but his friends will hang on every word.

The next part may surprise you. Having good friends that your child feels close with means he's *less* likely to have sex. Being the type of adolescent who has a circle of friends and is socially connected to others is a good thing in general and it makes your teenager less likely to have sex, perhaps because kids like these are already getting some of what they would be looking for in a sexual partner—namely, intimacy and companionship.

The Nerd Effect

Kids who are smarter, do better in school, and have plans for their future, such as going to college or pursuing ambitious careers, are less likely to have sex. It's long been believed that students with higher grades delay sex because they're focused on future goals and are more aware of what they have to lose from an unintended pregnancy. However, they're also less likely to engage in kissing and petting, so perhaps there are other reasons as well. They may have fewer opportunities (studying takes time and energy); parents who encourage their kids to achieve may also discourage them from dating; or maybe kids who get dates less easily turn to their studies. Of course, getting sexually involved can also take time and energy, and could be the cause of lower grades.

A recent study added a wrinkle to this story. It found that kids with lower intelligence are also more likely to delay sex. So it looks like it's the average kids, those who blend into the great middle, who are the most sexually active. Perhaps those with lowest intelligence are less accepted by their peers and have fewer opportunities for sex. Or perhaps their parents make more of an effort to watch over them and protect them.

While we're on the subject of education, it has also been found that kids who attend a parochial school or who attend a school with higher overall attendance levels (a marker for better schools) are more likely to delay intercourse.

It's not just classwork that matters. Kids who are more involved in extracurricular activities—in or out of school—tend to have sex later. Swimming, band, and the rest keep them occupied, provide monitoring, and give them opportunities to develop friendships. Maybe the soccer moms are on to something.

Having Faith

> We are bringing up our children in a home with values. We go to church every Sunday. They know that you don't have sex before you get married. If you just bring them up properly, they know what's right.
>
> —*Kathy, mother of three boys*

Religion may influence your child's choices, especially if your religion proscribes intercourse before marriage. But the effect isn't as strong as you might have predicted. Adolescents in families with religious traditions that frown on premarital intercourse are at best only somewhat less likely to engage in it.

Religious arguments for preserving virginity may be powerful for some kids and seem out of touch to others. What may be the deciding factor here is the extent to which your child has internalized the values of your religion and whether his role models live by these values. However, even when children are otherwise observant, they may not be when it comes to sex. We can't tell you how often an unmarried teenage girl comes into a clinic worried that she might be pregnant or have an STD. Does she know about condoms? Yes. Does she use them? No. Why not? Because they're against her religion. Adolescents, like adults, are quite capable of following rules selectively.

In one national study, children who considered religion and prayer important started having sex at an older age, though many still had it before marriage. In another, religious affiliation and attending religious events were associated with later sexual initiation for boys, but not for girls. It may be that these boys have sex later because of the religious values they've learned, but it's also possible that religious activities function much the way other organized activities function: as a form of monitoring and a way to engage youth in something that helps them feel good about themselves. Or parents who get their children involved in religious activities may supervise their kids better in general.

So if you put your teachings about sex in a religious context, this may influence your child. But don't depend on religion alone.

The Pledge

I've always had this idea in my head, the idea of waiting until marriage to have sex. I have thought this way since the 8th grade. I am now a junior in high school and yes, there is temptation everywhere! This Saturday I will have my True Love Waits ring ceremony. I am so excited! There are a lot of girls (friends) who are doing this also—a few guys too. This is special to me because I'm not great at a lot of things. I don't sing, I can't play sports and I'm not the smartest person. This is something that not all girls can do (that I know).

—*Asha, found on the True Love Waits website, www.lifeway.com/tlw*

One approach for preserving virginity that has grown out of a religious tradition is the public pledge some adolescents take to remain a virgin until marriage. The Virginity Pledge appears to have been first offered in 1993 through True Love Waits, an abstinence group that grew out of the Southern Baptist Convention. It has been estimated that by 2001, over 2.5 million adolescents had taken the pledge.

The virginity movement has more to offer than just a pledge. There are cards and rings. There are pledge Web pages, and pledge products your child can purchase (caps, T-shirts, mugs with slogans like "I'd rather break up than break out with Herpes"), pledge chatrooms, and pledge summer camps. There's even a musical.

Some kids become greater believers than others. A few years out of high school, Jane looked back on her Virginity Pledge: "I went to an all-girls school. They made us do the Virginity Pledge. I did it because, well, what was I going to do, say no? It was a joke."

Tina thinks better of it. "It wasn't relevant to me. I'd already had sex, and I didn't see anything wrong with it, but I think some girls take the pledge seriously. I think it helped them."

A study of the pledge found that teens who pledged started having sex an average of eighteen months later than those who did not pledge. The difference held up even when religious beliefs, family social status and income, and family structure (whether one or two parents live in the home) were taken into account. At seventeen years old, 65 percent of the pledgers were still virgins, compared to about half of the non-pledgers.

The pledge did not tend to work when just one teenager took it. Instead, groups of kids who pledged together seemed to benefit from mutual support. The pledge also seemed to be less effective once more than 30 percent of kids in a group or school took it, apparently because it no longer made the pledgers feel like they were part of a special group.

Learning to Abstain at School

You might wonder how the sexual education your kids get at school affects their decision to have sex or to abstain. The answer depends on the type of sex ed they are getting. Your child's school likely teaches one of two main types of sexual education curricula: abstinence-only education or comprehensive sex ed.

Abstinence-only education teaches that abstinence until marriage is the only safe and moral answer to the sexual questions of the teenage years. If it mentions contraception at all, it teaches that it is far inferior to abstinence in protecting teens from pregnancy and STDs.

Proponents of abstinence-only education argue that sex ed's purpose is to prevent sex outside of marriage and to reduce a student's risk of pregnancy and STDs, and that confining sex education to the encouragement of abstinence is the most effective way to achieve that goal. To teach about other aspects of human sexuality or other strategies to reduce risk, they contend, only encourages teens to have sex, which is dangerous and, in some minds, wrong.

Comprehensive sex ed (also called abstinence-plus) programs teach the value of abstinence, but add lessons in safer sex methods (including contraception and substitutes for intercourse) and any number of other sexual topics, like sexual decision making, the range of types of sexual expression, and abortion.

Proponents of this approach point out that despite any program's calls for abstinence, some teenagers will have sex. If we want to reduce adolescents' risk and protect their health, they maintain, we need to do more than teach abstinence. Withholding knowledge about sex doesn't prevent kids from having sex; it prevents them from having sex knowledgeably.

These competing claims have been the subject of less

research than you might have hoped. The efficacy of most abstinence-only programs has not been tested. The few studies that have been conducted have not shown them to succeed at their chief goals: to delay teens' initiation of sexual intercourse and to reduce frequency among those who have already begun. But because most of those studies have flaws, it would be premature to completely write these programs off as ineffective at delaying intercourse. New studies should shed more light on them.

Abstinence-plus programs have been better studied. Contrary to the fears of some, these programs do not appear to lead to earlier or more frequent intercourse or more sexual partners. In fact, some have the opposite effect—delaying sexual debut, decreasing the frequency of intercourse, or lowering the number of sexual partners. Some programs also increase students' use of condoms and other contraceptives. Others have little or no effect or only influence some of the behaviors.

Based on these data, the surgeon general recommended in 2001 that all U.S. schools pursue the more comprehensive approach to sex education. The American Medical Association and the American Academy of Pediatrics have done the same. And a major national survey of parents' opinions about sex education found in 2000 that the majority of American parents agreed.

The pledge was also more effective with fifteen- and sixteen-year-olds and less effective with eighteen-year-olds.

Which brings us back to the fact that even after pledging, quite a few adolescents still had sex during the next few years. And when they had sex, they were less likely to use a condom than kids who hadn't pledged—not surprising, perhaps, given that everyone expected them to remain virgins. The focus had been on teaching these kids not to have sex—rather than on making sure they knew about contraception. So if kids who've pledged break the pledge and have sex, they are less prepared to make it safer. On top of that, their first sex is usually unplanned, so they don't have a chance to seek out information about contraception.

From a health perspective, the eventual abandonment of abstinence tied with lower condom use raises a red flag. An eighteen-month delay in starting intercourse is impressive, but it's not the same as maintaining virginity until marriage. The bottom line message from research on abstinence programs in general is that children who only learn about abstinence will, in many cases, delay their sexual debut for a few months or a few years. Many still wind up having sex outside of marriage, so unless you believe it is never appropriate to use contraception, the evidence argues for teaching sexual safety, too.

Sobering Facts

We can't talk about abstinence without at least making reference to alcohol and drugs; they are so often participants in a child's sexual debut. Many teens make the decision to have sex in a fog of intoxication and clouded judgment. Some intentionally drink to gain the courage to make their moves or to have an excuse the next day—"I was so trashed, I didn't know what I was doing." Some may be plied with alcohol or drugs by a seducer looking to take advantage of them.

Not all kids are purposely using so-called mind-altering substances as a vehicle for having sex. They may be trying out several "adult" behaviors at once: drinking alcohol, smoking cigarettes, having sex. There's also the special case of Rohypnol, the so-called date rape drug, which knocks a child out so she can be taken advantage of without a struggle.

A lesson to teach your child: If she doesn't want to have sex, she shouldn't drink or use drugs. If she doesn't follow this advice, she'd better have a friend look out for her—not just to protect her from slipping into unwanted sex, but also from driving and other dangerous activities.

Not by Choice

Early sexual activity is sometimes coerced or forced.

In a national survey that included men and women, 7 percent of eighteen- to twenty-two-year-olds reported at least one episode of nonvoluntary intercourse—the rate for women was 12 percent, with almost half of them reporting the experience occurring before they were fourteen.

Parents tend to worry about girls being forced, but of course, as the numbers above show, boys can be forced as well.

The degree of fear and shame that can result from forced sex varies widely. Your daughter may be inclined to underestimate the effects. Assume she needs more help than she asks for, and if she will agree to it, get her some counseling, which can mitigate the emotional fallout of sexual trauma. Her clinician can refer her to a rape crisis counselor. If it just happened, she should be seen by a clinician to check for STDs and physical injury. The clinician can also check for physical evidence of the perpetrator that could be used in a later legal action. You, too, could be traumatized and might benefit from talking to a counselor.

If you're considering legal action, all states have statutory rape laws that specify a minimum age of consent for sexual intercourse, generally ranging from twelve to eighteen years of age. These laws are rarely enforced for consensual sexual activity.

Your child may not always be able to protect herself from being taken advantage of, but avoiding drugs and alcohol when she is in a dating situation, and avoiding partners who rely on them, can help. Intoxication is not a friend of consent.

Parents Matter

Finally, you will be pleased to hear that *you* can have a major influence on your child's decision to start having sex or to keep waiting. The rest of this chapter is dedicated to telling you how to do it.

As you will remember, monitoring is one of the trustiest arrows in your quiver: that is, knowing where your child is and whom he's with, knowing his friends and their parents, and knowing when he's coming home. Having an adult available to watch your child after school is an element of effective monitoring; so is just calling to check in if she's home alone. Well-monitored kids engage in less risky behavior of all types, and they start having sex later than their less-monitored peers.

All this makes good sense. If you need to stay at work late one day and you call your sixteen-year-old to ask what's up and would he please start getting dinner ready, he's not likely to get a girl pregnant that afternoon. But if he returns to an empty house day after day knowing that he won't hear from anyone until nightfall, and if when you do come home, you don't ask what he did that afternoon or look over the homework he was supposed to be doing, it may not surprise you to hear that he's more likely to get into trouble.

"If my daughter is going out with a boy," Lusita, an avid monitor, says, "I call his parents. I make sure they're aware I'm paying attention. That way, maybe they'll pay attention, too. I make sure the boy comes in when he picks her up. I want to meet anyone whose car she is getting into. I want him to know that I exist, that I care, and that I'm aware."

Remember, too, the power of closeness. As we explained in Chapter 2, adolescents who feel connected to their parents and family, who say they are loved and cared for at home, tend to have intercourse later than adolescents who are not as well connected to their folks.

Then there is the issue of parenting style, a topic in which by now you are an expert. As we have said, authoritative parenting (warmth plus high expectations) hasn't been tested for its effect on the timing of a child's sexual debut; but the kids of authoritative parents take fewer risks and take better care of their health than other kids, so we think it's likely that authoritativeness will, on average, delay your child's first sexual experiences.

Now for something harder (or impossible) for you to change. As is true with almost everything in our society, your socioeconomic status matters. If your income is higher, your kids will probably begin having sex later. Likewise if you or your partner has more years of education. We don't think children check your bank account before deciding to have sex. Rather, these indicators of social class may be markers for a whole host of characteristics that make it easier for children to delay having sex.

But all these influences that turn up in studies are just averages. Not all kids from families with high income delay sex, and not all kids from poor families have sex early. Your child is not preprogrammed.

Do You Approve?

You've got to teach them not to have sex before they get married. Any teenager can have sex. But then it doesn't mean anything. What do you have to offer your husband or wife if you haven't saved yourself?

—*Judith-Ann, on her seventeen-year-old daughter and twelve-year-old twin sons*

My concern is safety rather than is she having sex, or is she doing something against my values. How do you have safe sex if you want to have sex—that's what I want to get across.

—*Stan, on his fifteen-year-old daughter*

In considering how you might influence your child's decision about sex, a critical question is will she be more likely to wait if you tell her that's what you want? If you make it clear that you don't approve of sex in high school, will she listen? The answer is maybe.

There isn't nearly as much research on the subject as we would like, but there have been some interesting findings. In a large national sample of adolescents, researchers found that teens who say their parents disapprove of them having sex wait longer to have it.

This is a pretty satisfying bit of data, and it seems quite logical.

But as we said, research on talking to kids about sex can be something of a brainteaser.

Although kids' reports of their parents' attitudes correlate with when they had sex, their parents' actual attitudes do not. Interestingly, kids' statements about their parents' views just don't jibe with what their parents say, mostly because kids tend to underestimate how opposed to sex their parents actually are. So, in the research, the kids who said that their parents approved of sex were more likely to have had it; but in reality, their parents were quite likely to disapprove.

Now it may be that this mismatch is due to the fact that some parents just don't get their message across, and if they did, their kids would wait to have sex just like the others who heard their parents' message. If that's the case, our advice is simple: Tell your kids what you think.

But it may be that all the parents were equally communicative and all the kids got the message, but the ones who decided to have sex anyway rewrote history to justify their actions and decided that their parents really didn't mind. If this is the case, we don't quite know what advice to give.

What do we really think? We think both scenarios have some truth to them. Given that your opinion probably does make some contribution, we encourage you to express it. Repeatedly.

The Silent Treatment

Ask a sixteen-year-old girl, "Have your parents ever talked with you about sex?" and you're bound to get an answer like: "Never." "Not at all." "I can't imagine it." "They wouldn't be able to. I don't even think they know what sex is."

Try her mother: "Have you ever spoken to your child about sex?" The response may sound a bit different: "Of course. We both have." "All the time." "We had a wonderful talk."

Do children have amnesia? Do parents have overactive imaginations?

Maybe a little of both, although we have to say that if we were betting men, we'd bet the kids were right. Conversations about sex that have any substance tend to be so salient for kids that we think it's unlikely they'd forget them. Parents, on the other hand, are so eager to feel that they've done their job ("You learned about all that boy-girl stuff in school, didn't you?") that minor remarks, maybe even some unspoken thoughts about what they might say to their kid some day, can be remembered as full conversations.

There is an epidemic of noncommunication about sex. Call it denial. Call it holding onto the last vestiges of your child's so-called innocence. But don't call it a good idea. We have already mentioned that it is quite legitimate for parents and teenagers not to get involved in the details of one another's private sexual lives. But we also believe in the importance of teaching Lesson Four: sexual ethics and sexual safety for adolescents.

We're going to take you through that lesson, but let's pause for a moment to consider some of the reasons why you don't want to go there.

I Don't Want My Child to Grow Up Too Soon

If you're like some parents, you might be afraid to talk with your kids about sex because you just don't want them to grow up that fast. We understand. Learning about sex is a major milestone on the road to adulthood. How could you not feel that it represents a sign that your child is growing into his own life and out of yours? But, sadly, time and your kid will go on with or without you. Whether you talk with your kids or avoid the subject, they'll know about sex. Wouldn't it be better if you were involved?

I Don't Want to Promote It

Maybe you're afraid that if you talk about sex, your kids will think you're endorsing it. That's a common concern. We suggest that when you discuss sex with your teenager, you make it very clear to him just how you feel about it. Repetition helps. To make sure he isn't misunderstanding you, ask him to describe back to you what he thinks you've been saying.

If this concern has come up for you when discussing contraception with your teen, you may find Chapter 9 particularly helpful.

I Don't Know When to Start

Start young. As we said in Chapter 2, the lesson about sexual ethics and safety should begin by age twelve and should probably take the form of more than one talk. The older your child gets, the more likely she will have already started having sex or taken to heart the lessons of others. Better to inoculate her with knowledge and skills beforehand. The older she gets, the more difficult it may be to get her into an intimate conversation about this stuff.

As for the specific times to choose, we will leave that one to your instincts. Talking while driving seems to be a popular option. The setting is private, your kid can't escape, and you don't have to look each other in the eye.

If you find yourself procrastinating, consider setting a deadline. Carla got one courtesy of her monthly bridge game.

"Kit had just read an article that said you had to talk to your kids about condoms. We all had kids in junior high school, and not a one of

Tips on Talking

Seizing the Moment

Your life with your child is bound to present countless opportunities to open a discussion about sex. Your challenge: to take them. Here are some moments you might want to seize.

1. The latest teen soap is on the tube. Two characters are talking about having sex (if your kid watches teen shows, chances are this kind of opportunity to talk will come up, oh, every ten minutes). When the show reaches a commercial, ask your daughter what she thinks the characters should do.
2. Your son's reading will serve the same purpose. Ask him what's really going on in *The Scarlet Letter,* or what he thinks Romeo and Juliet were up to before the bird started chirping.
3. Make use of your extended family. When your daughter makes a joke about her older cousin being in love, ask what she thinks that relationship is like. Some families' instincts are to pretend the kids don't know about the unintended pregnancy or the gay uncle's new boyfriend. But they've probably overheard you, and these are great moments for teaching.

Exercises

Unless you run your home like a professional party planner, your daughter may think that you've been slipping into the liquor closet if you suggest that the two of you do some exercises together. Use this book as your excuse if you want to. Share in your kid's skepticism if necessary. We won't mind.

1. Go on the Internet together to look at websites that provide good information about sex and STDs and contraception. Learn as a team.

2. Trade roles. Get your kid to think up what topics he would discuss with his kid if he were the parent. You think up what topics you would ask about if you were the kid. Take it a step further and have the conversations with the roles reversed.

3. Sex, as you may have noticed, is not infrequently in the news. What STD had a sudden increase last year? What did the new study about condoms find? Pass your child the paper over breakfast and ask what she thinks.

Openers

If you're struggling to get the conversation started, try one of these.

1. "How's your sex ed class going? What topic are you up to now? How comfortable do the kids in the class seem to be?"

2. "In junior high school, kids sometimes start talking about dating and going out. Have kids in your school been talking about going out?"

3. "I'm reading this book for parents, and it says I should be talking with you about sex. Do you think other kids' parents do that?"

us had talked with them about any type of birth control. We decided we each had to talk to our kids before our next game. We made a rule that you had to use the word 'penis.' "

How did it go?

"It went well, really well. We were all happy we'd done it. . . . If Kit's son will just ask out my daughter, everything will be perfect, since I know he has protection!"

I'm Afraid It's Going to Be Too Awkward

Hey, you're a parent, not a sex therapist. Of course it'll be awkward. And you probably won't know all the answers. But, we hope you've learned, when you're genuinely trying, your kids can be very forgiving.

Jinhee gave up her fear of making a mistake awhile back. "I wanted to be a perfect mom who always knows the right thing to say, but that isn't going to happen. I make mistakes and say things I don't mean or that I shouldn't mean. I apologize when I'm wrong and try to do better the next time." Her kids are doing just fine.

It might help knowing that when asked privately, kids say they really value their parents' thoughts about sex. More than four out of five ten- to fifteen-year-olds think their mothers have a good understanding of the sexual problems and situations they face, and about three-quarters think their fathers do. Of those kids whose parents had spoken to them about sex, 87 percent thought their parents were helpful.

The parents who do make the effort tend to say it wasn't so bad after all. Sure, it can be scary. Sure, you can embarrass yourself. Sure, there can be awkward moments and moments of self-revelation that you worry will make your kid think less of you. But, with apologies to Nietzsche, that which does not kill you makes you stronger, and we haven't had any reports yet of death by talking.

He Just Won't Talk with Me

Most adolescents want some privacy. Even if your child is comfortable talking with you about sex in general, he may not want to talk about his own sex life. If this is the case, the challenge for you will be to find a way to discuss sex that lets your son feel you aren't invading his space. Talking about what other people—friends of his, television characters—have done or should do can be a more comfortable way for him to hear what you need to say. Talking with your partner or your friends about sexuality in your child's presence also works in a pinch.

If your relationship lacks a reasonable rapport on which to build, work on the underlying issues first. If you can't talk about what would be good for dinner, you aren't ready to talk about sex. You need to start with a solid-enough foundation.

And while you're working things out, try to find others your teen can talk with. Encourage her aunt to check in with her about sex. You can do the same for your niece and nephew.

I Don't Know What to Talk About

Here's your answer. The next four sections make up the bulk of Lesson Four.

Sexual Reasoning

In the early years after puberty, you can help your child begin to sort out the sexual situations she's bound to face sooner or later by helping her know her own mind. With your encouragement, she can start sharpening her ideas about sex long before she finds herself needing to make a snap decision in a dark corner of her boyfriend's basement.

Talk to your child about how she would like to act in various sexual situations before they occur. When she's going out with a boy, how far does she want to go? Does she want to do anything at all? What does she think her friends are doing, and how does she feel about their decisions?

Listen carefully as she formulates her thoughts. Encourage her to name the pros and cons of each choice, the pressures to choose sex in certain situations, and the consequences of saying yes or no. What would happen if she did have intercourse with him? What would happen if she didn't? She may have a ready answer for you, because she has talked through these issues with her friends, or she may never really have given her own ideas careful consideration.

Listen as she tells you, "Maybe a guy won't go out with me if I won't have sex with him." Or, "I'm never going to be one of those kids who feel pressured by anyone into having sex." Or, "I think I'd want to say yes."

Then give your perspective.

You can use these conversations to clarify your own thoughts, too. You don't need to figure out everything before you sit down together. It's okay to know that you want your child to wait for sex until he's older without knowing when the right time would be, as long as you acknowledge your uncertainty. One day you may sound to your son as if you expect him to wait until marriage for sex; a day later you may seem to be suggesting that sex on prom night would be fine. Acknowledging that you're uncertain about some things, and putting your heads together to figure them out, is much more valuable to your child than trying to present yourself as certain about these matters when you're not.

These decisions are hard. Your goal is not to get your child to reach the "right" decision in your first conversations. It's to help her learn that sex is something she will be making decisions about, and to move her toward developing the necessary reasoning skills. When you feel you *do* know what's best, it can be hard to balance your impulse to tell her what to do with her need to strengthen her decision-making muscles. If the risks are too high for what you consider a mistaken point of view, jump in and express yourself. But if they're low, maybe you should let her learn from her own experiences. Remember, at the moment the final decision has to be made, she won't have you there to help her.

Sexual Consent

Remember the statistics on nonvoluntary sex we discussed a little while ago? All teenagers need to understand that the decision to have sex should always be consensual. Based on surveys of their opinions about consent, boys in particular need to learn to accept it when a partner says no; but girls need to learn this, too.

You can make this part of Lesson Four a little more sophisticated by acknowledging the ambiguity here. Some people say maybe, or behave in a yes-ish way while speaking the language of no. Warn your kids that yellow lights are not the same as green ones. A partner who feels ambivalent about sex may agree to go ahead with a little urging, but afterward may feel regret and anger and accuse your child of taking advantage of his indecision.

You can also try to teach your child to give as clear a message about her wishes as possible to a potential partner. The earlier part of this lesson, the part about knowing her own mind, will help her make her thoughts more easily understood.

Tell your kids that they can communicate limits without conveying disinterest. If your son's date keeps suggesting that they spend time alone together, and he knows where that's going to lead (and he doesn't want to go there), he doesn't have to call it a night. He can suggest that they go to a movie or to a coffeehouse or someplace else where they won't be alone.

Finally, help prepare your child for the possibility that however clear she may be, some partners won't want to listen. Invite her to predict what this might feel like and to plan how she might react. She might decide to say no loudly and unflinchingly. She might want to cross her arms and pull away. Or she might conclude that in these circumstances her best approach will be to get up and go.

Sexual Safety

This crucial part of Lesson Four involves teaching your teenager before he's first had sex about the importance of using contraception every time to prevent pregnancy and STDs. We recommend making it clear that condoms should be used for every act of vaginal and anal intercourse, along with a hormonal method (such as oral contraceptives) or a female barrier method (such as a diaphragm). You can also propose unlubricated condoms and dental dams for oral sex. We acknowledge that this may be a losing proposition, and that you may prefer to recommend oral sex as a substitute for vaginal intercourse and settle for the lower but still-present risk. We describe these recommendations, and the way to get them across to your kid, in Chapter 9.

Fun Versus Fear

We assume that whether you feel that all sexual intimacy should be reserved for marriage or that sexual exploration should be encouraged during adolescence as a natural part of the developmental process, you want your child to have a healthy sex life whenever the time comes. If so, even as you lay out the need for sexual safety, don't forget to acknowledge to your child the joys of sex. Don't forget the part about sex being fun.

Focusing on sex strictly as a way of getting pregnant or contracting an STD or getting hurt or exhibiting moral weakness, without any discussion of what makes sexual intimacy enjoyable, can take its toll on impressionable adolescents. They may feel ashamed of their desires, let alone their actions.

Furthermore, this grown-up version of "Don't touch that; it'll fall off" probably isn't an effective way of getting a child to abstain from sex.

Fear has never been the most effective motivator. Though useful in the short run, its benefits tend to subside. If just before your son goes on a date, you show him a picture of a penis with a syphilitic chancre, he may swear off holding his girlfriend's hand, let alone having sex. But a month later, that photo is history, and even repeated viewings of that ill-fated penis will eventually lose their impact.

Your Moment of Truth

One thing she said to me was she was talking to one of her friends about sex and said, "I have to discuss this with my parents." And her friend looked at her like she had two heads. She said, "I would never take a big step like this without talking to my parents."

—*Marisol, on sixteen-year-old Alyssa*

At some point after all of this preparation, your child may decide to have sex. If all has been going well and you are very, very lucky, she may tell you.

Let's get back to Alyssa and Josh, the sixteen-year-olds who have been falling in love. After six months together (and a few years before that of having known each other), they began to feel that their trust in each other was so great, and their intimacy so deep, that the only step yet to take to fulfill their desire for connectedness was sex.

Alyssa's parents had prepared her well for this moment. They had taken the occasional opportunity to present their views about sex. They had told her about contraception and asked what her friends were doing (none of them had had sex yet). Alyssa knew a bit about their sexual pasts. Dave and Marisol had, in a number of ways, made it clear that sex was something they could discuss as a family. All of which may be why Alyssa went to her parents before she did anything with Josh.

"She came to us and said, 'Josh and I are getting very close and we're thinking about . . .' —well, she wanted to let us know that they were becoming physically intimate." Dave sensed what Alyssa was looking for. "She wanted our advice and our blessing. I think she trusted that we would understand and accept this, because we like Josh. But you know,

History Lessons

Maybe you've been worrying about this one: How do you advise your child to do something different from what you did?

Nancy decided to share her past with her daughter. "I told her that sex had been difficult for me. I slept with a bunch of guys in high school and college. It felt good in the moment, but I always felt bad afterward. Then I met her father. When we finally did have sex, it was incredible," she explained. "It was hard for me to tell her I'd slept around. It doesn't fit the image I have now. But I wanted her to know that I'd been there, that I'd done it all—so I know what I'm saying when I say it's better to wait until the guy is right."

Sharing your own experiences, whether admitting your mistakes or recounting the high points, can be quite effective. It can help establish an open dialogue, and it may diminish the chances that your kids will view your advice as uninformed or judgmental.

Skip found it productive to draw on his past to advise his daughter. "Let's face it. I remember what I was like. My job was to get sex. My question now is, how do I protect her from the junior version of me? I told her what guys are like, and when she laughed me off, I told her I was once one of those guys. That got her attention. It was like, no, really, I'm not kidding. They really are like this. And she listened."

Of course, you're not obligated to reveal your own history to your teenager. You have a right to your privacy. If he asks questions that you don't want to answer, you might try asking him how he would react if the answer was yes and if the answer was no.

It's also important to be sensitive to the fact that if you do decide to tell your child about your sexual past, it may be more than he wants to know. As we explained in Chapter 2, children of all ages may tend to avoid knowledge of their parents' sexuality. You may be shocked to discover how very much your kids have sheltered themselves from the facts of your sex life.

"A few years ago," Rosie, the mother of a thirteen-year-old son, says, "I was driving with Adam, and he blurted out, 'You and Dad had sex two times.' I didn't know what he was talking about. I was thinking he must have been listening at the door. But he meant two times ever, producing him and his sister. It sounds like a joke, but he was absolutely serious. I was stunned."

Here's the trick. Making it clear to your child that you know firsthand about sex is one helpful way, as Skip discovered, of establishing your teaching credentials. And the lesson that sex continues past the third decade of life is a good one to pass on. But you want to serve these goals while respecting your children's desire not to know too much or your desire not to reveal too much. You just have to find a balance that works for you and your child. Here's what Rosie tried.

"I asked him why he didn't think we would have done it more than twice and why he didn't think we still did it. He didn't know. He was still young and learning about sex, and it didn't seem to have occurred to him that we would have a sex life. I gave him a quick lesson in how sex is important throughout life, and I stopped being quite so secretive about our sex lives. Nothing big, but now I leave my contraceptive pills out on the bathroom counter rather than hidden in a drawer."

her mother has given her a lot of cautions about being sexually involved."

How did they react? As Alyssa remembers it, "My mother was extremely worried about my reputation."

But Marisol gave Alyssa a warning, not an order. "I first had sex when I was twenty-four, when I moved out of my mother's house,"

Marisol explains. "I knew I wasn't going to fit into my mother's concept of how I should conduct my life, so I chose not to have sex until I left that household. I didn't want to put Alyssa in the same position. I said this is what we think, but we will respect your choices. Through the entire process we were clear with her that we didn't feel she was ready to have sex."

As for Dave, Alyssa says, "my father was somewhat nervous." Dave, an undoubtedly liberal dad about sex in general, was nonetheless tense, and his tension got poured into concerns about safety. "He kept saying, just be safe." Dave, in fact, did more than talk.

"I went out to the store, and I bought her condoms. I told her about the signs of pregnancy." But he went further. "If she got pregnant, I told her, she would have to get an abortion. And if she didn't, we would help her get on welfare and set her up in an apartment, and she would get no more support from us."

Marisol tried to soften his admonition.

"I may think it's a reasonable thing for her to have an abortion, but I can't impose that on her. I did say, if you make that choice—to have the baby and to keep it—I will love the child, but I will not baby-sit. I will not raise it. You will have to deal with the consequences. She said, 'Ma, I really didn't want to hear all this. I get it, but it's more than I wanted to hear.' "

"It stressed me out so much!" Alyssa says. Still, she made a point of asking Josh, "If I were to get pregnant, would you be accepting of my having an abortion?" He said yes.

The stage was set for Alyssa and Josh to have safer, parent-accepted, but nonetheless discouraged sex. But Dave and Marisol weren't entirely ready to let go.

"They gave me the box of condoms, but then they set up all of these rules that essentially made it harder for me to see him. 'You can't go to his house in the evening, even if his parents are around. You can't be there alone in the afternoon.' And I was like, *contradiction*?"

Dave: "I think she came to us in part because she wanted us to hold her back a little bit. And we did."

"I was trying to make my relationship with them better by bringing this to them. But they treated me like a child" is how Alyssa saw it.
"So I went back to my old way of lying to them, and I slept over at his
house, telling them I was at a friend's. I probably wouldn't have slept
with him then if they hadn't made such a big fuss. It was more a rebelling
against them."

Well, who said this was going to be easy?

The Just-Right Rule

Should you follow Dave and Marisol's example and set some rules for
your child's sexual behavior?

"Kids need rules," says Danton, father of a fifteen-year-old girl. "It
provides comfort. We told her she can't have sex until she's been dating
a guy for six months. It relieves anxiety. She doesn't have to wonder
when, and she doesn't need to make a decision. We've done it for her."
(Message to Danton: It's not fair to make her break up with every guy
just before the six-month mark.)

Does Danton have the power to enforce such a rule? Not really.
Because Danton's daughter can have sex without his knowing about it,
his rule won't stop her unless she accepts it. That doesn't mean it won't
work. She might obey him simply because she feels it's wrong to defy her
father or because she trusts his judgment; but that won't be true for all
children, perhaps not even for all of Danton's children. In fact, one of
the biggest mistakes some parents make is thinking that they can control their kids' sex life.

Remember our discussion of induction and democracy? In
Chapter 7, we said that pretending to wield power you don't have can
undermine your authority as a parent. As we explained then, adolescents who want increased autonomy over their private lives will balk if
they don't get it. Just as Alyssa did. But as in Alyssa's case, that doesn't
mean kids don't want your guidance—or even your rules.

Alyssa's parents found out about her deception the day after she
slept with Josh. What could they do?

They grounded her. "We knew there was a risk in trying to police and repress this," Dave says, "but when she snuck around and went to his house, all hell broke loose."

Alyssa was forbidden from seeing Josh outside of school for a month.

"It was hard because we had just spent this night together. We felt so free, so invincible. Then we had to say, I can't see you. But the grounding gave me time to think of a different way to approach the situation and work things out with my parents."

Right after the grounding lifted, Alyssa and Josh both went on a school trip out of town. "We spent the night together in a hotel room. It was very free. But I didn't completely like being independent, because I felt unsafe. My friends were trying to abuse the freedom. To stay out until three. I was like, no. The reason my parents give me a curfew is because I need sleep. Still, I didn't like being housebound, either. I wanted a middle zone."

Dave had been right; Alyssa did want to be held back. And she also wanted to be let go. It took this family a few months to figure things out, but they did.

"I came home from the trip and told my parents, 'I don't want our relationship to be based on rules. I want it to be based on trust.' Eventually it worked itself out. I told them, 'I need more alone time with Josh.' They discussed it with Josh's parents and decided it would be fine."

If ever there was a time for induction and democracy, for warmth and high expectations, the afternoon your child comes to you and says she is thinking about having sex is it.

If you treat your child with respect, as an independent human being who needs to learn to make her own decisions and take responsibility for them, you will fare as well as possible at a tense time like this. If you present your views as doctrine, without an explanation of why you feel the way you do, and without giving your child the opportunity to express her views, your perspective may not be heard; or if heard, it may be rejected out of hand.

So ask for your child's thoughts on your rules. Give her a chance to weigh in. Consider modifying them if her ideas are reasonable. Or consider developing a set of guidelines together. Will she respond exactly as you hope? Not necessarily. But if she doesn't, you will all have something to talk about.

"Now Josh and I are allowed to be together for a few hours at home after school before my parents get home," Alyssa says. "It isn't open-ended. We know they are coming home soon. So that works out." Alyssa and her folks have found what they all felt was just the right amount of restriction, through what proved to be a fairly productive iterative process.

"You know," Dave says about Alyssa's experience, "it's happened a year or two sooner than I would have wanted, but I'd rather have it now with a kid who respects her than in two years with a jerk. We had a fear that it was going to create a qualitative change in our relationship," he said, "but it really hasn't. It's just another step along a continuum. She didn't make it hurt . . . too much."

Now for an Answer

We've left him hanging, our friend who asked, "How can I teach my daughter to have a healthy attitude toward sex, but prevent her from having any?"

The answer is don't try to prevent her. Just teach her. From the moment she enters your life, try to teach your daughter about her body, about pleasure and responsibility, about love, and about risk, and all the ways people like you and she think about sex.

Teach her how to think for herself and to make her own choices; and when she does, respect those decisions. They may not be yours. They may lead her toward sex when you would like to steer her away. Or they may pull her away from sexual opportunities you think would be good for her. But she gets to decide. All you can do is tell her how you feel, and after years of trying to help her grow into her own woman, realize that you are accomplishing your goal—even though, as Dave and Marisol found, that accomplishment sometimes smarts.

Chapter 9

"But if you do . . ."

THE ART AND SCIENCE OF ENCOURAGING SAFER SEX

Now, we've been following you and your child step by step to her first experience of intercourse since the two of you came home from the maternity ward. But we want to press the pause button right here. Because before your child has sex for the first time, there is something so important to talk about that it deserves its own chapter.

You may think it's fine for your daughter to have sex, or you may have been scouting out chastity belts online. Either way, you certainly don't want her to contract an STD, and you wouldn't want her to get pregnant before she's ready. If you think there's any chance she's going to have sex before marriage, we think she should know about contraception.

We have arrived at the technical part of sexuality. Up to this point, when you talked about dating, love, and sex, you drew on instinct and personal experiences. But with safer sex, you need to know the data. In this chapter, we'll talk about how to think about addressing the matter of contraception with your child. We also provide the details about each method in Appendix A so you'll have the information you need to give informed advice and answer questions.

"Don't—but If You Do . . ."

Let's say you don't want your child to have sex, at least not yet. Should you promote contraception? "If I talk to her about the Pill," you might wonder, "will she think I'm telling her it's okay to start having sex?"

And what about making contraception available? Some parents worry that if their kids have easy access to contraceptives, another barrier to sex will be broken down. They fear their kids will have more sex than if they had to make an effort to arrange protection, and given the failure rates of contraception, they would end up more, not less, likely to get pregnant or catch an infection.

On the other hand, as Stella, who bought her sixteen-year-old son a box of condoms, sees it, "it's not like these kids are so sold on condoms. They'll have sex when they have the opportunity. If a condom's there, they'll use it—I hope. But if it's not there, they're not going to turn down sex. I've made damn sure he knows how to take care of himself when the time comes. The stakes are way too high to ignore this issue."

As far as we can tell, teaching about contraception or making it easily available does not encourage adolescents to engage in sex. But it does appear to make them more likely to use protection when they do have sex. Some scientists even believe that learning about contraception may help to drive home the risks of sex and thereby discourage some teens from having it.

Now, the data to support this point of view are not definitive. We have, for example, evidence derived from studies of high school condom availability programs. These programs, which not only educate teens about condoms but also make them easy to get, have been shown to increase their rate of use by sexually active teens; but in no case, including a study of thirteen thousand students in New York, did the programs increase the rate at which kids became sexually active. Unfortunately, this research doesn't easily translate into what happens between you and your child at home, and the studies themselves have some limitations.

There are also data from studies of parent-child communication about contraception, which find that these talks don't increase the amount of sex adolescents have. Because of their limitations we can't say that these studies are definitive, but we can say that their findings make logical sense, that they correspond with our experience with teens, and that they are accepted as valid by most researchers.

What may make the difference in your child's interpretation of your advice is how you present it. The trick here is to talk about contraception in a way that conveys your reluctance about sex *and* your endorsement of safety. This may already be a familiar conversation for you, the don't-do-this-but-if-you-do-it-do-it-safely talk. (Remember "Don't drink—but if you do drink, don't drive. Call me, and I'll pick you up"?) You are trying to develop in your teenager the ability to make adult decisions, and adult decisions are complex. So your advice will have to be complex, too.

Obviously, you are not planning to toss your kid a box of condoms with a hearty "Have a blast!" You will fit contraception into a larger context. We will get to what methods you can recommend in a few pages, but when you reach the point of explaining how to use a condom, you also can invite him to talk about what sex means, whether it is appropriate for him at all now, and what place it will have in his current relationship. Take a balanced and reasoned approach like this, and we don't think you will have opened the floodgates of promiscuity.

You might try something like this:

> "You know I don't think you're ready to have sex. I think kids should
> wait at least until high school / college / marriage / they're in love. But
> I know that some of your friends are having sex, and you might decide
> to do it, too. So I want to make sure you know about contraception."

"My friends thought I was encouraging him to do it," Stella says. "I've thought about it. Maybe there's some truth to it. I told him he's too young, but who knows if he'll listen. Still, I'd rather take a chance that having condoms makes him a little more likely to have sex than put my head in the sand and think he won't have sex because he doesn't have a condom with him."

Which Method Is Best?

Not only do we think your teenager will benefit if you talk to her about contraception, we think she will be more likely to make wise choices if you help her pick which type to use. It's a complicated decision, and she will likely need advice from someone in the know. She could learn from her friends, her clinician, and the media. But who cares about her more than you do?

The selection of a contraceptive strategy is key. Your child needs to choose a method that works well all—or almost all—of the time. But she also needs to choose a strategy that she's comfortable with so she will use it faithfully, and one that she's capable of using correctly. Even the best contraceptive won't work if it's sitting on the shelf.

How hard is this or that method to use? Has her best friend tried it? Will it affect her pleasure? Her partner's? What are the side effects? How expensive is it? How difficult is it to get? How much planning does it require? You and your teenager can consider all of these issues as you decide which method she is going to make her own.

Let us make the selection process a little simpler for you from the start.

You want your kids to accomplish two things with contraception: to prevent an unintended pregnancy (if their partner is the opposite sex), and to avoid contracting an STD. Only condoms take care of the second goal. Both male and female condoms can significantly reduce (not eliminate) the chance of infection during intercourse, and since the likelihood seems pretty slim that female condoms are going to catch on any time soon (they are more cumbersome and expensive, but not without their benefits), we are going to make the following recommendations.

Your kids should use a condom every time they have intercourse (vaginal or anal).

And they should also use (unlubricated) condoms for fellatio. This one's going to be a challenge. Not many kids (or adults) appear to use condoms for oral sex. Some parents would rather their kids have fellatio without a condom than vaginal intercourse with (or without) a condom. But if you really want your kid to maximally reduce her risk of contracting an STD from fellatio, she should make sure the guy wears a condom.

For boys who are only having sex with boys, pregnancy isn't a concern, so they can stop right there. Condoms are enough: Condoms for anal intercourse and condoms for fellatio. Dental dams can also be used for anilingus. For girls having sex with girls, it's dental dams for cunnilingus and anilingus (the dental dams apply to heterosexual couples as well).

But for everyone else, condoms are not enough.

As they are routinely used by typical people in the real world, condoms fail to prevent pregnancy too often. To give your teenager the best chance of preventing an unintended pregnancy, she will have to combine the condom with one other method. The question to decide is which one.

The Ideal and the Real

One of the most important factors in selecting a contraceptive is determining how effective it is. Easier said than done. If you look hard enough, you can find almost any opinion you want.

Let's shed some light here. There are different types of effectiveness, and for some contraceptives, it depends a lot on the people using them. Also, there are good studies and not-so-good studies.

Sometimes we look at how well a contraceptive works if used perfectly. *Perfect use* means that your son uses it for every act of vaginal intercourse, and he uses it correctly every time.

But who's perfect? It's pretty common to forget to take the Pill every now and then. Or to discover you're out of condoms and tell yourself, "Just this once . . ." Who can say that she never ever left a diaphragm in the drawer because she didn't want to kill the moment? Even those who attend to their contraceptives with the reliability of an Eagle Scout occasionally make mistakes. Like putting the condom on backward, and then turning it around to wear it the right way.

For this reason, it's also crucial to know the success rate of a contraceptive in the case of *typical use*—what we can expect from the average person who occasionally makes mistakes and doesn't always follow instructions.

When picking a method, you and your teenager should first try to determine whether you think she would be closer to a perfect user or a typical user. Many adolescents are much closer to typical users, often falling on the more erratic side of typical. But that doesn't mean your

What About the Church?

> *Our religion is a very big part of what I say to them. We're Catholic. It's what I believe. I really want them to know that it's not okay to have a child without being married. . . . That is 100 percent because of my religious beliefs. I do believe in the Pill. I don't believe abortion belongs in government. It is not out of the question should one of the girls get pregnant. I'm a realistic and practical person.*
>
> —*Valerie, on her daughters*

If your religion proscribes premarital sex or contraception, you have an extra challenge when it comes to your kid's sexual life. Many of the parents we speak with are working on how to square, as Valerie saw it, a desire to be "practical" with a wish to respect their religion.

"When I say it out loud, it sounds so hypocritical. But does anyone really agree with all the church's teachings?" Gina asked. "I love the church. I go every Sunday. Am I a bad person because I had sex before I got married? I've told my daughter about condoms, because she needs to know these things. Look, you have to make compromises."

Some parents don't believe that there's anything to compromise about. Martha explains: "I don't know why I'd ever talk about birth control. It's just not relevant. My sons will not have sex before they get married. I know that because that's the way I raised them. They've gone to church since they were little. You teach them to avoid certain situations and what happens if you give in. If they asked about condoms, we'd find out why and explain that condoms are wrong."

Of course, there are ways to avoid pregnancy without contraception. We talked about abstinence in Chapter 8, and

Appendix A covers the periodic abstinence (or rhythm) method, although we can't recommend it for any but the most mature teens. Its demands are too great for most kids, who have unstable relationships and impulsive encounters, and it does nothing to prevent STDs.

daughter can't be a perfect user. Is there evidence that she could remember to take a pill every day without fail?

Does she floss every day?

Does she wear a seat belt every time she's in a car?

Does she turn in her homework on time?

If she hasn't demonstrated that she can be responsible about other personal habits, a contraceptive practice that requires remembering to do something every day or to plan in advance may be out of reach.

Reading the Rates

We have included a table on page 263 with success rates for each contraceptive method. Here's how to read it. Each method is followed by two percentages, one indicating the unintended pregnancy rate for a year of perfect use, the other for a year of typical use. These rates assume that unless a couple's method is abstinence, they are having vaginal intercourse eighty-three times per year, which is, in fact, the national average for all married adult women. Whether your teen has more or less sex than this, she is likely to be more fertile and less experienced with contraception than the average adult. It's not clear whether these figures are over- or underestimates for adolescents like her. But it's the best information we've got, and it's quite useful for comparing how well the different options work.

Let's look at what the table says about diaphragm use, as an example. With perfect use, 6 percent of women using the diaphragm as their only means of birth control for a year would get pregnant. Say there are

What Her Friends Are Using

In 1997, most ninth to twelfth graders who had sexual intercourse during the prior three months used some form of contraception the last time they had intercourse. Over half (57
percent) used a condom, 17 percent used the Pill, 13 percent
used withdrawal, 4 percent used another method, 15 percent
used no contraception, and 2 percent were not sure whether
they or their partner used contraception. (If they used condoms and another method, both were counted; if they used
more than one method other than condoms, the most effective one got the credit.)

Contraception use is higher among older teens. Older
girls are more likely to use the Pill but less likely to use condoms. Sex tends to become more frequent and regular, which
makes the Pill more practical. And older teens may find it easier to get to a clinician for a prescription.

But the decline in condom use as kids grow older
increases their STD risk. Condom use also declines as a relationship persists and if it is monogamous. Yet teen monogamy
is often serial monogamy, and not many adolescents (or
adults) get an STD checkup between partners.

100 couples using diaphragms for a year, and each couple has intercourse
the average number of times (83). That means 83 × 100 total acts of
intercourse, or 8,300 acts for all of the couples. That's a lot of intercourse. Out of those 8,300 acts, there would be 6 pregnancies, or about
1 pregnancy for every 1,383 acts of intercourse.

But that's with perfect use. With typical use, 16 percent of couples
will have a pregnancy over the course of a year. Why? Well, diaphragms
sometimes slip, but most of the shortfall occurs because people don't
always use them: the statistic includes women who say that the
diaphragm is their contraceptive but who don't use it all the time.

So here's what you need to ask—or rather, what your daughter needs to ask herself: Will she use a diaphragm every time? Will she use it correctly? Is she a 6 percent or a 16 percent kind of kid?

Finally, the principles of the ideal and the real apply to abstinence as well. Although abstinence from sexual activity (or at least abstinence from sexual activity that involves sperm getting anywhere near the vagina) clearly has a perfect use rate of 0%, its typical use rate is not known, but it's almost certainly not good. We don't know how often kids who choose to be abstinent wind up having sex anyway—and how many of them get pregnant. As we discussed in Chapter 8, kids who plan for abstinence and unexpectedly have sex may not be prepared with contraception.

Belts and Suspenders

As we see it, your teenager who is having intercourse will do best if she uses the "belt and suspenders" strategy for STD prevention and contraception (pregnancy prevention). Her condoms (every time!) are her belt, providing her STD prevention and contributing to preventing pregnancy. For her contraceptive suspenders, she has a choice of whichever method makes the most sense to her.

To complement the condom, the main methods we recommend (besides abstinence from intercourse) are hormonal methods (such as oral contraceptives and the myriad other ways of getting the hormones into the body) or female barrier methods (such as the diaphragm or the cap), although the latter have been much less popular with adolescents. As the accompanying table shows, hormonal methods are the most dependable, with perfect use pregnancy rates of less than 1 percent and typical use rates that are among the best. The IUD is also very effective, but we don't generally recommend it for teens (we explain why in Appendix A). Nor do we recommend sterilization, for obvious reasons.

Your child will get closer to perfect use with a contraceptive she finds easy to use, so it makes sense to think about which of these methods is easiest. The answer largely depends on your teen and her preferences. The diaphragm isn't too hard to put in (although some girls don't

Method	Typical Use	Perfect Use
Percentage of women experiencing an unintended pregnancy during the first year of typical use and the first year of perfect use of contraception		
No Contraception	85%	85%
Abstinence (from vaginal intercourse*)	?	0%
Condom, male (without spermicide)	15%	2%
Condom, female (without spermicide)	21%	5%
Oral contraceptive pills (The Pill)**	8%	0.3%
Depo-Provera (the injectable)	3%	0.3%
Lunelle (the injectable)	3%	0.05%
Norplant (the implant)	0.05%	0.05%
NuvaRing (the ring)	8%	0.3%
Ortho Evra (the patch)	8%	0.3%
Spermicide (cream, film, foam, jelly/gel, suppository)	29%	15%
Diaphragm (with spermicidal cream or jelly)	16%	6%
Cap (with spermicidal cream or jelly)		
Women who have been pregnant before	32%	26%
Women who have never been pregnant before	16%	9%
Withdrawal	27%	4%
Periodic abstinence (rhythm method)	25%	
Calendar method		9%
Cervical secretions (ovulation) method		3%
Sympto-thermal***	2%	
IUD		
ParaGard (copper T)	0.8%	0.6%
Progestasert (progesterone T)	2%	1.5%
Mirena (LNg IUS)	0.1%	0.1%

Method	Typical Use	Perfect Use
Sterilization		
Female sterilization	0.5%	0.5%
Male sterilization	0.15%	0.10%

*or from other activity in which sperm get near the vagina
**includes combined pills and progestin-only pills (minipills)
***a combination of the cervical secretions, calendar, and basal body temperature methods
Adapted from Hatcher et al., *Contraceptive Technology,* 18th rev. ed. (New York: Ardent Media, 2003). This is an excellent and thorough text on contraception.

like the idea of inserting it in their vagina) and even the cap, which some find more difficult, can be managed, but they don't work unless you use them. Your daughter has to remember to take one of them with her. If she has sex often, inserting a diaphragm may start to seem like a nuisance; or she may get so quick with it that she doesn't even give it a second thought. Barrier methods are probably best for a girl who doesn't like taking a hormonal contraceptive (because of fear of side effects, for example) or who doesn't have intercourse often and so doesn't want to use a contraceptive that's working round the clock in her body.

If she opts for the Pill, on the other hand, your daughter won't have to worry about having it with her or fussing with it at the moment of truth. On the other hand, some kids might have a harder time with the consistency the Pill demands. If she has sex only rarely, the daily effort required to remember to take a pill may not seem worth it.

Notice, though, that the typical use rates for Depo-Provera, Lunelle, and Norplant are very close to their perfect use rates. Once you've got the injection or the implant, you can't mess up. Yes, you have to remember to repeat your Depo or Lunelle shot on schedule (every three months or one month, respectively), but that's not nearly as hard as remembering to take a pill every day. These are the methods we recommend for teenagers who have sex frequently and who have a hard time keeping focused on the mundane but critical details of prevention.

The patch and the ring are so new that we don't yet know how teens will take to them, but given that they only need to be replaced once a week, it's possible they'll be a good compromise between a daily pill and a monthly shot. Your daughter should check for the latest information.

As we discuss in Appendix A, nonoxynol-9, the main spermicide available in the United States (in the form of creams, films, foams, jellies/gels, suppositories, and tablets), doesn't provide protection against HIV and may even increase the chances of catching HIV or other STDs, especially if it is used a lot. Therefore, we don't consider it a preferred suspenders to use with condoms, although (because it does contribute to pregnancy prevention) it's usually better than no suspenders at all. Still, nonoxynol-9 is best reserved for use with a diaphragm or cap.

Check out Appendix A for the facts about each method so you can decide which ones you want to recommend. And also encourage your daughter to talk with her clinician for guidance on which methods will be best for her.

"Mom, the Condom Broke": Emergency Contraception

Even if you've talked through the issues of contraception with your daughter, and even if she and her partner planned in advance, accidents can happen. Condoms break, diaphragms become dislodged, and girls who swore they would wait until next year suddenly find themselves smoking the proverbial cigarette and wondering how they ever lost control.

If your daughter finds herself in such a situation, she could use emergency contraception (EC), a catchall name for several methods that prevent pregnancy after vaginal intercourse and that are more commonly, but not altogether accurately, known as the morning-after pill. EC neither needs to be taken by the next morning nor consists of a single pill. For that matter, it doesn't necessarily come in the form of a pill at all. (We describe the specific types of EC in Appendix A.)

The standard approach to EC involves taking hormone pills—the same type of hormones that are in oral contraceptive pills but in a much higher dose. EC may work in several ways. If your daughter takes the pills before she ovulates, they may stop or delay her ovulation so that the egg won't be fertilized with sperm. If she has already ovulated, the pills may inhibit the egg or sperm from moving through the fallopian tube, inhibit fertilization, or inhibit implantation. But they do not appear to disrupt or harm an established pregnancy (a fertilized egg that has already implanted).

Your daughter will take two doses twelve hours apart, and she needs to take the first dose within seventy-two hours of having intercourse. Sooner is better. If she takes the second dose a little early or a little late, it's probably fine. If it's soon after intercourse, timing the first dose so that she doesn't have to wake up in the middle of the night for the second dose is probably fine, too. Even after seventy-two hours have passed since intercourse, the pills may still prevent some pregnancies, although there's little research to show how well.

EC pills require a prescription, although the medical community is encouraging the Food and Drug Administration (FDA) to make them available over the counter. Your daughter can talk with her clinician about getting a prescription to hold onto just in case she needs EC some day.

You may fear that EC will make your daughter more likely to take chances. The studies show that giving women EC to keep just in case does not discourage them from using their regular contraception. Nevertheless, your daughter should know that the success rate of EC is significantly lower than the rates for the Pill, the diaphragm, or the condom. So EC is not recommended as a form of regular birth control. Also, it doesn't protect against STDs.

If your child or your child's partner ends up needing EC, there's clearly something to talk about. You may want to discuss why their regular contraception failed or why they didn't use any. Obviously, as hard as it may be, it's wiser to ask gently (*"I'm sure this is upsetting. What do you think happened?"* or *"Had you considered using contraception?"*) than to accuse (*"What the hell were you thinking?"*). Sometimes adolescents have done everything just right — they stored the condom correctly, checked the expiration date, and so on — and it just broke. Other times they ignored their better judgment, possibly under the influence of alcohol or a manipulative partner. Regardless, your child will probably be doing her own soul-searching. It may be easier to have a productive discussion after the immediate fear and any side effects have passed.

One possibility, easily forgotten in the race to get EC, is that your daughter didn't use contraception because she wanted to get pregnant or wasn't sure. Even if that wasn't her goal, the sudden possibility that she could be on the verge of a pregnancy might arouse mixed emotions. Time is precious, but discussions with you or others, including a counselor, could help her figure out what she really wants. She should feel comfortable with her decision to take EC. If it is your son whose partner is considering EC, he may be having similar feelings.

Teaching Your Teenager About Contraception

And now, it's time for a little talk.

Perhaps your child will invite you in for an intimate discussion about contraception. Charu's did. Sort of.

"I was walking by Ray's room—he was fourteen then—and I heard something like 'You pull out right before you come, but if you aren't fast enough, she can douche.' I swung open the door and blurted out, 'You've got to be kidding. That's not even close!' I wasn't even sure who was in there with him. It was, to my horror, my younger son, Joey, who was twelve. Then came the cover-up: 'We were just joking,' 'We were practicing lines from a play.' "

Charu once taught eighth grade.

"I told them to make a list of the top ten ways to prevent getting a girl pregnant, and then we'd talk about it. I came back a while later. The list included condoms and the Pill, and that was it for real methods. I could tell I had my afternoon cut out for me. We disposed of the withdrawal method rather quickly. Having sex after masturbating—to use up your sperm—crossed that one off, too. It never occurred to them that you could refrain from intercourse and do other things instead. They'd never heard of diaphragms or much else. Ray believed that a girl couldn't get pregnant her first time. We definitely talked through the logic of that one."

If you are lucky enough to be presented with an opening like this for a talk about contraception, seize it. It will spare you the awkwardness of having to bring the discussion up artificially. Then again, awkwardness may not be an issue if you get as frightened as Belle did.

"I was reading an article about a teenager who had the AIDS virus, and I was thinking how sad that was. It didn't seem related to my life at all, just sad. Then it said that he wanted to be an architect, which is what Corey wanted to be at the time. And it hit me that this boy in the article was only a year older than Corey. When Corey got home, I didn't waste any time. I told him to get in the car and I took him to the drugstore, and we went through the condom section."

Belle had Corey pick out three types of condoms, which they took home, opened, and stretched over a cucumber. "I told him he could do the live demonstration on his own."

Afterward, Belle felt reassured that she had gotten her message across. "He could see the concern I had without my having to lecture him. I didn't say 'don't you dare' or 'you'd better listen to me.' I know my son—a lecture would have turned him off completely. But he understood how serious this was."

You may not need to make a special effort to start a contraception discussion if you've been open all along. Tex and his wife created a lifetime of learning opportunities for their kids.

"I don't get what the big deal is," Tex says. "You just present contraception as a part of life when they're growing up. We don't hide my wife's pills. They're on the counter. When they've asked what they're for, my wife's told them. She had to go off them for a while, so we used condoms. The box was next to the bed. My kids are growing up taking it for granted that if you have sex, you use contraception, unless you're trying to have a baby. It's just a given."

When to Talk

The goal is to introduce the subject of contraception before your child is likely to have sex. You want your child to use contraception the very first time he has sex (unless he's already with a healthy spouse or partner, and if the partner's the opposite sex, ready to have a child). Using contraception for the first time can set a good pattern for the future. It's easier to begin with good habits than to break bad ones.

Waiting until you think your child needs the information can be tricky. It's so easy to guess wrong. Many parents, if they talk to their kids about sex at all, start long after the kids have become sexually involved.

The best approach is to time your talk to puberty, a milestone that's impossible to miss.

Before he reaches puberty, you can say a few words if contraception comes up. Answer his questions in a clear, simple way. If he finds your Ortho-Novum in the medicine cabinet, you can explain that you use it for making love because it's not the right time for you to have another baby. If he's interested in understanding more, you can add that the pills temporarily stop you from releasing an egg that could get fertilized and grow into a baby.

Once he reaches puberty, you can discuss contraception in more detail. If you believe in the use of contraception, present it as a routine part of sex whenever sex comes up. If you don't support its use, you can explain that some people use it for premarital sex or for sex within a marriage, and then explain why you don't approve of it.

Then as soon as group dates, flirting on the phone, or scented notes begin, it's time to provide specific details about the contraceptive options. If you get an eager listener, now is a good time to help her make a decision about what she will want to use. Share what you have learned, then encourage her to investigate. She needs to learn how well the methods work, what's involved with using them, and what the side effects are. She can talk to her clinician and to friends to see what they prefer. If she has a partner, they should filter all this through their own values and preferences and see what works for them.

Weighing the Risks

It is often said that adolescents consider themselves invulnerable, that they don't think bad things can happen to them. That's a bit simplistic. Teens don't routinely jump off buildings. But there seems to be some truth to the notion that they don't always consider the consequences of their actions, particularly if the consequences are not immediate. They may not be good at understanding probabilities, either, so they might not be able to evaluate the difference between "likely" and "definitely" or "rarely" and "never."

But each adolescent is an individual. You know how yours thinks and whether he makes careful decisions. We think it's a good idea to help your son think about consequences in a realistic way. "If you have sex without a condom, you'll get AIDS" isn't going to work if his friends don't use condoms and don't seem to have gotten HIV. (Of course, people can go years without symptoms, so his friends might not know that they have it.) If you tell him his girlfriend will get pregnant if they have sex, and they've already had sex without her getting pregnant, they might decide they must be infertile or protected in some special, supernatural way.

Be honest. Tell your daughter she won't necessarily get pregnant any one time, but she might. The important thing is for her to understand that if she routinely has sex without an effective contraceptive, she stands a good chance of getting pregnant. Even if she uses a condom, there's still a chance—but it's a lot, lot less.

Similarly, teens may need help thinking about the chain of events that can be set in motion after they make a decision. They may think more about the short-term impact of having sex ("He'll love me more" or "This is going to feel so good") than about the impact over the rest of their lives if they get pregnant. If they think sex without a condom isn't so bad because they can just take antibiotics or have an abortion, have they thought about what happens if their partner doesn't want an abortion? What happens if they don't get any symptoms so they don't know they need an antibiotic? What if they catch something that antibiotics can't cure?

Even if your teenager is aware of the risks of pregnancy or STDs, in the moment, those risks might seem less important when balanced against the absolute promise of immediate gratification or the embarrassment of figuring out how to put on a condom for the first time. That's why preparing in advance—deciding how he wants to handle enticing offers, learning about contraception, and so on—is so important.

Practice Makes Perfect

Whatever type of contraception your teenager decides to use, she needs to use it correctly. That means she needs to practice before she finds herself caught up in the heat of the moment. If she's never inserted her diaphragm except for the test run in the clinician's office, will she do it correctly while her boyfriend's scrambling to get his pants off? If he's never put on a condom, will he figure it out the night he loses his virginity?

If you want your child to use contraception properly, teach him how. Hey, would you let him borrow the car without teaching him to drive first?

In case you're a little rusty on your condom skills, or never learned, we have included a set of instructions (see page 272). You can buy a box with your son or daughter and figure out together how they work. Have him put two fingers together and roll a condom over them. Or pick up a zucchini and show him how it's done. He can try blowing it up like a balloon to see just how strong it is. If he happens to get one that breaks, use it as a lesson that they're not foolproof.

If he insists, "Of course I know how to use a condom," let him show you. Have him put one on a banana with his eyes closed, as if he's in a dark room. He can start by taking it out of the package. (Getting the condom out of the wrapper isn't always easy, and he needs to learn how to do it without tearing the condom.) Make sure he unrolls it correctly. If he tries to put it on the banana inside out, tell him to throw it out and start over. He should also practice on his penis, on his own time. If he's smart, or a little horny, he'll take the hint to masturbate with it on to see how it feels.

Practice. Practice. Practice.

Vince didn't have to ask his sixteen-year-old son. "I was taking out the trash, and I noticed a condom. I couldn't believe it. It was there, clearly used." Vince had mixed feelings. "I was kind of happy for him. I was never bold enough when I was his age to go all the way. But there was something about him doing it in the house that bothered me." He confronted his son, who informed him that he had never had sex. He'd been masturbating with a condom to see what it was like. "I guess that's what happens when a straight-A student discovers sex."

After the condom incident, there was more of a dialogue between Vince and his son. "Once you've stumbled into discussing masturbation with your kid, there's nothing left to hide. So now he asks me for advice about sex."

The same goes for diaphragms, caps, and rings. If you don't know how to insert one (and we have no appropriate piece of fruit to propose learning on), your daughter's clinician can teach her (and you). Just make sure she understands what her clinician said.

Taking a pill requires no particular technical know-how, but remembering to take it can be a challenge. You might give your daughter some tips, like tying pill taking to some part of her routine she never forgets, like taking out her contacts or brushing her teeth.

Confronting Your Kid's Resistance

Of course, even teenagers who know which contraception to use, and are proficient in how to use it, have been known to leave the little miracle of modern science sitting in a drawer. There are as many reasons kids don't use contraception as there are kids. Here are some reasons you might hear, and some responses you can try:

"She'd only slept with one other guy before me." Ask him how many people that first guy had slept with. And is he looking to become a father.

"He was the valedictorian, so I wasn't worried." Remind her that little gonococci and hepatitis B virions are equal-opportunity infectors.

"I didn't want my parents to know, but I had no other way to get to the doctor." If you've discussed contraception with your child, you've already taken a major step toward overcoming this common stumbling block. Tell her you'll make a doctor's appointment and then offer to stay in the waiting room.

"I wasn't planning on having sex that night." If your child has been sexually active or is considering having sex, tell him to make sure that he has contraception with him when going out with his girlfriend or boyfriend. Some kids don't want to prepare because they feel conflicted about having sex or they worry what others will think if they are found carrying contraception. If your daughter feels shy about admitting that she's got a condom in her bag, she can explain, if anyone asks, that she always takes it with her, whether or not she hopes to have sex. That way, she'll have it when she needs it, whether that's next week or next decade.

How to Use a Condom

1. Check the expiration date. If the condom has expired, don't use it.

2. Make sure the package isn't damaged. Store condoms in a cool, dry place, away from direct sunlight. Yes, you can put some in the glove compartment before a date, but bring in the extras afterward. You can store one in a wallet for a little while, but over time, the latex will wear out. If there is any doubt about how it has been stored, throw it out.

3. Open the package just before using the condom. Be careful not to tear it.

4. Unroll the condom directly onto the erect penis. Do not unroll it before putting it on. Do not fill it with air or water to check for holes; this can make it more likely to break. A few drops of lubricant inside the condom can increase sensation. But be sparing. Too much lubricant can make the condom slip off. Put it on before the penis gets near the vulva, the anus, or the mouth. If the penis is uncircumcised, pull the foreskin back before putting the condom on.

5. If the condom has a reservoir tip, pinch the air out before putting it on. If there is no reservoir, squeeze the end of the condom to create a pocket that can fill with ejaculate. Condoms are strong enough that they'll probably be fine even if you don't squeeze, but why take chances?

6. When unrolling a condom, the ring should be on the outside, facing away from the skin of the penis. Roll it all the way down to the base of the penis or as far as it will go. If it goes on inside out, don't redo it. Discard it. It may have come in contact with sperm, bacteria, or a virus.

7. Only use water-based lubricants with latex condoms, because oil-based lubricants will break down the latex. Oil is fine with polyurethane (plastic) condoms.

8. If the condom breaks or falls off during intercourse but before ejaculation, replace it.

9. While withdrawing the penis after intercourse, hold the base of the condom in place so that it does not come off. The condom will be less likely to come off if you pull out while still erect.

10. Never reuse a condom. Throw it out in a safe manner where a child won't find it.

She can make it quite clear that it's neither an invitation nor a guarantee, just a safeguard. She can also blame it on you: "Dad doesn't let me go on a date without protection."

"I don't like the way it feels." Your son wouldn't be the first to say that condoms decrease sensation, although some consider it an advantage because they don't ejaculate as quickly. Tell him to try different brands. A small amount of lubricant inside the condom can help. But if it still doesn't feel as good, it's a trade-off. Outside of a lengthy and reliably monogamous relationship (not exactly the hallmark of adolescence), not using a condom means risking an STD. For boys who have trouble maintaining erections with a condom, switching to the female condom is an option. A diaphragm that doesn't fit right can be uncomfortable, too. Let your daughter know that it can be refitted. As for hormonal contraceptives, if she is troubled by side effects, she should talk with her clinician about changing the dose or selecting another brand.

"It kills the moment to stop to put on a condom or insert a diaphragm." We have two answers to this. First, yes, it does interfere in a moment of wild abandon, but as your son may have learned when he was four and you found him masturbating in the supermarket, sexual pleasure comes with rules and responsibilities. The second answer is, don't think of it as an interruption. Eroticize it. Your son's partner can put the condom on him or sexually stimulate him while he puts it on himself.

"I've heard they can mess you up." There seems to be a steady flow of sci-fi rumors about contraception: Norplant rods migrating through the body; diaphragms vanishing into the uterus. When your child hears of something that happened to a "friend of a friend," she should have some healthy skepticism. It can take a lot of factual information to convince her that such rumors are not true. Keep in mind, though, that these stories take hold for a reason. There is something scary about taking a medication or putting an object in your body, especially when you don't really understand how it works. Even more so when you're being discreet about it and don't feel you can talk with your regular clinician or your family.

"It's his responsibility."

"It's too hard to get, and it costs too much."

Let's spend some time on these last two.

Whose Responsibility Is It?

Adolescents often assume that the boy brings the condoms and the girl takes care of anything else. Let's change that. Let's say from here on out they both take care of everything.

"My friend thought it was odd that I was telling my daughter that she had to have condoms with her when she went out with her boyfriend. She said, 'That's the boy's job.' I said, 'His job is to get lucky.' " Miriam, whose daughter is sixteen, has a sense of her role, too. "My job is to make sure she knows how to look after herself. She's the one who's going to get pregnant. She'd better do whatever she can to protect herself. I don't allow any damsel-in-distress BS in my home."

The bottom line is that they should both bring the condom. (Actually, they should both bring more than one since condoms can break.) Or they should both discuss that they aren't going to have sex until they are ready to take responsibility for using contraception and using it properly.

Unfortunately, things aren't always that simple. Your daughter may want to use condoms, but she may find that the boy refuses. Tell her to anticipate some resistance, which she should try to explore should it come up. It may be that her partner doesn't know how to put on a con-

Having a Comeback

If your teenager is worried that his or her partner will say no to contraception, you can try role-playing a scene together. You be the date.

Throw her a curveball: "What? Don't you trust me? I'm clean." She can answer, "Well, I'm certainly not going to trust you now. You may be clean, but you don't know if I am. So what if you got something from me and gave it to your next girlfriend? And what if you got something from your last girlfriend and gave it to me?"

When he says, "I'm too big for condoms," she can say, "Sounds like you're too big for me. If you can manage to squeeze yourself into a condom, then I'll know you're the right size." Or, if she's feeling more generous, she can say, "We'll get you the extra-large variety."

When she says, "Don't worry. It's not my fertile time, and I'll get an abortion if anything happens," he can say, "The fertile time isn't so exact, and what if you change your mind about an abortion. I don't take chances like that." Or he could say, "That's fine for you, but I'm not comfortable with abortion. I know it would be your choice, but I wouldn't want you to have one, so we'd better take precautions or just do something else."

When he says, "I've never had sex with a guy before," he can say, "I haven't either, but it's not worth taking any chances. It's easier and safer to just use a condom every time."

When she says, "But I love you," he can say, "If you loved me, you wouldn't pressure me to do something I'm not comfortable with."

When he says, "I'm leaving for the front tomorrow, and I might never return," she can say, "I don't sleep with guys who steal their lines from World War II movies."

dom, or that he's been told that real men don't use them. She can work through these issues with him.

True, your daughter can't make the boy use a condom. All too many girls fear they will be rejected if they say no to sex without a condom, and they're not willing to break up over that. Girls will often put up with a lot in a relationship—boys will, too, although not usually over contraception—but this accommodation involves taking a serious risk for her health and her future. At the least, she can protect herself from pregnancy with the Pill or another female-controlled contraceptive method—often surreptitiously. Needless to say, a girl in this situation needs to do some real soul-searching about what is best for her. You can help by trying to talk with her about her priorities in a relationship.

We talk about abuse and power relationships in Chapters 8 and 10, and about how to deal with the boyfriend you don't like in Chapter 7, but the first step in empowering your children is to give them the information they need to decide what's best for themselves. Teach your sons and daughters how to treat others well and how to look after themselves. And intervene if you feel your child is being put at serious risk—love, and dependency, can be blind.

Who's Going to Get It?

Of course I gave my son condoms. I don't want him getting a girl pregnant. It doesn't matter whether he uses these or gets his own. It means he's on notice. He has no excuse for not using condoms.

—*Clint, on his sixteen-year-old son*

Time to get practical. Who's going to get the contraception? Kids can't use it if they can't get ahold of any, and getting ahold of it isn't always easy for a teenager.

Some forms of contraception require a prescription, which means going to a clinician. Does your daughter have a way to get to her clinician, especially if she's afraid or embarrassed to tell you? Can she get to a clinic by bus? Is there a clinic at her school, and did you sign the consent form for her to get care there? Better to avoid all this subterfuge by working out with your child in advance just how she is going to get the goods.

Get as involved in this process as feels comfortable for you and your child. You can make the appointment with the clinician or just give her the number. Drive her there or lend her the car. Pick up her prescription at the pharmacy or remind her to do it. The challenge is to show your support, give her the privacy she needs, and most important, make sure the job gets done.

Condoms don't require a prescription, but that doesn't mean they're

---

Condoms and Clinics at School

Some high schools make free condoms regularly available on campus.

There are those who contend that condom availability programs create a sexually permissive atmosphere at school. Students will think, they maintain, that their teachers and administrators are endorsing teen sex. However, the few studies on condom programs, although they have some scientific limitations, have indicated that the programs do not increase sexual intercourse but do increase condom use among some sexually active students. If anything, rather than create an atmosphere of free love, they seem to encourage more restrained attitudes about sex, probably by increasing awareness of and discussion about AIDS, STDs, and pregnancy.

Some schools go even further by offering teen health clinics on (or near) campus that offer all sorts of health care, including providing contraception and testing for STDs and pregnancy. School clinics can make it easier for adolescents to get care without the typical impediments of cost, access, and privacy. Consent from you is almost invariably required for use of reproductive health services.

School personnel may also have a lot to offer. School nurses, guidance counselors, and school psychologists can provide advice to you and your kid. The sweet old nurse who looks like your grandmother may keep a stash of maps to the local Planned Parenthood clinic next to the immunization cards and Band-Aids. School librarians may help your teenager find some useful books or direct your child to some good websites. Favorite teachers and coaches can also be a resource, as can school administrators.

Some schools also offer relevant extracurricular activities. There may be an organized group of students who teach other students about HIV and sexual risk prevention, based on the notion that peer educators' appeals may be especially compelling and credible to kids. Studies show that these programs can be effective, particularly for the peer educators themselves. Not a bad reason for your kid to sign up.

easy to get. It can be embarrassing for your kid to buy them. Even if a clerk is daydreaming about her vacation, your son may be sure he saw her smirk when she price-scanned his condoms. You know he's terrified she'll blurt into the PA system, "Price check on Trojans, twelve-pack. Ribbed."

Some pharmacies keep the condoms behind the counter, so your kid will have to ask for them. This helps prevent shoplifting—not uncommon for a pocket-size product people feel embarrassed to purchase—but it also discourages adolescents and shy adults from buying them. Most pharmacists will take their job seriously and provide contraceptives in a professional manner and possibly offer advice on proper use. But your daughter may get one who takes it upon himself to give her a lecture about why she's too young to have sex.

Which leads us to an important question: Should you provide condoms yourself?

If you feel torn about what to do, you are not alone. Again, you may fear that giving your teenager condoms is sending a permissive message. It may reassure you to know, as we discuss on the next page, that condom availability programs in schools have been shown not to make teens more likely to have intercourse.

Then there is the issue of boundaries. How comfortable do you feel participating in this part of his life? Not everyone wants to get so involved in the specifics of their child's sex life.

If you have resolved these questions, you next face the fact that somebody has to pay for this stuff.

Should you pay, let your kid foot the bill, or split the cost with him? If you pay for everything else, this may be one more item on the list. If your son has a job that covers some expenses, perhaps this should be one of them. Even if you don't approve of his having sex, you might want to pay anyway to make sure he's got protection; or you might feel he needs to take responsibility and pay for it himself.

Louisa is nonchalant about buying her daughter condoms: "What's the big deal? I just ask what she needs, and I buy it. It's no different from her maxipads and conditioner. And if she's going to the store, she picks up whatever I need. Isn't that why we're so glad when they get their license? Then they can drive to the store, too."

Louisa adds: "Am I happy she's having sex? No. Am I happy she uses condoms? You'd better believe it."

The Protection Perspective

When it comes to stopping the spread of STDs and preventing unintended pregnancies, sex really can be made much safer. Having read this far, you now know how to help your kid master that task. And so this seems like a good time to point out one more thing. Stopping the spread of STDs is a compelling goal, of course, but that doesn't mean that sex needs to be cleaned up in some broader sense. Your child can and should diminish the risks of unintended pregnancy that come with intercourse, but that doesn't mean that the sex she has shouldn't or won't feel risky in other ways. Because sex isn't only about safety.

Paying attention to sexual protection is a practical approach to one aspect of sex that calls out for practicality—an arena in which caution, planning, and predictability are not only beneficial but essential. But as a point of view on sexuality as a whole, the protection perspective will only illuminate one corner of what your teen is going to discover.

Even with all the germs taken care of and the sperm neatly segregated from the eggs, your child's discovery of sex, whether on a first date or on his or her wedding night, is bound to be messy, imperfect, and unpredictable. Hopefully, that's the way it will be the next time and the next time and the times after that. And hopefully, that will be part of the fun.

Chapter **10**

And so it begins

PARENTING YOUR SEXUALLY ACTIVE CHILD,

FROM THE FIRST TIME ON

It's happening.

It's happening right now while you are reviewing the quarterly sales report you've been waiting all day to get your hands on. Fiddling with a paragraph, you have a vague sense that you left the chicken in the freezer. You consider asking your daughter to start defrosting it, but she's at tennis practice. You'll pick up something on the way home. You'll finish this first.

Your daughter isn't at practice.

Did you know that the first time a teenager has intercourse, it is more likely to be in the summer than at another time of year? Did you know that girls are more likely than boys to consider themselves in love with their first sex partner?

Lately your daughter has seemed pretty taken with a boy in the tennis league. She was telling you last week how interesting he is, how he has been teaching her about philosophy. She seemed sad that he'll be heading back to college at the end of the summer. There was something in the way she looked when she described him, you remember while waiting for the printer to spit out the pages, that made you think they might be having sex.

You were right.

It's happening right now in his bedroom, for the first time.

Did you know that most girls' first time is with a boy one to three years older than they are? That boys are more likely to first have sex with someone their own age or younger?

Did you know that your daughter has been planning this for about a month?

Did you need to know? Did you *want* to know?

Here you are in the office, finishing something important to you, and there she is at her boyfriend's, starting something important to her; and though you don't know what's happening, you have had seventeen years of telling her everything you wanted her to know and listening to every little thought that popped out of her head. She's about to start her senior year of high school, and you're already getting used to the fact that you don't keep tabs on each other like you used to.

Should you? Could you?

How would you know? This is a first time for both of you.

The First Time

"Jessie was fifteen, and she had had a boyfriend for a year," Liz explains. "I suspected that they would probably be getting intimate at some point. I picked her up from his house one day, and I just looked at her and I knew. I asked her, 'Did you have sex with Chris today?' She was mortified. She said 'How did you know?' "

How *did* she know?

"I can't tell you. It was just the way she looked at me. Maybe the way she avoided my gaze. I just knew."

How did she feel?

"It scared the shit out of me."

If it had been your daughter asking, "How did you know?" two hours after she first had sex, how would you feel?

Maybe you'd be fine about it. Maybe you'd think it's great that she has had this experience. Or maybe you support, in theory, the idea of teens having sex, but there's something about your own daughter doing it that jars you.

Maybe you are opposed to the whole concept of sex before marriage or sex before adulthood, and you would have felt devastated or furious if it had been your daughter.

Or maybe it's already been you, and you know exactly how you felt.

When she was sixteen, Candy came home at three in the morning to find her mother waiting up, fuming. When Candy said yes, she did have sex, and no, she didn't think it was any of her mother's business, her mother, seized with rage, swept Candy up in her arms, all 105 pounds of her, held her suspended in a moment of utter perplexity, and then dropped her on the couch. It was the only thing she could think of doing.

Some parents throw their kids out of the house, stunned that their child could have so utterly repudiated their values. The prospects for these kids can be grim. Some parents leave home themselves—not literally, but they retreat into a kind of wounded silence. They can't put their complicated feelings into words.

Marty could, at least when talking about his daughter Heather.

"When Heather was dating a guy at school—she was fifteen or sixteen—I had to be informed by my wife that she had had sex with him. I was a little upset at first—I kind of wanted to pull my hat down around my ears and not hear about it."

What exactly was that feeling?

"Loss of innocence as the father, my loss, because there is suddenly an adult sexuality. Watching her blossom into a young woman and the awareness that seems to go with that, you kind of block it out and you hope she makes intelligent decisions and you try to shield her from making adult choices. And then all of a sudden she has made that choice. If you ever thought about it, you knew it was inevitable. But for me, there is just a loss of innocence."

For Marty, that wasn't all.

"Heather has been overweight. That has limited her opportunities. One of my concerns was that being overweight, she would have less of an ability to find love or loving, and that included sex. When I heard, I had all of those other feelings, but I also had a twinge of relief that—this may sound bizarre—she had at least understood the sexual embrace of another human being. That she had shared herself. It was a very mixed set of feelings."

What Was It Like for Her?

You have to wonder, because you may never really find out, what was it like for your kid?

In a survey that asked boys and girls to rate their first experience of intercourse, most boys said it was "pleasant," "fine," or "terrific." Most girls checked off "neutral," "disappointing," or "a disaster." This finding, which strikes us as a helpful thing for kids—especially girls—to hear before they have sex, tends to hold up. Boys are more likely in most surveys to describe their first time as a good experience. Girls are more likely to feel let down.

This may have something to do with the fact that in this typically fumbling encounter, it is believed that boys are more apt than girls to have an orgasm. It's also the case that girls more often say that they decided to have sex for reasons of love, while boys more often say that they did it because they were aroused—and first times turn out to be a whole lot better at satisfying a desire for release than for love. (Other reasons that both sexes check off on surveys include feeling ready, feeling that most kids their age are doing it, and being drunk.) Girls more often say that their partner pressured them, while boys more commonly say that their peers pressured them. So when it's over, girls may feel that they've given something up, while boys may feel that they've gotten something. Traditional language even supports this view: girls lose their virginity; boys get lucky.

It turns out—and you might want to pass this on too—that girls, and their boyfriends for that matter, are more likely to describe their first experience as having been pleasurable, and less likely to say that they felt guilty, when the sex took place in the context of a close relationship.

Planning also helps. Girls who have planned their first experience express less regret afterward. And when a couple plans ahead, they are more likely to use contraception. Still, although first sexual encounters are typically unplanned, most teens do indeed use some sort of protection. A 1995 study found that 70 percent of teenagers used condoms the first time they had intercourse.

Carlo, who was sixteen and in love and who did plan his first sex ever with his girlfriend of nearly a year, had this to say about it: "It's not as easy the first time. It's not as if—people make it sound as if it's easy and that it automatically feels good. But it's tough the first few times."

Physically tough or emotionally tough?

"Physically tough."

Or Emotionally Tough

Undoubtedly, when some kids have sex for the first time, they realize what all the fuss is about. Your daughter may wish that she hadn't waited so long. Even if she decides she's not crazy about the guy, she may still know she likes sex—really likes it. The horse may definitely be out of the barn. And if she *is* crazy about him, the horse may be clear to the next county by now.

Or things might not work out so well.

"It's not pregnancy or VD that scare me, although I realize they're important. It's whether she's emotionally ready." Nelson is talking about his daughter, who is seventeen. "I can teach her about condoms. I don't know how to teach her to handle her emotions. I don't know if she can handle it when she thinks she's in love with a guy because she sleeps with him, and he moves onto the next conquest."

What about Nelson's son, who is fifteen?

"I'm not as worried about him. I don't know if this means I'm sexist, or if the world is sexist, or my son and daughter are just different. But I don't think he'd be as emotionally vulnerable if he had just had sex. I think it will be more of a physical thing. He would be happy in the backseat of a VW Bug, or in the custodial closet at school. But Katie probably dreams of a bed of rose petals and a boy whispering 'I love you' into her ear. They are very different."

Nelson may be right about two things—Katie *may* be dreaming of rose petals, and his thoughts may be informed by a kind of attitude toward women that itself can color a girl's first sexual experience. As we discussed above, girls are more likely than boys to report feeling down after their first sexual encounter, and they do discuss sex more romantically, but this may well be, at least in part, because the world has been telling them that girls who have sex are loose or worse, and that if girls have sex it had better be for love, not lust. It could be that boys' first experiences of sex are better, that they can enjoy Nelson's imagined quickie in a custodial closet, because they don't have to schlepp all this baggage in there with them.

It could also be, in the end, that boys' and girls' experiences are much more similar than the research shows, but boys feel that they are expected to say it was good, and girls feel that they should express regret.

Be that as it may, it is pretty clear that the first time can leave your kid walking on air or skulking around under a cloud. Kids who believe that they shouldn't have done it, who have grown up with strong negative messages about sexuality, will probably feel worse. This sort of guilt consumed Lawrence, a gay teenager from a family in which being gay was not a good thing.

"I came home and took a really long shower. I felt dirty. My mother made my favorite meal for dinner—meat loaf. I remember eating in front of the TV and feeling criminal."

For Lawrence, and for a great many teenagers, although they may never tell their parents what happened, what they imagine their parents would think if they knew plays a major role in shaping their reaction to their secret sexual debut.

But even teens who think their parents would be happy for them have their own mixed emotions. It could have been a truly bad experience, because it was with the wrong partner, at the wrong time, in the wrong place, or because coercion was involved.

And, as Carlo pointed out, your kid's first experience of sex can be physically tough.

A girl may find penetration painful (see our discussion of the hymen; for a comprehensive resource on pain and other female sexual problems, we recommend *For Women Only: A Revolutionary Guide to Overcoming Sexual Dysfunction and Reclaiming Your Sex Life,* by Jennifer Berman and Laura Berman). If it hurts a lot, she might be afraid to try again. A boy still learning how intercourse works may lose his erection, or reach orgasm very quickly, or not be able to come at all. If his partner is understanding, it may not be so bad; but if his partner laughs or teases him, he could be humiliated.

Growing It Back

We've been hearing for years that if you haven't had sex in six months, you revert to virginity. There's always a cousin of a friend of a friend whose hymen grew back. In case you're wondering, it won't, although we still think Oscar Levant was on to something when he said he knew Doris Day before she was a virgin. Why?

Because as a society, we put so much weight on the notion of loss of virginity that making subsequent choices may seem irrelevant. If your daughter thinks that everything is tied up in her being a virgin, what happens when she loses her virginity? Does she feel she has no reason to abstain from sex in the future? Does she feel her sexuality isn't worth protecting anymore?

Obviously, just because your daughter isn't a virgin doesn't mean that she can't say no, make choices, or choose to wait until marriage or love or whenever feels right for her. But it may not be as obvious to *her* that *anyone* can abstain from sex, whether they've had it before or not.

Nothing you do is likely to take away the notion of first intercourse as a rite of passage, a defining moment in your child's life. But you can help her realize that it's not the only important event. She has every reason to make a decision each time the opportunity to have sex arises.

The Hymen

Despite its diminutive size and apparent lack of physiological purpose, the hymen has played a fairly prominent role in sexual politics. Named for the Greek god of marriage, it's just a little bit of tissue that surrounds the border of the vaginal opening, but some folks make a pretty big fuss over it.

Loss of virginity is said to "break" the hymen, or, in less reverent lingo, "pop the cherry." Indeed, the penis usually just stretches the hymen rather than actually breaking it, although it sometimes causes a small tear. The hymen may be stretched well in advance of intercourse, and some girls just naturally have a hymen that's looser.

Except in very unusual circumstances, using a tampon or having a pelvic exam will not break the hymen. For that matter, even having intercourse doesn't always do that much to it.

If your daughter's hymen has not stretched already, her first experience of intercourse may hurt as the penis stretches it. There may also be some blood. This isn't the case for all women, but it's a real possibility. Warn her about it. If your daughter is planning ahead for intercourse, she can use her finger to stretch the hymen for a few weeks beforehand, inserting her finger and moving it around to widen the opening. (Sometimes the hymen is too tight for her finger to loosen it or for the penis to get through. A clinician can help it along.) She should also ask her partner to enter slowly and gently—all the more reason to have sex with someone she knows and trusts.

Pain can also occur after the first time or from other causes, such as the girl's vagina not being adequately lubricated. Boys may be so eager to get a move on that foreplay may last about as long as it takes to say, "I'm coming!"—not much time for the girl to lubricate. Your daughter can purchase lubricants at the pharmacy, or teach her guy the joys of slow, seductive lovemaking. If pain persists, she should see a clinician.

The Lay of the Land: What American Adolescents Do

As we said before, adolescents are having sex. Knowing what other kids are doing might help put your own teen's sex life in perspective. Here's a thumbnail sketch.

We mentioned in Chapter 8 that there has been a recent decrease in the percentage of kids who have had intercourse. But once they start, they seem to be having it as often as ever.

In 1999, one-half of high school students reported having had vaginal intercourse. A little less than one in ten high school students said they had started before they were thirteen, and by the time they became ninth graders, nearly 40 percent had. By twelfth grade, almost two-thirds had had intercourse. So if your child has sex before he graduates from high school, he is squarely in the majority. If he has it in middle school, he is in a small but significant minority.

Some teenagers try sex once and then don't do it again for quite a while. It's not as readily available to all of them as you might think. And even when sex *is* readily available, some decide that once they've satisfied their curiosity, they want to wait for the "right girl" or the "right boy." Or they'd just rather wait until they are older.

But for most kids, the first time is soon followed by the next time and the time after that. Among high school students who have had intercourse, nearly three-quarters have had it in the past three months. They may not have it every night or even every week, but it's not a rare event, either. As best we can tell, they tried it and they liked it and they're not giving it up.

And many aren't having sex with just one partner. A third of high school students who've had intercourse have had it with four or more different people. That's true regardless of what grade they're in—more evidence that once they start, they keep going back for more.

Teen sex is not all about intercourse. There's plenty of other stuff going on. For example, a national study found in 1995 that about half of unmarried fifteen- to nineteen-year-old males had been masturbated by a female, about half had received fellatio from a female, nearly 40 percent had performed cunnilingus, a little over half had had vaginal intercourse, and about one in ten had had anal intercourse with a female. All told, about two-thirds had engaged in at least one of these activities.

Sexual activity with partners of the same gender is rarely explored in national studies, but this study of boys was an exception. It found that 5.5 percent had some sort of sexual activity with another male. What the study doesn't tell us is how many consider themselves gay, bisexual, or heterosexual. Research asking adult gay men to look back finds that many didn't engage in sexual activity with other males while still in high school, either because they were closeted (to themselves or others) or because they didn't know how to find interested partners.

When Your Child Has a Disability or Chronic Illness

When it comes to sex, kids with disabilities and chronic illnesses are, first and foremost, kids—they are curious about sex, they want to explore it, and they dream of falling in love.

The few studies on the subject have found little difference between the sexual activities of chronically ill adolescents and other teens. This is especially true when the former have fairly typical puberty and their illness has not prevented them from regular social relationships with peers.

But *your* experience of your child's sexuality may well be colored by his condition. For some parents of disabled kids, sex is the last thing on their minds. Some don't notice the signs of their child's budding sexuality. And some don't want to.

"I don't think I ever dealt with sexual issues with her," Spencer says of his daughter, a mildly retarded young woman in her twenties. "She seemed so naïve. I wasn't worried that she would get pregnant, because she was never alone. I guess something could have happened at school, but I don't think she was ever apart from her class.

"I'm more worried now. She lives on her own in an apartment, and she has a job delivering the mail in a big law firm. We never thought she'd be independent, so I'm happy, but I'm afraid someone could do something. Maybe that would be good, as long as it wasn't forced, but I don't know if she'd want to. I don't know what she knows."

Bob's son is a senior in high school. His right leg was amputated above the knee when he was a child and fell out of a third-story window. "I talked to him about everything I talked to my older son about. I always wanted to convey to him that I thought he could do anything he wanted. Once I asked him whether he was concerned about his leg and how girls would react—that was before I knew he was gay—and he said he was. We talked about it, like about how it might make some girls interested in him out of curiosity, and some girls might stay away for fear. That was a few years ago. He's been dating a boy from his school for the past few months. I'm not real worried about his leg because he doesn't seem to be."

But it's not necessarily so straightforward for all kids, especially if they have a more severe illness or disability. They may be physically unable to explore their own bodies. If they don't get much privacy, they may not be able to do much that's sexual or romantic, be it alone or with a friend. They may be isolated from other kids and miss out on social opportunities. They may not be able to get to a store to buy condoms. Kids who are infertile may think they don't need to worry about contraception, but they can still get STDs.

However much you might like to simplify your disabled child's life by tabling issues of sexuality, keep in mind that her sexuality will arrive invited or not—and thank goodness, because it may well provide her with satisfaction and fulfillment. Talk to her clinician and her teachers for advice. If she has a condition for which there are support groups or chatrooms for parents, bring the issue up there. And then talk with her.

She needs all four lessons in this book. She should learn about bodies, sex, puberty, contraception, and everything else. Yes, she may get hurt just like any other girl, or worse. But she can also be loved and cherished and desired. And she can love.

As for substance use, one-quarter of high school students drank alcohol or used drugs the last time they had intercourse, which raises concerns about whether they used protection correctly.

How are they doing along those lines?

As we described in Chapter 9, the last time high school students had intercourse during the past three months, 57 percent used a condom, and 17 percent used the Pill. The 1990s saw an increase in condom use, but a concomitant decrease in oral contraceptive use—from a health perspective, a mixed blessing. These teen contraception habits translate each year into about 3 million cases of STDs, about one-quarter of all new HIV infections, and about 1 million pregnancies (three-quarters of them are unintended, and about one-third of the pregnancies end in therapeutic abortions).

Hooking Up

KATIE: *I think of it as kissing.*

LOREN: *I think of it as, like when . . . 'cause . . . I don't know what I think of it as. It's usually something you think, it's like with no feelings involved. I would never say to Isabella, "Did you hook up with your boyfriend?"*

ISABELLA: *I think it means something different to everyone.*

—Katie, Loren, and Isabella, best friends, all fifteen years old, giving their definition of hooking up

All of this detail on what teens are doing sexually is bound to be obscured when your son, if he tells you anything, says, sure, he's hooked up with a girl or two. What, you may wonder, does that mean?

Your very uncertainty, of course, is a major purpose of the vague term *hooking up.* It works for teens today the way *sleeping with* may have worked for your generation. Nobody really knew exactly what you did, but they sure managed to let their minds wander.

When younger teens talk about hooking up, they are more likely to be thinking of kissing or making out than the older kids, who may well mean intercourse (or, I want my friends to think we had intercourse even though we didn't). Hooking up may also suggest oral sex to kids across the age spectrum.

There is, though, one meaning that keeps coming up when we talk to kids about what they consider a hookup. It's "casual."

"It's no big deal. It's just a hookup. It doesn't mean anything," explains Cindy, a high school sophomore. Do you want to get more involved? "No, why? It's not like that."

Whether they are talking about kissing or intercourse, teens consider the hookup a kind of no-strings-attached, one-night stand—except that it probably happened during the day behind the gym, in the living room when you weren't home, or at a party. Kind of like a junior quickie, there is no implied commitment, no obligation, no need to send roses or call the next day. In fact, the meaning of hooking up is well clarified by that other famously vague phrase of teens. Hooking up, whatever it is, is not "going out."

Pornography

Should you one day go searching under your son's bed for the quilt he used last winter and instead turn up a well-thumbed copy of *Hump* magazine, you will have some thinking to do. Is it wrong for him to be reading porn at age seventeen, or fourteen, or twelve? Is it harmful? Should you disapprove?

Any number of experts will line up to answer these questions for you. Some will say that teens who use pornography become casual, even callous, about sex—that they develop chauvinistic and objectifying attitudes about women and unrealistic expectations about what they look like and what they do. Others will say that viewing pornography has no known negative effects on children of any age.

Unfortunately, the research available hasn't resolved this debate. So you'll need to decide for yourself what you think about your son's use of pornography. Here are some ideas that may help.

First of all, your child is not unusual. Most teens have seen a pornographic magazine or video (not to mention a website) before they leave high school.

Pornography certainly seems to fill a need. It can open a door to satisfying sexual experiences for teens too inhibited or isolated to enjoy them with others. Although it's been known to stir up the desire to search out sex of the non-solo variety, some kids say they've also found it to be a tool for maintaining abstinence — a trusty companion when self-restraint is painful and even cold showers fail to dial down the heat. And, unlike the real thing, the excitement of pornography comes without any risk of STDs or pregnancy or breaking someone's heart.

If you neglect to talk with your kids about sex, for better or worse, porn can provide a hard-to-come-by practical education in the mechanics of sex.

Still, your son's issue of *Hump* ought not be his only source of information about the way the sexes interact. You can help place pornography's lessons in context by sharing your perspective on it with your teenager. Tell him you know that he has probably seen porn (no need to embarrass him by revealing what you saw under his bed), and ask him how realistic he thinks those depictions of men, women, and sexuality are. Tell him what you think is left out or distorted (for example, that most women don't have breasts that size, or that most men's penises are not that large).

If there is something indisputably good to come from your teen's use of pornography, it would be a discussion like this in which you engage your child's moral reasoning in the contemplation of a sexual issue and offer him your thoughts on the matter.

We should note, though, that there's porn, and then there's PORN. On one hand, there are naked women and men in various poses; and on the other, there are women being humiliated and demeaned by men. We don't know whether the latter provides a release for men who would otherwise abuse women, or whether it encourages such men. But even parents who have no problems with porn in the abstract may find that some of it is more than they can tolerate.

Some parents also don't want their kids to purchase

pornography because they don't want them to support what they consider an exploitative industry.

If you really want to make an impression and minimize the role of porn in your kid's sexual education, get him in touch with a competing perspective on sexual pleasure. A good sex manual will give your teen some of the titillation he is looking for and the how-to information he needs in the context of a healthy perspective on sexuality and relationships. Ideas about sexual positions will be combined with important reminders about responsibility and contraception that you won't find in porn unless you squint, and no one will have been exploited in the book's production (unless you count the underpaid editorial assistant). *The Complete Idiot's Guide to Amazing Sex* by Sari Locker is an informative beginner's guide appropriate for teens.

Older Guys, Younger Girls

I was on a cruise with my mom, and I met this guy, Perry, and he was really great. He was like twenty-three. It was really nice with him, because he would talk with me, and he was interested in what I had to say—not like the guys who were my own age. They are all so immature. Perry was sensitive. I wanted to explore things more. I'd decided that this was my week to go crazy, so I let him know that I was available.

—*Cindy, age sixteen*

When teens get involved with much older partners, it isn't always a bad thing. Some of these experiences are recalled as wonderfully romantic, and surely some of these couples have had long and happy relationships. But the idea does make us a bit uncomfortable, and we suspect it may have a similar effect on you.

Here, principally, we are thinking about younger girls with older guys, the more common pairing. In one national study, one in four 15-

to 19-year-old girls said their most recent sexual partner was a man four or more years older. The same was true for only one in twenty boys.

Older partners can be attractive because they have money, a car, status. Girls may find that they enjoy interacting with men more mature than boys their own age. And it may be harder to deflect their advances. They may know better how to charm a young girl and make her feel special.

Why worry? Because a younger girl will be less experienced than her partner and possibly less in control than she'd be with someone her own age. Sex may escalate faster than she would choose. It has been found that as a likely result of this dynamic, teenage girls with partners six or more years older are more likely to get pregnant than girls seeing boys closer to their own age.

When Josie was fifteen, a twenty-two-year-old man asked her out. "It was exciting. He had a full beard, and I thought that was really, really nice. I couldn't believe he took me out when he could have asked out any of the girls. He had his own car, and he took me to a real restaurant. I was a virgin, and though I acted mature, I didn't know what I was doing." Her date brought her back home. "We were kissing good night on the porch, and all I could think about was what would happen if my father opened the door. That image told me I shouldn't be going out with this guy."

How would she feel if her fourteen-year-old daughter dated a guy that much older? "Not good. But the situation is totally different, because we talk about this sort of thing, which I never did with my parents. And I will invite in any boy or girl she goes on a date with for a few minutes." For some thoughts on discussing these matters with your besotted teen, see Chapter 7.

Home Bodies

The other day we were talking about what the kids get up to after school and are they "hooking up," and one of the mothers in my car pool said something like, "I don't mind if they do it, but not in my home." I was stunned! I mean, if they are going to do it, I want it in my home.

—*Shelley, on her fifteen- and fourteen-year-old daughters*

If they're going to have sex, I'm not going to make it any easier for them by letting them do it here, and to be honest, I don't want to know about it.

—June, on her seventeen-year-old son and his girlfriend

If you have succeeded in establishing an open dialogue with your kid about his sex life, you may soon face the sometimes unsettling question: "Can we do it here?" Obviously, if your kid is going to have sex, he has to do it somewhere, and home would seem like a better place than parked between two Dumpsters outside Chuck E. Cheese. Still, some parents don't find themselves entirely prepared for the possibility of chatting over pancakes with their son's new girlfriend.

What should you do?

Well, what makes this a tough one is usually the fact that even if your child has your (perhaps grudging) acceptance of his sexual life with his girlfriend, you may not be ready to endorse the affair wholeheartedly. Inviting the two into your home for an intimate evening, while you are there knowing (or imagining) exactly what is going on, can feel like more of an embrace of their lovemaking than you want to offer.

It may also be closer than you want to get to your son's sexuality, which you may find easier to consider in abstract terms than in Sensaround.

Then there is the issue of his kid sister.

When Inga's son Anders made it home for spring break his senior year in boarding school, he brought his girlfriend with him. "He was eighteen at that point, hardly a child. It was sort of assumed that they would stay in the same room. Which they did."

Inga kept an eye out for her fifteen-year-old daughter Suzanne's reactions.

"One day Suzanne called me at work and said, 'Anders and Claudia took a shower together. It was really scary!'

"Now Suzanne is a pretty direct kid," Inga says, "so when she said it was scary, we took it literally. I think what was happening was that she was getting a little overexcited by it all. So we asked Anders to throttle back on the public displays of affection. I also told him that when we were together watching television it wasn't appropriate for the two of them to disappear for three hours. I mean, I wouldn't do that with their father.

"I'm not prudish about sex," Inga explains. "I think the kids *should* have sex. But when Suzanne said essentially it was too in her face, then I felt okay, this is getting out of control."

If your sexually active child isn't having sex at home, he will find a way to have it, but where? Will he resort to a semipublic setting where he could get in trouble? Will it be that much harder to get a condom on in his girlfriend's car, or to remember to bring one? Will he therefore skip the condom? It seems to us, although we don't know of any research on the subject, that your teenager is more likely to use contraception if he's in a safe and controlled environment, one where he will have had at least a little time to set things up for the occasion and where the atmosphere isn't one of subterfuge.

And, hey, maybe *this* will inspire him to clean up his room.

Some parents who see encouraging their children to bring their sex life home as a powerful kind of monitoring don't even wait for them to ask.

"I think I took the rebellion out of it by saying if you are going to have sex, you should do it in your room," Sandy, mother of a sixteen-year-old, says. "I'd much rather she do it here. At least if they were having sex in my house, I'd know where they were. He couldn't abuse her. If she said no, it would be harder for him to force himself on her. I think she probably actually did something only once or twice, but my permission allowed us to get past all the secrecy."

Sandy based her decision not only on safety issues but on what she saw as the importance of maintaining honesty at home. "I didn't want her sneaking around behind my back. It's so easy to do that, and then you keep doing it and it undermines your relationship with your parents."

If you let them have sex at home, you may find yourself helping them more than you expected.

Take Alaida, a mother with a seventeen-year-old daughter, Cecily. They both felt that Cecily's first sexual experience with her boyfriend might be more comfortable if it took place in her own bedroom. Cecily and her boyfriend picked a date, Alaida agreed (she would be home that night), and the plan was put into action.

The next morning there was a quiet knock on Alaida's door. "Cecily came in, crawled into bed with me, and said, 'Mommy, the condom broke.' "

No, this is definitely *not* your granddaddy's parenting.

Boo-boo Kiss

The question for you and your teenager here is just how involved are you going to get in the ebbs and flows of her sex life, which is looking more and more adult and deserving of privacy, but which is still, let's be honest, more than a little wet behind the ears.

Maybe you'll pitch in when she's in distress, a time when your teenager is probably about as receptive to your help as she is going to be these days—and when you may find it's just too rough to sit on the sidelines.

Few things are more painful than watching your child suffer. "If I had my way, I'd put her in a bubble and never let her date" is the sort of thing we hear a lot. Your daughter radiates joy when she starts going out. It's difficult not to get caught up in the excitement. Three weeks later, they break up, and the look of devastation on her face as she stares into her toast is heartrending. "I don't know what to do," one father worries. "I don't know how to help her. It doesn't matter who did the breaking up. It's nearly always this bad."

"Her boyfriend broke up with her, and suddenly Mr. Perfect was Mr. Jerk. I'd pegged him from the start," Payel says of her fifteen-year-old's ex, and we have no doubt she did. "I tried to help her see what I saw. I asked questions: 'Has he dated before?' 'What happened to those relationships?' 'What do you talk about?' No effect. So now I pick up the pieces."

Well, there is some preventive work you can do. As we discussed in Chapter 7, it's not your job to choose your child's dates. But you can soften the blow by tempering her expectations. If she starts each date thinking he's The One, she'll be let down each time it doesn't work out. Of course, she can get excited, but help her think of going out as a chance to check out a guy, with the awareness that most won't turn out to be The One. Some kids will actually listen to this stuff. Others will be so infatuated that reason will have to wait until after the fall.

And when that happens, you can move into action in the way only a parent like you with a proven track record of boo-boo magic can. You don't need to say much about what happened to be supportive. A warm hug and a kiss do wonders. Remind her how wonderful she is. It's amazing how helpful it is to be a little kid with a mommy or daddy who adores you at times like these.

Then again, some kids don't want to crawl back into the nest. They react to a breakup by trying to act the part of a stoic grown-up. You can cozy up to these kids, too, as long as you don't expect them to cry on your shoulder—at least not right away. Remember special days out together, just the two of you? If she's game, one of those would do well right about now. An afternoon out shopping, hiking, or shooting hoops can help you get closer with these strong, silent types.

Closer, Closer . . .

Maybe you'll get more involved. Maybe you'll steer clear of the details of your son's sex life but find your way into some intimate and frank talks about love.

"We focus on relationships," Keenan says of his seventeen-year-old son. "I tell him stories from my past. I tell him how I chose his mother, or rather how I got her to choose me. I don't mind him having a good time, but there is nothing more important to me than him settling down with a woman who makes him truly happy. I'm not sure he really understands the difference yet, but we're working on it."

Maybe your kid, like Keenan's, will open up to you about what's going on with his girlfriend. But what about sex, the *sex* part of sex, pleasure, and the have-you-tried-this-yet kind of talk? What if your daughter comes to you as Grace's did and says, "Mom, I've been try-ing and Wes tells me I just can't get it right. How do you give a blow job?"

Are you up for that?

Pointers?

It took me years to learn how to make a woman feel good. Why do we waste so much time? No one teaches you these things. Where was my big brother? Where was my father? Why don't we teach our kids this stuff?

—*Ed, father of a ten-year-old son, Bradley*

You taught your kids how to throw a ball, how to choke up on the bat, and how to catch. Should you teach them how to have sex? Where to touch? How to please a partner? And if you don't teach them, who will? Kids these days seem to get their know-how from some combination of rumor and fantasy, pornography and sex manuals, friends, more experienced partners, fumbling, and a little bravado. How well do they learn? Well, how well did you?

Let's listen to Meryl, the mother of fifteen-year-old Sunset, explain her point of view. "I think I have an unusual perspective. Years ago, when I was only a few years older than my daughter is now, I taught my own mother about orgasms." Really? How'd that happen? "It was part of a you-don't-know-anything moment. But we both suddenly realized that she didn't know what I was talking about. I remember looking her in the eye and asking what sex felt like for her. She could only talk about feeling close to my dad."

Meryl was inspired to take action. "I told her how to bring herself to orgasm so she would know what it felt like. She had had no idea what she was missing. And it worked—she actually taught my father how to give her an orgasm."

Meryl is determined that her daughter won't miss out. "I decided I wasn't going to take any chances with Sunset, and I taught her all about her body and what feels good. I've made sure she knows she needs to have pleasure, and if the guy isn't interested in that, get rid of him."

Ed has made a similar vow for his son Bradley. "I'm going to teach my son about the practical aspects of sex. I don't want him learning from friends who don't know what they're talking about. This is an important part of life. I want him to hear it from me."

Charles had a plan to make this easier with his fourteen-year-old son. "I started by telling him a story about me and how I'd totally made a fool of myself with this girl on prom night because I didn't know how to have sex. This is a little embarrassing, but I didn't know how to put it, you know, in, so I was just pushing against her and nothing was happening. She just said forget it. So I told him this story, and he said, 'Good, now I don't have to feel like the biggest geek in the world. You already hold that title.' After that he wasn't afraid to ask me questions, and he asked a lot of good questions."

If Meryl's and Ed's and Charles's kids are happy to hear about sex and techniques from them, then more power to them. Their talks can get as specific as they like.

Still, not everyone feels that once a child's sex life becomes a reality, getting close to those private embraces, however inept they may be, is a good idea. Harry's parents apparently fell into this category.

"I've let them know everything," Harry says at sixteen. "I feel very comfortable with my parents—more with my mother than my father. She's always asking me if there's anything I need to talk to her about. I felt good talking to her about sex."

What do they discuss?

"Just not being a selfish lover. It feels fine, because she seems pretty open about it. I told her when I was thinking about having sex. She said she was grateful I told her. But then she said she didn't want to know any more details. We haven't talked about sex since I started having it."

Harry and his mother are not unusual. Their situation is one reason why in Chapter 2 we encouraged teaching your child about the pleasures of sex before he's ready to have it with others. Because once he actually embarks on a sexual career with partners, you or he may feel quite certain that those pleasures need to take place in private—in the same way you may feel it is important to keep details of your own sexual explorations private from him.

But what about Ed's uncertainty and Meryl's mother's life without orgasms?

In this most untraditional of parenting conundrums, we would like to check in with one of the most established parenting gurus we know of: Dr. Spock.

In his classic book *Baby and Child Care,* pediatrician Benjamin Spock described the proverbial game of catch between father and son. He discouraged fathers from being too focused on their boys' technique with a ball. "Feeling approved by his father," he wrote, "helps him more than being coached by him."

Let's consider this analogy for a moment. For a boy to play a great game of baseball, he will need to know a world of technical skills, like how to slide into home plate. His mother or his father could teach him that, and so could a Little League coach, just as well.

But who better than his parents to teach the boy that it's important for him not to hurt himself because he is so valuable? That it's fine, even exciting, to take a risk like stealing home? That he needn't feel ashamed of failing if he gets tagged out? These are the lessons good parenting provides, and they are easily taught without any reference to the fine points of sliding.

And if those lessons are taught, isn't it likely that the boy, if he gets a chance to play, will take a few of his own stabs at sliding into home plate and ultimately figure it out?

Meryl's mom would have known about orgasms if her own mother had explained how to get them. No question. But there is also a good chance she would have found out on her own if her mother had communicated early that her body was fun to explore, that sexual fulfillment should be a part of her life, and that women deserve to know about sexual things just as men do.

Chances are, if she had been given a basic grounding in the value of looking for them, she would have found her orgasms.

Your Call

All of which is to say, if talking technique with your sexually active teenager feels like more than you bargained for, or more than he wants, or if it seems perfectly natural to the both of you, feel free to follow your instincts. Respect each other's boundaries and teach what you're comfortable with. But try not to skip the basic message that your child's body and its pleasures are good.

Eva and her son found a dialogue that worked for them. "I didn't give him a play-by-play. I think a lot of this you just learn by discovery and exploration, and I wouldn't want to take away the joy of that. What I did teach him was that there is so much to discover. Also, that it's not just his genitals that are sexual, that parts of his body that he never associated with sex may be quite sexual with the right person. I told him to be bold, to try things, to take chances so he'd be open to experiencing pleasure."

No matter what you teach your child, he will of course do most of his learning on the job. You can give your child specific ideas about what feels good, how to please a partner, even what techniques to try. You can give more general advice, like encouraging him to explore what he likes and then to ask for it, or informing him that real sex is rarely as smooth as it is in the movies. You can tell your child to always be sensitive and affectionate with his partner, to ask her what she wants, and to attend to her pleasure as well as his own.

But if you do, you might also bear in mind that not everyone is looking for this kind of sex. Warmth and cuddling may not in fact excite your child, whose goal may be to find someone with as rough a point of view on sex as her own. The day that happens, the day she finds that man or woman, she might well ask herself, "Why didn't my parents tell me about this?"

But then again, she might just as well feel the satisfaction of having discovered something wonderful all by herself.

You Made It

Well, even after conceiving, bearing, birthing and rearing her, even after watching her and talking to her for almost 20 years, I would have to say, no, I don't know [my daughter]. She comes fully equipped with her own self, which is other than mine, and is in some ways entirely outside my experience.

—*Jane Smiley, "Mothers Should,"* New York Times Magazine

Congratulations. You made it.

You made it through red-faced diaper changes, hoping she'd finish rubbing herself before your mother came back into the room. You made it through the time she walked in on you and, since the lights were off, you just sent her back to bed without getting up off your husband, but then couldn't have sex for two weeks. Through "Mommy, where's my penis?" and "How does Daddy's seed get in there?" and "Why can't I take a bath with him anymore?"

You made it through "Why can't I marry you?" all the way to "Why are your boobs so small?" The growth spurt, the tampon, the crush, the breakup, the condoms, the cucumber, and the diets, and you never, never made a joke about her boyfriend's hair. That she knew of. You've been advising, worrying, comforting, and cajoling for a long time now. Maybe even pushing, conniving, and, on rare occasions, intervening.

So where did it all get you?

It got you here, driving home with an almost finished sales report and a bag of cheeseburgers and fries in the passenger seat, a middle-aged businesswoman on her way home to have dinner with her daughter who got home an hour ago after having sex with her boyfriend, and who used a condom like you taught her, and who can't really be called a child anymore, because she's so grown up.

Flash forward a few more years. She's just graduated from college and moved into an apartment she found without you, although she asked you to help her fix it up. She had a boyfriend the last two years of school, but they split up recently. She sort of explained, but you still don't really understand why. She seemed okay about it. She has her first job. These days, she seems more than ever to have become the person she is going to be; more explicitly, more emphatically, herself.

What now? Where exactly in her life do you fit in?

Well, of course, she still needs a lot of help.

There is, believe it or not, a little more to adulthood than developing a mature romantic and sexual life. But even on the sexual front, there is still room for you to keep up the reminders about decision making and protection, to offer some comfort when things don't work out and some advice about love when they do.

Still, your position is changing, and it will continue to change.

With a child, you're clearly in charge, and with an adolescent, you still have a great deal of responsibility, even if she's beginning to share it with you. But by the time your child starts slipping into adulthood, her needs for you are just not what they were. You feel more and more like peers, but you will never be equals. In fact, you may feel that your differences were never so pronounced, because now they aren't based simply on an age gap, but rather on the fact that as adults you are different kinds of people. As Jane Smiley observed, writing about her twenty-year-old daughter, she is someone other than you. Her reaching this stage in her sexual development has made that pretty clear.

Since she was born, your child's sexuality has been a robust sign of life. Now, like then, it's a sign that she is establishing a life that will endure beyond you, that may surpass the limits of your imagination, because she will make it her own.

Yes, she has come this far from a small creature who spent her days sleeping, eating, and crying and was completely dependent on you. She's not yours in that way anymore.

Oh, well. You still have that new apartment to help her fix up. And maybe while you're helping her hang the curtains, she'll fill you in a bit more about her breakup, and you'll have a few words of comfort. Maybe a few months later there'll be a new guy you'll get to meet. She might even ask what you think of him.

And consider this: Someday, perhaps in the not-too-distant future, she may have kids of her own. And when that happens, if that happens, well, then, you two are *really* going to have something to talk about.

Part III

Risks

Chapter 11

Bugs in the system

AIDS AND OTHER SEXUALLY TRANSMITTED DISEASES

YOU KNEW SOMETHING WAS WRONG when your daughter came in the door. She avoided your gaze, gave a monosyllabic answer or two, and disappeared upstairs. You figure you'd better check on her. You knock. No response.

"Can I come in?"

"If you want to."

She's flipping through a magazine.

"Whatcha reading?" you ask, never sure what to say to get her talking. She cries.

Her boyfriend told her he has gonorrhea.

You (a) didn't know she was having sex with him, (b) can't believe she didn't use a condom, (c) instantly feel furious although you're not exactly sure at whom, (d) don't remember what people do for gonorrhea, and (e) now have four new reasons for not knowing what to say.

You sit on the bed and put an arm around your crying daughter and say the only thing that comes to mind.

"Damn."

We hate STDs, too.

If you have ever found yourself in this position, the material in this chapter and the appendix on specific diseases (Appendix B) may be all too familiar.

If you haven't, read on. You don't need to know all the details about every different STD and how they're treated. But you might want to become familiar with how they are spread, how to prevent them, and what types of symptoms warrant going to a clinician.

Do you really need to worry that your child might contract one? Or is the talk about STDs exaggerated to scare kids away from sex?

The answer is yes—to both questions.

On one hand, because we so rarely openly explore the topic of STDs, we tend not to think about their risk as much as we should. STDs are at epidemic levels among adolescents in the United States, but they don't get discussed all that often. Then there is HIV, which was once a cause of hysteria, and is now, with new treatments, a matter of complacency among teens and sometimes even their parents. We seem to go from one extreme to the other, perhaps because we can sustain peak levels of tension for only so long.

With all you hear and read, it's hard to know what to think about HIV and other STDs. Add to that the fact that we are talking about your child's health, in some cases his life, and it's a wonder anyone can make any sense of it at all.

We're going to try to make some sense.

Could Your Kid Get One?

Where we used to live, I'm sure I would have thought about it. I just didn't think I needed to worry about that sort of thing here.

—*Cassandra, mother of a sixteen-year-old girl with herpes*

STDs are remarkably common among adolescents. According to government estimates, every year, about one out of four sexually active teenagers contracts an STD and about two-thirds of all STDs are diagnosed among people less than twenty-five years old.

Here are the stats on just two of the many STDs. In 1998, about two hundred thousand cases of chlamydia were reported among fifteen- to nineteen-year-olds in the United States, but because so many cases are never diagnosed, let alone reported, many, many more teens are believed to contract chlamydia each year. Not a lot of data are available on how many people get human papilloma virus (HPV), but it's estimated that there are 5.5 million new cases a year (including adults). Strikingly, 75 percent of fifteen- to forty-nine-year-olds are believed to have been infected at some time in their lives, and 15 percent of them are believed to be infected at any one time.

The statistics are dramatic, and some STDs can be pretty awful. But if you're like many parents we know, you might be asking, what do national statistics have to do with my child? Does my son need to worry about getting a disease?

Well, it is true that STDs affect some groups more than others. They discriminate on the basis of sex—or more succinctly, they prefer women. Primarily because of biology, as we'll explain later, it's easier for a woman to contract most STDs from an infected man than vice versa. Women are less likely to have symptoms and less likely to receive a correct diagnosis. Therefore, they get less-timely treatment and more serious complications. There are also regional differences in the prevalence of certain diseases. And there are differences among various racial and ethnic groups.

But your child's risk depends largely on what type of sexual activity she engages in and how often, whether her partners are infected, and what actions she takes to reduce her risk.

How They Spread

STDs are a vastly diverse group of organisms, including viruses, bacteria, and tiny little beasts. Their unifying theme is only their mode of spread: sexual contact.

Mind you, as we discussed in Chapter 8, sexual contact includes more than just vaginal intercourse, so even virgins can get STDs. Oral sex doesn't spread STDs as easily as vaginal and anal intercourse, but it is nevertheless a way to catch diseases like chlamydia, gonorrhea, herpes, and HIV. Kissing can spread some (like herpes), and just touching can, too (HPV, crabs, and scabies). Indeed, your teen can catch some of these diseases without any sexual contact at all. Hepatitis B and HIV can be spread by sharing needles. But as for toilet seats and doorknobs, when it comes to STDs (the common cold is another matter), some sort of intimate contact between two people (usually their body fluids, but with some STDs, only their skin) is required.

STDs open doors for each other. People who have an STD that causes sores (such as herpes or syphilis) or irritation (such as trichomoniasis) are more easily infected with other STDs, like HIV, that need to find a route into the body.

Why Do Adolescents Get So Many STDs?

There are several reasons.

First and foremost, teens have intercourse and when they have intercourse, they don't always use a condom.

And they don't tend to settle into relationships for very long, often moving on to new partners before the symptoms of disease emerge. Multiple partners, sequential or simultaneous, create multiple opportunities for catching a disease and spreading it to others.

Many adolescents drink alcohol and use drugs and so have impaired judgment in social settings that leads to greater sexual risks.

And they are biologically more susceptible to STDs. The inner surface of your adolescent daughter's cervix is still maturing. The cells are not as tough as they will be by the time she reaches adulthood, so bacteria and viruses can more easily infect her.

Most adolescents with an STD never have symptoms, so they don't go for treatment. When they do have symptoms, they all too often ignore all but the most unbearable ones, hoping they'll go away. They're more likely to get care if they can get to a trusted clinician or a confidential clinic. The longer they wait, the more damage an STD can do, and the more opportunity it has to spread to others.

How Serious Are They Really?

Different diseases have vastly different implications for your child's health. Crabs, for example, can be annoying, but they are ultimately rather trivial. Many STDs, though, are serious. Chlamydia and gonorrhea can develop into pelvic inflammatory disease (PID), which not only causes pain but can also cause scarring that may leave women infertile or at risk for an ectopic pregnancy or miscarriage. STDs rarely cause infertility in boys, but they can sure cause a lot of pain.

Many STDs (like syphilis, for example) can harm a developing fetus and cause abnormalities or prematurity.

The virus clan has among the worst consequences. Herpes, although less deadly than some viruses, causes painful blisters that can recur throughout life, but new medicines are helping control the symptoms. Although most people recover from hepatitis B, it can be rapidly fatal or cause liver cancer years later. HPV is usually minor, but it can cause cervical cancer a small percentage of the time.

And then there's HIV. For men, HIV is responsible for more deaths than any other STD, but among women, cervical cancer (usually due to HPV) causes the most deaths.

Fearing HIV

How concerned should you be about HIV? This is a tough one, because in considering HIV risk you are multiplying the very small likelihood that your child will become infected by the very large impact of an infection.

There's no magic formula to calculate the risk. Most adolescents won't get HIV, even if they have lots of unprotected sex; but some will, and it's difficult to know who they will be.

All else being equal, if your son is having sex with boys, he is probably at greater risk. If your daughter is having sex with a guy who uses injection drugs, she's at greater risk, too. If you live in a community with a high HIV rate, any of your sexually active children may be at risk. In a city like New York, an epicenter of the epidemic, your child would have a higher chance of infection than in a community less affected by HIV. But of course, that doesn't mean that teens in small towns are all free from risk.

Precautions against HIV are similar to precautions against chlamydia, gonorrhea, and many other diseases. So if fear of HIV inspires kids (or others) to be more careful, the benefits accrue as a reduction in the spread of many diseases. From a public health perspective, it doesn't matter what motivates people to reduce their risk, as long as they reduce it.

But there's also a risk of focusing too much on HIV. We worry when HIV is the only reason given for sexual risk reduction. In an environment in which kids see none of their friends getting sick (teens with HIV often aren't diagnosed until much later), they may not believe risk reduction efforts are important. We think it better to teach your children the diverse reasons for risk reduction, including other STDs and unintended pregnancy, rather than depending on the fear of HIV alone to motivate them to make the healthiest choices.

What Can You Do?

On the prevention front, we have discussed nearly everything you can do to reduce your child's risk of getting an STD in Chapter 2 (monitoring, closeness, authoritative parenting, and communication), Chapter 8 (teaching about abstinence and less-risky ways of being intimate), and Chapter 9 (teaching about condoms). The only other strategy is making sure your child has had his hepatitis B vaccine series (most babies get it nowadays).

But there's something more you need to think about. You don't only want to prevent your child from getting an STD; you also want to prevent the negative consequences if he does get infected.

Gene was caught off guard when his seventeen-year-old son Carl wanted to talk about something but seemed unusually nervous. Carl said that he had a rash around his genitals, but he was going to be okay. Gene didn't understand why Carl was making such a big deal out of it. "He seemed to be taking this so seriously. I'm thinking, 'Why is he making such a big deal about jock itch?' And then he told me." Carl had thought he'd had herpes. He'd found a public clinic in the phone book and taken a bus. The doctor had assured him it wasn't herpes, showed him a photo of the real thing (which looked very different), and prescribed some cream.

"I wasn't sure how to react. I was proud of him for being industrious enough to figure out where to go. But I felt bad that he had to go through all that without me to help. I had to think about why he didn't come to me in the first place." Gene asked Carl to come to him the next time he was worried about something.

Why didn't Carl go to his father right away? "I don't know. I guess

I was embarrassed. I knew he wouldn't get mad, but he has a disappointed look he gets that is worse."

Your kid's main defense against some of the worst consequences of STDs is getting to a clinician soon after an infection. Your challenge is figuring out how to make this happen. Here are a few suggestions.

First, because telling you may be an impediment to his getting treatment, try to establish a way for him to see a clinician without your knowing. The trick is to make sure your child has a doctor, nurse, or clinic he can find, get to, and pay for without involving you.

Second, your child is obviously the first person who will notice any symptoms if she has an STD (that is, if she's lucky enough to have symptoms). Give her basic information about STD symptoms so that she'll

Reasons to Go to the Clinician: STD Symptoms

1. No symptoms, but had sex with someone who finds out he/she is infected.
2. No symptoms, but has been sexually active, and is due for his/her next annual or semiannual STD check.
3. Pain or itching on or around the genitals.
4. Burning or pain when urinating, or having to urinate more often than usual.
5. Discharge from the vagina or penis — could be white or yellow, could be watery or thick.
6. Swollen genitals.
7. Rash on or around the genitals — bumps, blisters, warts, sores, redness. Could have similar symptoms around the mouth or anus if had oral or anal sex. Could have a sore throat without other symptoms of a cold.
8. Atypical vaginal bleeding (including bleeding with sex).
9. Any bleeding from the penis.
10. Pelvic pain.

know to react. Pain in the genitals, for example, or a discharge should be checked out. So should unusual bumps. Likewise pelvic pain or abnormal vaginal bleeding or (if she has anal sex) anal symptoms. She might notice a rash or some stains on her underwear from a discharge. We list the common symptoms of STDs in the accompanying box.

Third, let your child know that if he discovers that a sexual partner of his—past or present—has an STD, he should always get checked by a clinician.

Finally, because most teens with STDs never get any symptoms, establish a pattern of routine screening for your child.

Getting Screened

Sexually active teens should get regular STD screenings—at least annually, but given the epidemic spread of often asymptomatic diseases like chlamydia (up to 85 percent of cases in girls are asymptomatic), potentially every six months.

You and your child can discuss routine screening with her clinician. He can also tell you whether testing is covered by insurance, and, if not, how much it will cost. Public health clinics in your area may be able to provide free or reduced-cost screening.

Pelvic exams provide a good opportunity for your daughter to get tested for various STDs. Pap smears performed during pelvic exams can detect cervical HPV infections. In fact, regularly scheduled testing can pick up most of the important STDs your daughter or son can contract, including chlamydia, gonorrhea, and HIV.

When the Diagnosis Is Positive

For most infections, your child will be prescribed some medication. Some diseases can be cured with a single dose, but some require a week or more. Even if your son's symptoms go away before he's used up his medicine, he should finish the full prescribed course. Really. Remind him. These diseases can be quite sneaky. The symptoms may go away, but the bug may still be active. If the clinician says to come back to make sure the STD is really gone from his system, your son should do that, too.

While receiving treatment, he'll need to abstain from any sexual contact that could transmit the infection. His partner also needs treatment, or they'll risk passing the infection back and forth.

If the disease is not curable, there may be things your child can do to limit its impact, such as taking medicines that keep it at bay. He also needs to learn how to prevent spreading it to others. He may need counseling to deal with the effects of having a frightening infection, not only HIV but also chronic hepatitis or herpes. Support groups and Web-based resources can help. If the infection is serious, you may also want to get counseling or support for yourself.

We don't mean to state the obvious, but if there was ever a teaching opportunity, this is it. Your daughter needs advice on how to prevent STDs; she needs to think concretely about why this happened and how to prevent it in the future. She may have resolved to never, ever let this happen again. And she may mean it. But over time, if she's like other kids, she'll forget. An occasional refresher talk about STDs may not be a bad idea.

Of course, this will only be a part of your reaction to your child's diagnosis, the bulk of which should be simple, unconditional support.

Protecting Others

In addition to taking care of himself, your teenager, if infected, should make sure to get word of his infection to any partners he could have infected and any partners who could have infected him. They will need

When a Prepubescent Child Has an STD

When a prepubescent child has an STD, it is necessary to consider sexual abuse. Some STDs, such as chlamydia, gonorrhea, and syphilis, can be transmitted by the mother at birth, but if acquired after the newborn period, these infections are almost always evidence of sexual contact. Other STDs that may appear in prepubertal children, including HPV, are not necessarily spread through sex.

to be examined by a clinician. Clinicians may treat his partners even if they have no symptoms or positive lab tests—it's just not worth taking a chance. His doctor or nurse can tell him how far back in time to go in notifying his former sex partners.

If your son doesn't feel comfortable telling his sexual partners, the public health system in many states will notify them about possible exposure to STDs without revealing his name. Although the process is confidential, if he gives the name of a girl who's been sexually involved only with him, she will of course guess whom the call is about.

Protecting others may also involve protecting a fetus or newborn baby. Some STDs can be transmitted from a mother to her unborn fetus or to her infant during the birth process or breast-feeding. For diseases that can be cured, like gonorrhea and syphilis, treating your daughter protects her baby. For diseases that cannot be cured, like HIV, she can take medicines while pregnant and she can give the baby medicines after birth that reduce the chances he will become infected. In some circumstances, the clinician will recommend a cesarean section to prevent the baby from contracting the disease. We'll talk about prenatal care in Chapter 12.

A Disease Is a Disease Is a Disease

"Did you hear? Jennifer has a strep throat. I always knew this would happen to her. She takes buses, goes to the grocery store, even uses public bathrooms. Don't tell anyone I told you, but I heard she once shared a Coke. You get what you ask for."

"It's a shame. He was such a nice boy. But he was too friendly. Everyone wanted to shake his hand. He just never learned to say no. If you shake hands with one boy at a party, you're really shaking hands with everyone else he's shaken hands with. And now he has diarrhea. This will ruin his reputation."

Your child will probably be embarrassed about having an STD. You may be embarrassed about it, too. There's a certain stigma that tends to come with STDs. Perhaps it's a holdover from the endemic shame of sexuality. Your child feels that she's gotten nature's verdict: it *was* dirty to do it. She may think it reflects poorly on her judgment in selecting a sexual partner (as if she could tell). She may think she got what she deserved for breaking the safer sex rules. She may simply feel ashamed of anything that calls attention to the fact that she has genitals. And a sex drive.

You may be able to confront these stigmas rather forcefully.

"I'd never expected to tell her. I'd never even thought about it. It just came up," Emma, the mother of sixteen-year-old Chrissie, says. "Chrissie was laughing about a classmate she'd heard had herpes. There wasn't a trace of sympathy in her voice. I had to say something."

About a week later, Emma told Chrissie that she wanted to tell her a story. "I was nervous. I felt like I was about to open myself up for judgment and ridicule." Emma had gotten herpes when she was in her twenties. Her husband knew, but it wasn't something she discussed with anyone else. "I waited about a week, so she wouldn't realize I'd overheard her that day. I told her in the context of talking about condoms. I wanted to instill a little humanity in her. It made it real for her."

Just so you're not caught off guard, we should let you know that in some teen circles, stigma is definitely not a problem when it comes to certain infections. An STD can be a badge of honor: proof that a kid has had sex. All the more reason to include STDs as part of your effort to school him in the mysteries (and maladies) of sex.

Chapter **12**

With child

Handling intended and unintended pregnancies

"Mom, dad, I'm pregnant."

Does any other announcement provoke such a vast array of reactions? From dread to anger to fear to relief to joy. In a perfect world, a pregnancy would always be a cause for celebration, but we don't live in a perfect world, and not all pregnancies are desired. Teen pregnancies, in particular, are associated with more than their share of sorrow and regret.

Throughout the last three decades of the twentieth century, about a million women younger than twenty became pregnant each year in the United States. About half of them gave birth to a live baby, just over one-third had an abortion, and the rest had a miscarriage or stillbirth. Unfortunately, about 80 percent of adolescent girls who became pregnant were not trying to become pregnant.

There have been some encouraging developments of late. The 1990s saw a decline in the percentage of teens who got pregnant. This is good news, and it will be even better news if the trend continues. But the fact remains that each year, many, many adolescents become pregnant when they are neither ready nor interested in being a parent.

Some didn't think they were capable of getting pregnant. Some weren't able to get contraception, and some didn't know how to use it correctly. Some were forced to have sex. And some just got caught up in the moment.

Some wanted to get pregnant. Some didn't, but weren't disappointed to learn they were.

Although the rate of adolescents' sexual activity is similar in the United States and many other industrialized countries, the teen pregnancy rate is much higher in the United States than in most of these countries. There may be many reasons for this discrepancy, but lack of education about sexuality and lack of availability of contraception are thought to be among the most important.

In this chapter, we'll take you through the main considerations you and your child will face if your daughter or your son's girlfriend gets pregnant.

Finding Out

There was something in the way she looked at me. I went to the bathroom and checked the box of pads I'd bought a month ago. It hadn't even been opened. That made her about three weeks late for her period.

—*Floy, on her seventeen-year-old daughter*

She'll know before you will. The most obvious clue that your daughter is pregnant will be that her period is late. Her breasts may start to feel tender, and her nipples may become sensitive. She may feel tired and nauseated and find that she needs to urinate often. Much later, around the sixteenth to twentieth week of the pregnancy, she may begin to feel the baby move.

She may not tell you. But you may notice other clues. She may be skipping school, feeling depressed, acting angry for no apparent reason, or doing other things that show something's wrong. Even if she weren't pregnant, these things would catch your attention, but don't forget to add pregnancy to the list of possible explanations.

No one will know for sure until the pregnancy test.

Rabbits don't have to die anymore. Pregnancy tests measure the hormone human chorionic gonadotropin (hCG), which is produced within one day of the fertilized egg implanting in the uterus. This hormone increases for about the first two months of pregnancy. The actual test is called a beta-hCG test. The clinician can test your daughter's urine or her blood. Urine tests can detect a pregnancy as early as ten days after fertilization, or about four days before her next menstrual period is due; blood tests may detect a pregnancy a day or two earlier, but she probably won't get to her clinician that soon, so the urine test is usually all she'll need.

Your daughter can also get a home pregnancy test without a prescription. Some tests can detect a pregnancy as early as the clinician's test can, even before she has missed her period, but other home tests take a little longer. These tests are quite accurate if she follows the instructions carefully. However, given their anxiety, many adolescents perform the test incorrectly, such as testing too early in the pregnancy, so some pregnant girls mistakenly think they are not pregnant. Your daughter should test herself again if she performed it on the early side and it was negative.

At sixteen, Helen may have had a fairly typical experience with the home test. "I just started crying. I don't know why. The instructions were easy, but I was too scared of doing something wrong." Her brother wanted to get in the bathroom and heard her crying. "Bobby started shouting, 'Mom! Mom! Helen's crying in the bathroom.' Then there's the knock on the door and suddenly she's in the bathroom and the pregnancy kit is there, and I'm sobbing, and she takes it all in, and she gave me a huge hug, and I just cried on her shoulder."

Helen's mother read the instructions for her. She'd already missed her first urine of the day (the one that this test required for accuracy, although not all home tests do), so her mother took her to the clinic where they could do a more sensitive test. It was negative, to the relief of both of them. "After the test said I wasn't pregnant, she talked with me about what had happened."

The Waiting Game

The earlier your daughter finds out she's pregnant, the better. If she wants to carry the baby, she should start prenatal care right away and give up cigarettes, alcohol, and drugs. And if she doesn't want to carry the baby, her abortion options will be greater if she finds out earlier.

But girls don't always take the test as early as they should. There are many reasons for a delay. Your daughter might not want to know if she's pregnant. As long as she hasn't taken the test, she can tell herself she might not be. Or, she may not realize her symptoms could mean she's pregnant, particularly if her periods are usually irregular and she attributes her nausea to a virus.

And even if she's thought about the possibility, she may not know what to do. She may not trust her clinician, or she may be afraid he'll be too expensive—she may not know about free clinics or home testing. She may also fear someone (like you, perhaps) will figure out she's pregnant if she's spotted at the store or the clinician's office.

Patty, fifteen at the time, thought she might be pregnant, but she was afraid to go to the drugstore to get a pregnancy test because someone might see her. Her friend Toussi offered to help. They may have seen one too many detective movies.

"We sat outside the store for about fifteen minutes to make sure no one we knew went in. Toussi brought hats for us to wear, and we both wore sunglasses. I stayed by the door as a lookout, and Toussi checked all the aisles to make sure we didn't miss anyone. Then she filled a basket with shampoo and magazines and she slipped the pregnancy test package underneath everything and got in line to pay. Toussi told me she wimped out with the clerk and made a comment about hoping her mother really was pregnant because she wanted a little brother." Patty turned out not to be pregnant.

"I think the whole stealth thing distracted me from thinking about how scared I was."

It is possible, of course, to avoid some of the cloaks and daggers in dealing with a possible pregnancy by having an anticipatory talk with your daughter as she becomes sexually active.

Ellen told her daughter about her own pregnancy scare as a teenager. Ellen had waited for three months thinking she was pregnant, afraid to tell anyone. Then her period came. She had been afraid her father would kick her out if she were pregnant. "I think it broke down a wall. How hard can it be to come to me with a problem if I've already told her I was human once, too. We have a good relationship anyway, but I wanted to make it easier for her to talk to me about anything—not just pregnancy. I figured if I've opened the door with a pregnancy scare, there's not much she should be afraid to tell me."

If She Isn't Pregnant

If your daughter wasn't trying to get pregnant, a false alarm is an excellent time for her to learn (or relearn) how to prevent it from happening again. The same goes for your son.

You might think the experience of a false alarm would make a girl extremely careful afterward. That may be true for your daughter, but about six out of ten adolescents in one study who had a negative pregnancy test became pregnant within one and a half to two years.

Ectopic Pregnancies

Most pregnancies that aren't terminated end in a healthy baby and a healthy mother, but complications can occur. *Ectopic pregnancy* is one such uncommon but dangerous complication. It can present problems early, before your daughter's been to the clinician or even knows she's pregnant.

An ectopic pregnancy occurs when the fertilized egg implants somewhere outside the uterus, usually in one of the fallopian tubes. In adolescents, the most typical reason is scarring in the tubes from prior PID.

An ectopic pregnancy can be very difficult to diagnose. The most common symptoms are irregular menses, vaginal bleeding, and pelvic pain. If your daughter has an ectopic pregnancy, she needs urgent medical attention. If it's not treated, the pregnancy can rupture her fallopian tube leading to serious complications. Urine pregnancy tests can be negative, and the clinician may need to do several blood tests and an ultrasound. An ectopic pregnancy can be treated, however, and most women who are treated in a timely fashion can get pregnant again.

Of course, you may want to be gentle when making your point—
your daughter and her partner may be quite shaken. They should consider what decisions led to the pregnancy scare, and what steps they could
have taken to avoid it. If they were using contraception, were they using
it correctly? Should they change methods? They may have been using
reliable contraception correctly and ended up in the small group of couples who get pregnant anyway. But most adolescents (and adults) who get
pregnant unintentionally were using contraception incorrectly or not at
all. Your daughter should learn how to prevent any more pregnancy scares
either by using contraception properly or by refraining from intercourse.

If she wasn't trying to get pregnant, she will probably be quite
relieved. But it's not always so simple. Even if she felt completely
unequipped to be a parent, your daughter may still feel a sense of loss.
There may have been a thrill in thinking her body was capable of creating a new life. She may have been distressed, but the attention she
received from you and others may have helped her feel important or
loved. The same may be true for your son if there was a chance he was
going to be a father. Instead of celebrating with your child, you may find
yourself comforting her or him through a grieving process—surprising,
perhaps, but understandable.

If She Is

Upon learning she is pregnant, your daughter may feel shocked, elated,
angry, petrified, or proud, or she may experience a seemingly contradictory combination of emotions. She may respond by ignoring the pregnancy and hoping it will just go away, or by learning everything she can
about being pregnant and how to do it right.

Some girls feel that they couldn't be pregnant and decide the test is
wrong. A positive test is almost always correct, but a clinician can confirm
it. Just as it's risky to delay a pregnancy test, it's also risky to delay acting
on a positive test. It won't go away, with the exception of a miscarriage,
and hoping for a miscarriage is not, in most cases, a winning proposition.

Sooner or later, your daughter will have to figure out what to do.
What will she decide?

What Now?

My dad poured himself into his work when I was in high school. He escaped from everything that was going on in the house. When I got pregnant, he just avoided me. He didn't know what to do. My mother did the same thing. They talked about sending me away, like to a convent where I could go and have the baby. But I was excited! I thought it was just the best thing. I was excited, and I still am.

—*Patricia, thirty-one-year-old mother of three*

The decision about how to respond to an unintended pregnancy is the biggest decision your teenager has ever faced. She will need advice and support.

Her choices include having and raising the baby (with or without the father's involvement), having a family member (hers or the father's) raise the baby, giving it up for adoption or foster care, or having an abortion.

Whether your daughter has always known that she would keep the baby if she became pregnant, or whether she decided long ago that she would abort if her contraception failed, the reality of being pregnant may change how she views a lot of issues, and she may rethink her earlier ideas.

She needs to think about her values, what will be best for her, and what will be best for the baby. She should also consider the impact her decision will have on the rest of her family and on the boy and his family. Even if she decides that what's best for her is different from what's best for everyone else, she should be aware of the implications for them.

Some questions she should answer if she is considering having the baby: Is she comfortable with people knowing she is pregnant? Does she prefer to live with an out-of-town relative once she is showing? How will she pay the medical expenses? Does she have habits that could harm her developing fetus, such as smoking cigarettes? Will she go for prenatal care?

Will she raise it?

As well you know, raising a child requires love, money, patience, time, commitment, more patience, more love, and work. Your daughter needs to make sure she can handle the physical, emotional, and financial aspects of raising a child. She needs to understand that having a baby is a full-time job—that babies need constant attention, even when she's having a bad day. This is a subject on which you are an expert—let her know what it's like to be a parent. She should also know just what kind of support to expect from you and other family members, what role the father and his family will play, where she and the baby (and possibly the father) will live, how she will support herself and the baby, and what the impact will be on her and the baby's future lives.

If she is considering giving the baby up for adoption, does she think she'll be able to part with him? How does she think she'll feel in the future? What will it be like to know that he is out there and that she can't see him? Would she want to arrange to be in his life in some small way?

Finally, how does she feel about abortion? She may want to know the details about how it is done, whether it will hurt, what the risks are, and how she may feel afterward. Her reactions may surprise her (and you). She may believe in a woman's right to choose but feel abortion is not a choice she could make. She may have been a strong opponent of abortion, but now decide to have one when faced with the prospect of a child. The conflict between her moral views and her personal desires may be great and add to the emotional trauma.

Who has legal authority over what happens depends on which state of the country your daughter is in. Regardless of the law, there are many potential participants in this decision. In addition to the two potential parents and their own parents, other family and friends may have something to offer. Your daughter's clinician can tell her about the health aspects of her options. Her religious adviser can help her think about her decision in the context of religious values. A counselor from school or an organization like Planned Parenthood can also help.

Planned Parenthood's mission is to provide nonjudgmental care and support for all options. Some clinics that do not perform abortions may provide comprehensive counseling to help your daughter decide what's best for her. However, some organizations may actively discourage abortions or not mention them as an option. If you and your daughter agree with their position, such settings may be fine. But if she has any doubts, your daughter may prefer to go to a clinic that will support her in considering all of the possible choices.

It may help your daughter to talk with other adolescents who have faced the same choice and made various decisions. It can also help to talk with adults who made such decisions when they were adolescents. And then there's you.

Your Role

I reminded myself to stay calm—this was harder for her than it was for me. I decided I should wait for her to come to me. I tried to wait, but I didn't last ten minutes. So I put some cookies on a tray, and I brought them up to her room and sat down next to her on her bed and put my arm around her. She knew I knew. I just said, "I love you," and we sat there.

—*Floy, on her seventeen-year-old daughter*

Are you having some feelings about this?

Tracey assumed her daughter Callie had been taken advantage of. "I called his mother, Elizabeth. I'd known her for years—not well, but we'd say hi when we'd see each other. I started off calm, and then I found myself screaming at her for what her son had done to my daughter. I can't believe I did such a thing. What if she hadn't known yet?" It came out later that Callie had said she had a diaphragm in, which wasn't true. "Callie didn't even have a diaphragm! I owed Elizabeth a big apology. She understood.

"I had all this anger. It would have been easier if I could have blamed someone other than Callie. But I didn't have that luxury."

You may be flooded with feelings, and whatever your daughter decides, this pregnancy will unalterably affect your life. But here's the kicker. She's going to make the decision. And even if you have a strong sense of her values and ambitions, you may not be able to predict what she'll want to do about her pregnancy.

You may know exactly what you think she *should* do, and you may want to tell her—command her—to do it. You may not want to wait for her to decide, and you may not want to risk her making what you consider the wrong choice. But there may be consequences to trying to impose a decision.

If she is like most girls, it will be best for her to think this through and come to her own decision. Even if she reaches the same decision that you came to, the process of getting there can help her accept whatever happens. The potential consequence of having you or someone else dictate the decision is years of resentment and regret. She may agree that your choice was best, but she may never forgive you for taking away her autonomy. That doesn't mean she won't need your advice and, depending on the state where you live, your permission.

Some parents who disagree with their daughter's decision will try to block an abortion. Although they can legally stop it in some states, it is uncommon for a court to deny an adolescent's petition to have an abortion without parental approval. A blocked abortion can have serious negative consequences for the mother, her relationship with her baby, and her relationship with you.

"I've never believed in abortion. I'm not the type to be out in the streets protesting, but I don't think abortion is right," says Margaret, whose daughter got pregnant at seventeen. "But my daughter said she was going to have one, and I didn't know what to do. She could see that I was devastated—this was even worse than her being pregnant."

Margaret sought advice from her own mother, who told her to go with her daughter to get the abortion. "She said I belonged at my daughter's side. I had to accept that this was April's decision, not mine. My mother had always been against abortion, too, but she was adamant about this. She told me I would never forgive myself if I abandoned April when she needed me most. Having gone, I can tell you this—I can't imagine her going through it alone."

Don't Make Me a Grandmother

Or you may be approaching your daughter's pregnancy from the other perspective, desperate for her not to bring this child into your family.

"As I saw it, there really was only one option," Lisa explains about her daughter's decision. "There was no way she could have a child this young. She had her whole life ahead of her. Carry a baby and put it up for adoption? Was I supposed to ship her off to my sister's for the rest of the school year? I know this isn't politically correct, but really—there was no choice here. This is not a community where tenth graders have babies. I knew from the start she had to have an abortion, and that we had to keep this as quiet as possible."

Lisa's daughter did not agree. She wanted to learn about all of her options and talk with others, including the boy. "I took enough psychology in college to know I had to pull back," Lisa observes. "If I insisted she have the abortion, she'd want to have the child as an act of rebellion. I let her know what I thought, but I also said it was her decision. She met with a counselor at the women's clinic and talked it over with friends—I really don't know what life experience they were drawing on to give her advice—but that's what she wanted to do." After about a week, her daughter decided to have an abortion. "That week was hell on me," Lisa adds.

If you find yourself in this position, you have even less power than the parents who want to prevent their children from having an abortion. No parents can legally compel their child to have an abortion or to give up the baby for adoption.

The best approach, the only reasonable approach we can think of, is simply to express your views and the reasons for them, and to explain what sort of support you are willing and able to give with each of her options. You can make it plain, for example, that if she keeps the baby, you will not help take care of it. If this is true, it is information she will need in making her decision.

The Invisible Man

It's easy to forget the impact on the father. If it's your son whose girlfriend is pregnant, he is in a delicate position. He may have the same emotions and reactions she has. He may be excited, afraid, confused. But she's the one who will carry the baby or go through an abortion. He may be just as invested in the baby as she is, but he has no legal authority about what happens before it is born. He can't make her have an abortion or stop her from having one. He cannot make her get prenatal care or stop smoking. He has no power beyond the power of persuasion. But if she carries the baby, once it is born, he will have all sorts of legal rights and responsibilities, perhaps more than he is ready for.

He certainly will have more influence over his partner's decision if he stays involved and tries to be supportive—if he makes himself available for her to turn to when she wants to talk about her choices.

It's not uncommon for the fathers in teen pregnancies to be in their twenties. Don't count on older men to act more responsibly than younger ones. They may run for cover even faster when they hear a baby's on the way. Still, just because a man's twenty-three, that doesn't mean he doesn't love your daughter and doesn't want to be a father to his child. It may not be the typical scenario, but it happens.

Becoming a Teenage Mom

> I was well-educated. Came from an upper-middle-class family. I was pretty secure. I was very solid. I think that's why it worked.
>
> —*Donna, forty-year-old mother of two, who had her first child at sixteen*

Let's look at each of your daughter's options in a little more detail, starting with keeping the baby.

As you may have suspected, having a child as a teenager appears to reduce the future prospects for both the mother and the child. Your daughter may be less likely to finish high school or college. She may develop new dreams and goals, many of which revolve around her role as a mother, but her old plans may no longer be viable or important to her. The children of teen mothers are also more likely to do worse in school and are more likely to have early pregnancies themselves, although if the teen mother continues to live with her parents, things usually turn out better for the baby.

That said, it also appears that the impact on the mother may be less than is popularly believed. If you just compare teen girls who have babies to teen girls who don't, the former certainly do worse in terms of education, income, and family life. But the question is what would their lives have been like had they been the same person without having the baby? It looks, on average, like their lives may not have been very different.

This is a hard topic to study. Teenagers who have babies are different from teenagers who don't, so it's hard to find a group of girls without babies that is otherwise the same as a group with. We can match them by family background, family wealth, race, and religion, but we can't match them for inner drive, sense of responsibility, or personality. Maybe the girl who wants to become a lawyer is less likely to have sex or more likely to use a condom or more likely to have an abortion because she knows a baby would derail her plans.

At forty, Donna owns a women's clothing store, has a husband who's a teacher, and has two daughters, one twenty-four and one twenty-two. "I kind of take offense sometimes when people jump to the conclusion that when any young woman has a child it is automatically a bad thing. It's great being a forty-year-old woman and having two young women who are your daughters."

How was she affected by having two children before graduating from high school?

"I did great. It's never held me back from anything I wanted to do. And both of my daughters are wonderful young women. I have never regretted getting pregnant or having children."

If you were to see Donna say this, you would know two things. One, this is an incredibly buoyant and energetic woman. And two, she really means it. Our guess is that this energy and confidence is what got her through the kind of challenge many seventeen-year-olds from her wealthy suburban high school couldn't have imagined.

"Jenny was born in October of my junior year. September of the following year I went back to high school. I would go two nights a week. I was fortunate that they had an alternative program at night. When I was a senior, I had Nan. Nan was in my arms and Jenny was at my side at my graduation. I started college the next fall. When the kids were babies, I worked delivering papers at night. I would stop the car and breast-feed when I needed to. It took me eight years rather than four to get my B.A., but then I went on to get my masters in business."

All of which is to say, the impact on an individual girl may be very different from the average impact that turns up in a study. Some girls really would have gone on to fulfill ambitious personal and career goals had they not become a parent. Conversely, if your daughter decides to have a child, that doesn't mean that she can't pursue her dreams. An individual woman can definitely beat the odds. She won't be the first teen mother to go back and complete her high school degree, go on to college, get an excellent job, and support her child.

When it comes to the health and development of the newborn, the studies are again limited and have murky and sometimes conflicting results. All things being equal, it looks like having a teen mother has at most a small negative impact on the baby's health, especially if she gets good prenatal care. It's not biology that's the problem. What really matters are the mother's income and education and circumstances. Teen mothers don't usually have much income. They tend not to complete their education, and they often get poor prenatal care. None of these bodes well for the baby.

Raising a child will be easier if your daughter has your encouragement. Adolescent mothers whose parents are involved and supportive are more likely to return to school and achieve. Of course, not all teen mothers, maybe not even most, wind up as content as Donna. But even if your daughter isn't quite as resilient as she was, you might keep in mind Donna's assessment of her teenage life: "If you are given support— and I was given a lot—and if people have a positive attitude toward you, things can work out wonderfully."

Adoption

Not many teens choose adoption, but it is an important option for girls who are not comfortable with abortion and yet do not feel able to raise

Prenatal Care

If there is any chance your daughter will have the baby, whether she will keep it or put it up for adoption, she should get prenatal care immediately. This is important for her health and the baby's. Many pregnancy complications can be prevented with timely prenatal care. She will be checked for anemia, high blood pressure, STDs, and other infections and conditions that can harm her health or the baby's health. She will learn that she shouldn't smoke, drink alcohol, or use drugs during her pregnancy because they can harm the baby. One of the best ways she can demonstrate that she is responsible enough to care for a child is by giving up her substances for it. She should check whether any medicines she's taking could harm the baby.

Good prenatal care will also include advice about other things your child should do while pregnant, such as taking prenatal vitamins that contain folate to reduce the chance of birth defects (it is even better to start taking these before pregnancy). A summary of common recommendations can be found at www.plannedparenthood.org.

a child. There are plenty of prospective parents who are eager to adopt and provide a loving home for a child.

State laws govern adoptions, so we will have to speak in generalities here. There are various types of adoptions. In a *closed adoption,* the names of biological and adoptive parents are kept secret. Later, if the biological parents develop medical conditions relevant to the child's health, they can share the information through the adoption agency. Once the child is eighteen years old, if she and one of the biological parents both sign up with a reunion registry, their names can be shared with each other.

In an *open adoption,* the biological and adoptive parents are known in some way to each other, whether by exchanging names or meeting in person. The biological parents often get to choose among potential adoptive parents. Sometimes the biological parents play an active role in the child's life, through letters or occasional visits. However, the adoptive parents have all the parental rights.

Adoptions can be arranged through a public or private agency that screens potential adoptive parents. Some agencies may cover your daughter's prenatal expenses (so may some adoptive parents) and provide a place for her to live while pregnant. Adoptions can also be arranged privately through an attorney. It is illegal for someone to pay your child to give up her baby. A private adoption may not have as many support services, such as counseling, associated with it, but your daughter's clinician or her religious advisor can make a referral. Such services can be very helpful in thinking through the implications of the decision and in preparing to give up a child.

Both biological parents must consent to the adoption, unless a parent cannot be located or is declared unfit. If the father is not married to the mother, he may need to establish paternity to exert his parental rights. A parent cannot give final agreement to turn over the child for adoption until after the baby is born. The length of time before the adoption can be finalized varies across states. No matter what was agreed to before the baby's birth, biological parents have a right to change their minds afterward. If one parent wants to give up the child and the other does not, a judge will decide. Adoption must be approved by a judge, usually after the baby has been with the adoptive family for a period of time. Sometimes there is also a grace period after the adoption is finalized when the biological parent can petition to get the baby back. But by and large, adoption should be considered a permanent transfer of parental rights.

Foster Care

Your daughter can place her baby with a foster parent who has been approved by an agency. The biological parent(s) are expected to take the child back in a reasonable amount of time, perhaps after high school. The state usually provides medical coverage and some funds for expenses. The state has temporary legal responsibility for the child, although biological parents may be able to make major medical or educational decisions. Foster care can be provided by a relative or family friend, but some states limit funds for relatives. When there are not enough foster families, children are placed in institutional settings.

Usually both biological parents need to approve placing the child in foster care, although a judge can circumvent the father. If biological parents do not visit their child regularly and plan for his or her future, the agency may take away their rights and put the child up for adoption.

Another approach is for a family member to take care of the child informally until your daughter has finished school or has settled into a job and is ready to assume responsibility. If the caregiver lives with your daughter and her child, then transitioning back to your daughter may be easier for the child. Depending on the relationship of the caregiver to your daughter, a legal contract may help. Regardless, both parents usually have a right to take back the child from an informal situation, unless they lose those rights by not staying involved.

Abortion

An option that incites conflict, frustration, and ambivalence, abortion is the second most common end point for all teen pregnancies.

Your daughter, if she is considering aborting, may need to take some time to make a decision she feels comfortable with, but she can't mull it over for very long. As her pregnancy progresses, abortion options decrease (for example, medical abortions are usually not performed after the ninth week), abortions become more expensive, and the risks of surgical abortions increase. So do the legal restrictions.

Abortion is one of the most common surgical procedures performed in the United States. Although adolescents have fewer complications than adults when they have abortions during the same week of pregnancy, in practice adolescents have their abortions later and so have more complications. Teens have later abortions for several reasons. It takes them longer to learn they are pregnant and to seek health care. In some states, your daughter can't have an abortion without your notification or permission—sometimes both parents must give permission.

Abortion Methods

There are two types of abortion, surgical and medical. The choice of abortion method should be made in consultation with your daughter's clinician. The range of options for the type of abortion declines with advancing gestational age.

Surgical Abortion Methods
Dilation and Curettage

For years, dilation and curettage (D & C; also sometimes called Suction Curettage) has been the most common form of abortion used in the United States, with over 95 percent of abortions performed with this method.

Dilation is typically required and can be accomplished with several methods. A laminaria (made from seaweed) can be placed in the cervical opening to slowly expand it. It generally works within six hours (although it may take longer) and causes little or no pain. Osmotic dilators are quite similar except that they are manufactured synthetically, may cost more, and tend to work faster. A mechanical dilator can also expand the cervix and may be used in conjunction with a laminaria or osmotic dilator.

Following dilation of the cervix, a thin tube connected to suction or a syringe is passed through the cervix to extract the products of conception (the fetus and placenta) from the uterus. (Local anesthesia can be used.) The procedure takes about ten minutes. Some cramps may occur (like menstrual cramps or stronger) during and after the abortion. The clinician may also prescribe antibiotics to prevent infection.

Dilation and Evacuation

Also known as D & E, this is the procedure most typically performed in the second trimester, especially from thirteen to sixteen weeks gestation. It is similar to a D & C, except greater dilation of the cervix is needed to make sure that the larger products of conception can be removed. Forceps are often required for complete removal of the products of conception. The removal procedure takes ten to twenty minutes.

Local anesthesia is usually all that's needed for the procedure, although general anesthesia may be recommended by the clinician or requested by your daughter.

Medical Abortion Methods

Several medical abortion methods have become available in the United States in recent years, and it is expected that over time they will be used more and more in place of surgical methods. Medical abortions are generally performed in the first seven to nine weeks after the last menstrual period. They often feel similar to a miscarriage, with a lot of cramping and possibly some nausea and vomiting. They may also cause some belly pain and diarrhea. There is usually a lot of vaginal bleeding during the first few hours and then there may be a little irregular bleeding, including some blood clots or tissue, for a month or longer. If a medical abortion is incomplete, a surgical abortion can be used to complete the process.

Medical abortions are generally safe, although they should not be used by someone who has severe anemia or certain other conditions. IUDs should be removed first.

Methotrexate

Methotrexate is a medication that is given as an injection to interrupt a pregnancy. It is used in conjunction with Misoprostol, which causes the uterus to contract and empty. This method involves three visits to the clinician, first to get the Methotrexate, then seven days later to get the Misoprostol (by

pill or suppository), and finally about two weeks later to confirm
that the abortion is complete. Methotrexate has about a 90 percent success rate in early pregnancy. The abortion is usually
complete within eight days.

Mifepristone

Also known as RU-486, Mifepristone blocks the hormone
progesterone, which is needed to maintain the lining of the
uterus. As the lining breaks down, the pregnancy ends. It suc-
cessfully interrupts about 95 percent of pregnancies.
Mifepristone comes as a pill taken by mouth. It is given in a
three-visit sequence (it includes the use of Misoprostol), similar to Methotrexate. The abortion is usually complete within
eight days.

(In other states, she can do as she wishes without your knowledge.) So,
there can be a delay if your daughter is afraid to tell you or if you (or her
other parent) can't be found, although a judge can waive the need for
one or both parents' involvement. The cost can also cause a delay, which
only increases the cost more. An uncomplicated first trimester surgical
abortion will probably cost at least several hundred dollars, and the price
goes up quickly as the pregnancy advances. Insurance sometimes covers
abortions, and some clinics offer reduced fees.

Your daughter may need to travel an hour or more to find a clinic
that performs legal abortions or that will even tell her that abortion is
a legal option. Your daughter's own clinician should be able to refer her
to someone who can discuss her options. However, if your daughter is
not comfortable with her clinician, she can contact Planned Parenthood at 1-800-230-PLAN or at www.plannedparenthood.org, or the
National Abortion Federation Hotline at 1-800-772-9100 (in Canada,
1-800-424-2280).

After an Abortion

Most women do not suffer from long-term emotional problems related to the abortion. Such problems are more likely to occur when a woman aborted a wanted pregnancy for health reasons or because of major problems in her life, when she was conflicted over having an abortion, or when she already had emotional problems. To put things in perspective, women tend to have fewer emotional problems after abortion than after childbirth (obviously not a reason to have an abortion).

In the short term, women may have a variety of reactions. If your daughter is like most girls, she will probably feel a sense of relief. She may also feel sad and depressed and have lingering feelings of guilt at having gotten pregnant in the first place. She may mourn the loss of her pregnancy. Let your daughter know you are there to support and help her. She may benefit from some counseling.

As for physical effects, abortions have fewer complications than childbirth and many surgical procedures. Complications can occur, and it is important for your daughter to discuss them with her clinician to make an informed decision. After having an abortion, your daughter should check with her clinician if she has signs of infection, such as fever, chills, a vaginal discharge that smells foul, belly pain, cramping, aching in her lower back, or persistent or heavy bleeding.

Women who have first-trimester abortions do not have more pregnancy complications or difficulty getting pregnant in the future. Less is known about the impact of later abortions, but women with uncomplicated later abortions also probably have no future pregnancy problems.

Your daughter can get pregnant again within about ten days of having an abortion. So, if she continues to have intercourse, she will need to use contraception to prevent unintended pregnancies. Her menstrual cycle should resume in about six weeks.

After your daughter's abortion, you may need to mourn a loss, too—the loss of the baby, the loss of your child's innocence, or the loss of your authority over your child, particularly if you disagreed with her decision. If you need to protect your child's privacy, you may be limited in where you can turn. If you can't discuss the situation with a relative or a friend, you may want to consider a therapist or your religious advisor. Do not underestimate the potential impact on your feelings. Whether you agreed with your child's decision or considered it a repudiation of your moral code, such an experience can take its toll.

A Common Goal

Although there are clearly wide-ranging opinions on abortion, there is probably one goal for which there is consensus: that the announcement that began this chapter—"Mom, Dad, I'm pregnant"—would always be a happy one. We wish we could tell you how to guarantee that your daughter would never have an unintended pregnancy or that your son would never be an unintended father. We can't, of course. But you do know how to reduce your child's chances of facing this particular challenge. And now you know, too, what to do if an unplanned pregnancy arises in your family. That's good, because if it does happen, your kid is going to need a knowledgeable, committed person like you on her side.

Appendix A

CONTRACEPTIVE METHODS

HERE IS A REVIEW of the various types of contraception and the latest information about their benefits and side effects. We also provide estimated costs, which may range widely. Some health insurance policies may cover the costs. A table showing the pregnancy prevention rates of each type of contraception appears in Chapter 9.

As further research is conducted, better information on contraceptives is becoming available and new contraceptive methods are being developed. Always consult your child's clinician for the most comprehensive and up-to-date information and for advice tailored to his or her own health status and needs. You can also find recent information on the website of the federal Centers for Disease Control and Prevention (CDC) at www.cdc.gov.

Abstinence

Abstinence isn't exactly a form of contraception, but when practiced properly and consistently, it sure is effective. It's cheap, it doesn't require a prescription or visit to a clinician, and it's always available. We discuss abstinence in Chapter 8, but we will review some key points here related to contraception.

If your child's reason for being abstinent is to prevent pregnancy, then he or she will only need to abstain from vaginal intercourse. (Actually, there is the occasional "virgin pregnancy" when sperm fall near the vaginal opening and are able to swim up the vagina. This is rare, but it can happen, so the male partner should aim away from her vulva when he ejaculates.)

Abstinence for the purpose of preventing STDs involves a much longer list of proscribed activities. As we discuss in Appendix B, genital warts, crabs, and scabies can be transmitted simply by touching or lying against each other unclothed, whereas HIV requires the exchange of body fluids through such acts as vaginal or anal intercourse. So when it comes to STD prevention, there is a continuum of risk that your adolescent needs to think about.

Abstinence for religious purposes or personal views may vary and will, of course, depend on the particular religion or moral code your child is following. In general, though, abstinence motivated by religion will usually exclude all forms of intercourse and possibly any sexual activity that involves ejaculation.

Because of the multiple potential definitions of abstinence, it's best, as we discuss in Chapter 8, to clarify which definition you are using when talking with your kids. Otherwise, even if your kids are trying to follow your advice, they may be engaging in activities you presumed they knew to forgo—or they may be refraining from activities that you consider reasonable options.

One approach to abstinence is outercourse, which consists of variations on mutual masturbation. Many public health advocates are promoting this approach as a way to have sexual intimacy and satisfaction without some of the associated health risks. (The outercourse slogan is "On me, not in me." A little blunt, we suppose, but you have to admit, it gets the point across.)

Setting a rule to abstain from all sexual intimacy may not work for some adolescents; once they slip and engage in some activities, they may feel like they failed, throw in the towel, and just keep going all the way to intercourse. So a measured approach—where their goal is to engage in some but not all forms of intimacy—may be more manageable. For others, this kind of approach won't work. It's either all or nothing for them, so nothing is the best way for them to maintain abstinence.

Upsides

Abstinence doesn't depend on remembering to bring anything along on a date (except willpower and the ability to say no) or to take a daily pill or to go to get a regular shot.

Abstinence is the most effective way to prevent both pregnancy and (depending on just what is being abstained from) STDs.

Downsides

If adolescents are taught only about abstinence but not about contraception, they may not know how to reduce the chances of having an unintended pregnancy or contracting an STD if they do not remain abstinent.

The Male Condom

Condoms prevent pregnancy by blocking sperm from entering the vagina, and some types of condoms block transmission of many STDs as well. Indeed, the male and female condom are the only types of contraception that substantially decrease the transmission of STDs.

Most male condoms are made of latex (including 97 percent of condoms sold in the United States). Although their effectiveness has not been demonstrated conclusively for each STD, studies with people who are using condoms as well as studies in laboratories have shown them to provide substantial protection against some diseases (especially HIV). Scientists infer from these studies that condoms similarly protect against other diseases and so recommend condom use against them as well. Indeed, condoms do not *guarantee* protection against any type of STD. (Among other reasons, condoms can break.) They reduce the risk of catching or spreading STDs, but they don't eliminate it. Also, of course, condoms only protect against STD transmission involving the penis. Many STDs can be transmitted through other routes, such as between the vagina and the mouth or from skin to skin.

Lubrication makes latex condoms less likely to break and more comfortable for vaginal and anal intercourse. (Unlubricated condoms make more sense for fellatio.) Only water-based lubricants should be used with latex condoms as oil can weaken the latex. Oil-based lubricants to avoid include Vaseline, baby oil, cooking or salad oil, massage oil, cocoa butter, cold cream, and many moisturizing lotions. If a girl is being treated for a vaginal yeast infection, the medication she puts in her vagina is probably oil-based, so she cannot count on latex condoms until she has completed the treatment. (She can instead use polyurethane condoms, which we describe below, because oil doesn't harm them.) There are many effective lubricants that are water-based, such as K-Y jelly and products designed specifically for use with latex condoms. For a twist, try egg whites.

Some men who are bothered by the reduction in sensation that can occur with latex condoms prefer lambskin condoms (also called natural membrane condoms) made from a lamb's intestine (for anatomy buffs, they are made from the part of the intestine called the caecum, with one condom coming from each lamb). Although sperm cannot pass through natural membrane condoms, small viruses can. So lambskin condoms are useful for preventing pregnancy but not for preventing the spread of HIV, herpes, or hepatitis B. These condoms only make sense for long-standing monogamous couples that do not need to worry about STDs, and therefore we don't recommend them for most adolescents. As for the diminished sensation, a few drops of lubricant inside a latex condom can help make their use more pleasurable.

Another type of condom is the polyurethane condom, also called the plastic condom. It is thinner and stronger than latex condoms and can be used with oil-based lubricants. Research is still being done to determine how well plastic condoms protect against STDs, but expectations are high that they are protective.

Some condoms come with spermicide on them. There is no evidence that the spermicide on the condom is useful for pregnancy prevention, because not much is on the condom and if the condom breaks or slips off, the sperm may not even come in contact with the spermicide. A vaginal spermicide is much more effective for preventing pregnancy. However, the major spermicide available in the United States, nonoxynol-9, does not protect against HIV and other STDs, but rather may increase the chances of becoming infected. We discuss spermicides in more detail below.

Condoms are relatively cheap. A plain latex condom costs 25 to 50 cents or more, a lubricated one costs the same or up to double, and a plastic condom costs one to two dollars.

Upsides

Except for the female version, male condoms are the only contraceptive proven to prevent STD transmission, making them indispensable to your sexually involved teenager. They are also easy to carry around and don't require a prescription.

Downsides

First, unlike with some forms of contraception, you have to decide to put them on each time. Many adolescents who consider condoms their means of contraception do not use them every time they have intercourse. Also, some boys put them on after they've already started intercourse, on the assumption that they only need it during ejaculation. Not only can the girl get pregnant from sperm in his pre-ejaculate, but they can both contract STDs before he puts on the condom.

And second, condoms can break. Condoms generally break less than 2 percent of the time, and most breakage doesn't seem to be due to manufacturing defects. We're told that quality control in condom production is pretty intense. Most breakage and slippage of condoms is due to people using them incorrectly. Fortunately, many of the breaks occur before intercourse has begun, but not all.

What to do when a condom breaks? If your son hasn't ejaculated yet, he should first withdraw (remember, there may be pre-ejaculate in the condom that could impregnate his partner) and then remove the condom immediately. He shouldn't continue with intercourse without putting on another condom. If he has already ejaculated, he and his partner should wash off the penis and vagina, anus, or mouth with soap and water to reduce the possibility of getting an STD. A woman can consider emergency contraception, which we discuss later in this appendix. A woman or man who has been exposed to HIV in this situation should contact a clinician immediately about taking medication that can prevent infection.

Finally, although it's rare, some people are allergic to latex. They can use plastic condoms, or if STDs are not a concern, lambskin condoms. An allergy can cause irritation, itchiness, a rash, or in extreme cases, difficulty breathing and shock—similar to what happens with allergies to medicines and foods. If your child gets any of these symptoms from blowing up a balloon, he or she may be allergic to latex. Check with a clinician. A little itching around the genitals could also be from the lubricant. He or she can try a different lubricant.

The Female Condom

The female condom was developed to give women more control over contraception and STD prevention. It consists of a polyurethane pouch—kind of like a clear plastic sock—with a thin ring at both the open and closed ends. It can be inserted up to 8 hours before intercourse. Your daughter uses the ring at the closed end to insert the condom into her vagina and anchor it so that it covers her cervix, similar to the way she would insert a diaphragm. The ring at the open end remains outside her vagina against her labia. The inside of the condom is prelubricated, and extra lubricant is provided for use on the outside of the condom.

Current recommendations are to use each condom only once, although there is some expectation that future studies may find that reuse (after washing) is safe. Unlike the latex of male condoms, the polyurethane is not damaged by oil-based lubricants.

Male and female condoms should not be used together because they can stick to each other and pull off.

So far, female condoms have not become a standout in the contraceptive cornucopia. They were only approved by the FDA in 1993, so they're relatively new. At present, many pharmacies don't carry them. They're more likely to be found in sex specialty shops.

Female condoms cost two to three dollars apiece.

Upsides

Initial studies did not look at the ability of female condoms to prevent the spread of STDs, but it is believed that they are effective—potentially more effective than male condoms because of less leakage from pinholes and tears. And the polyurethane that rests against the labia may provide an additional barrier to prevent contact between the base of the penis and the labia.

Some women like the female condom because it gives them a sense of control that they don't have with the male condom. They can take charge of inserting it correctly and making sure that it is not damaged. Some also like the way it feels and that, unlike all the other methods under their control, it can be used for both pregnancy and STD prevention. If a boy is uncomfortable wearing a male condom, or loses his erection, he might do better if his partner wears a female condom.

Downsides

A lot of women have trouble with the female condom at first and may even need a few months of practice to master proper use. Your daughter should definitely test one out before using it for sex. She also needs to make sure to use enough lubricant, or else it can slip out.

Some women complain that the female condom squeaks during sex. The sound is like air rushing out of a balloon, probably because air is squeezed out of the condom during sex. The unexpected noise can be a buzz-kill.

Some do not like the way it looks, with the ring hanging out of their vagina, and some find the inside ring uncomfortable.

Dental Dams

These five-inch-by-five-inch (some come larger) squares of latex (the same material as latex condoms) can be used for cunnilingus and anilingus to create a barrier between the tongue and the vagina or anus. (They are not strictly contraceptives because they are not used to prevent pregnancy, but we include them here because they are recommended for STD prevention.) A condom sliced lengthwise and opened into a square or a piece of plastic wrap can be used as a substitute.

Dental dams cost one to two dollars apiece.

Upsides

These dams are believed to protect against STD transmission during cunnilingus and anilingus.

Downsides

Dams can decrease sensation for both parties.

They have not been adequately studied, and some clinicians worry that saliva or other body fluids can slip around the edges of smaller dams.

Oral Contraceptive Pills

Most oral contraceptives (OCs) contain two hormones—estrogen and progestin—that suppress ovulation (prevent release of the egg), thicken cervical mucosa to prevent sperm from getting through, and block implantation of a fertilized egg in the uterus. These are called *combined OCs*. Another type of OC that adolescents use less often contains only progestin. It is called the *mini-pill*. We focus on the former but say a bit about the latter as well. All OCs are informally referred to as the Pill.

OCs usually come in a packet that includes all the pills your daughter will take for a full 28-day menstrual cycle. Each pill is numbered sequentially to indicate the day of the cycle on which to take the pill. It's only necessary to take the hormones for 21 days each cycle. Therefore, pills come in two types of packets: 21-day packets, which she stops taking for a week before starting a new packet, and 28-day packets, with an extra 7 days worth of pills with no hormone in them. These other pills are called reminder pills. With the 28-day packet, your daughter just keeps taking pills every day of the cycle, so she doesn't need to remember when to start a new cycle.

OCs need to be taken every day. This can be challenging for teenagers, or for that matter, for women of any age. Your daughter will probably find it easiest to remember if she works taking the pill into her daily routine—perhaps she could take it when she brushes her teeth. If your daughter misses her menstrual period but did not miss any pills, it's unlikely that she is pregnant. If she misses two periods in a row, she should get a pregnancy test.

Your daughter should have an open discussion with her clinician about the pros and cons of OCs and her ability to use them correctly. Most girls don't experience the side effects we detail below, but girls who know about side effects in advance not only can make more informed decisions but also are more likely to stick with OCs once they start taking them—it's easier to deal with side effects if they are prepared for them.

Daily pills cost anywhere from one hundred to three hundred dollars per year, depending on which type of OC a woman uses and whether she purchases generic pills (and of course, where she purchases them). Some clinics make them available for much less.

Upsides

If you haven't dealt with OCs in a while, you should know that today's have many fewer side effects than those of a generation ago.

OCs are a contraceptive method that can be entirely under your daughter's control if she prefers not to tell her partner or does not feel she can.

They have some additional health benefits, such as reducing the chance of endometrial cancer, ovarian cancer, benign breast disease, ovarian cysts, fibroids, ectopic pregnancy, PID, and anemia. They can reduce menstrual bleeding, menstrual cramps, and mittelschmerz (pain at the time of ovulation). And, perhaps the most popular extra benefit for adolescents, they can reduce acne. Clinicians sometimes prescribe OCs as treatment for particular conditions independent of pregnancy prevention. Many girls are happy to hear that OCs will not diminish their ability to become pregnant in the future.

A girl with irregular periods will have regular periods while taking OCs, but the periods may become irregular again once she stops. OCs also let girls avoid menstrual periods during special occasions like a high school graduation or a vacation by extending the number of days they take the "active" hormone pills or by skipping the pill-free week altogether.

Downsides

OCs do not protect against STDs, so adolescents will also need to use a condom for that purpose.

OCs are among the most researched medications we have, and

they are very safe for most users. However, they do have potential side effects, and your daughter should know about them.

Side effects include headaches, missed periods, spotting, breakthrough bleeding, breast fullness and tenderness, cloasma (darkening of the skin on parts of the face), and decreased sex drive. Some girls get nausea, which usually resolves after the first few cycles. OCs can make depression worse, but they are more likely to improve it. Your daughter may have heard that OCs will make her gain weight. Although some girls gain weight while taking OCs, as many seem to lose weight, and it's not even clear how much the weight change is affected by OCs.

OCs can increase the risk of deep vein thrombosis (a blood clot) and other heart or circulatory system diseases, but usually only in women who are over fifty or who have some other risk factor or related condition. The combined effects of smoking and using OCs can greatly increase the risks. Although women who have reached thirty-five or forty should not use OCs if they smoke, adolescent girls who smoke may take OCs.

There may be a small increased risk of cervical and liver cancer, but researchers are still trying to figure it out. Despite earlier concerns, the latest research shows that there is no increased risk of breast cancer. Women who take OCs are more likely to get a benign liver tumor called a hepatic adenoma, but this tumor is rare even among OC users.

Some symptoms that indicate it's time for your daughter to contact her clinician include severe belly, chest, or leg pain; severe headache; difficulty breathing; blurred or limited vision; difficulty speaking; and depression. Her clinician may want to be contacted about other symptoms as well.

Different formulations are more likely to cause one or another side effects. Some side effects will vary with your daughter's health habits and medical history. Girls with certain medical problems should not take OCs: specifically, girls with a history of clotting problems; very high blood pressure; and some types of liver disease, heart disease, or cancer. Some other medical problems don't keep a girl from using OCs

Emergency Contraception

We discuss emergency contraception (EC) in general in Chapter 9, but here are some details about specific methods.

The Preven Emergency Contraceptive Kit includes four estrogen-progestin pills. Your daughter takes two pills within seventy-two hours of intercourse and two more twelve hours later. If she is in the fertile period of her menstrual cycle (which lasts about six days), her risk of pregnancy drops by about 75 percent, from 8 in 100 to 2 in 100.

About half of women who use these pills experience nausea, and about one in five vomit (symptoms shouldn't last more than a day or so). If your daughter vomits within an hour of taking the pills, she may need to repeat the dose. She can take an antinausea or antivomiting medicine an hour before the first dose. Less common side effects include fatigue, headaches, and irregular bleeding.

The kit includes a home pregnancy test so your daughter can make sure she is not already pregnant from earlier sex (although the pills won't hurt an existing pregnancy). Her next menstrual period may start several days later or earlier than expected. If it doesn't come within three weeks of taking the pills, she should take a pregnancy test.

Plan B is another type of EC. It uses progestin pills without any estrogen, and your daughter takes one pill initially (within 72 hours) and one more twelve hours later. Plan B is more effective than Preven, reducing the chances of pregnancy during the fertile period by 89 percent, from 8 in 100 to 1 in 100. It also causes much less nausea and vomiting.

Regular oral contraceptive pills can be used as EC if taken at a high dose, and many have been approved by the U.S. Food and Drug Administration. As with Preven and Plan B, the first dose should be taken within seventy-two hours, and the

second dose should be taken twelve hours later. Approved
pills include Alesse or Levlite (one dose is five pink pills);
Aviane (one dose is five orange pills); Levlen or Nordette (one
dose is four light-orange pills); Lo/Ovral, Levora, or Low-
Ogestrel (one dose is four white pills); Ovral or Ogestrel (one
dose is two white pills); Triphasil or Tri-Levlen (one dose is four
yellow pills); and Trivora (one dose is four pink pills). Your
daughter's clinician can advise her about this option. Other
medicines could affect her EC dose, so she should tell her clinician if she's taking any.

A final option is the copper IUD. If inserted within five
days of intercourse (and possibly later), it appears to act as EC
by preventing implantation, thereby reducing the chances of
pregnancy by more than 99 percent. We mention the IUD so
you'll be fully informed, but it is generally not recommended
for adolescents (see the section on IUDs later in this appendix).

Additional information is available at the Emergency
Contraception Hotline at 1-888-NOT-2-LATE and Website at
http://ec.princeton.edu.

but mean that she should check in with her clinician more often. OCs
can interact with other medications (including some standard antibiotics), so if your daughter goes to a clinician who did not prescribe the
OCs, she should mention them.

Missed Pills and Back-ups

Your daughter should only choose OCs if she really feels up to the
responsibility of taking regular pills. However, even the most conscientious people make mistakes, and things do happen that interfere with
daily routines. Your daughter's clinician should tell her what to do if she
misses a pill, but here is some general advice:

If she misses taking a reminder pill (one of the pills without any hormones), not to worry. She should just throw away the one she missed and keep going with the packet. The reminder pills are really just place holders to count the seven days when hormones are not necessary.

If she misses a hormone pill or takes it twelve or more hours late, she should use a backup method for the next seven days.

If she is less than twenty-four hours late, she should take the pill, and then take the next pill at the time she would have taken it if she hadn't gotten off schedule. If it's exactly twenty-four hours late, she should take both the missed pill and the pill that is currently due. If it's been more than twenty-four hours, meaning now she's late for a second pill as well, she should take one missed pill now and the next pill at the regular time and throw out any additional missed pills.

If she misses a pill during the third week (days fifteen to twenty-one), she should finish the rest of the hormone pills as usual, but then she should skip the fourth week's pills (in other words, she should not use the non-hormone reminder pills). Instead, she should start a new packet as soon as she finishes the third week of hormone pills.

When your daughter first starts taking OCs, unless she starts on the first day of her menstrual bleeding, she will also need to use a backup method during the first seven days because the OCs will not prevent pregnancy right away.

And she will need to use a backup method when she stops taking OCs altogether. Many pregnancies occur because girls forget to start using another form of contraception when they stop their OCs.

The Mini-Pill

The progestin-only pill is known as the mini-pill. Most adolescents who want to take OCs will use the combined pills because they are more effective. However, some girls cannot take combined pills because of side effects such as nausea, breast tenderness, severe headaches, and high blood pressure.

Many of the benefits as well as risks are the same as those described above for the combined pill, which is not surprising given that they both have progestin. These pills reduce menstrual blood flow (sometimes to nothing), menstrual cramps, menstrual pain, mittelschmerz, and pain associated with endometriosis. They decrease the risk of endometrial and ovarian cancer, and PID. They do not contain estrogens, so they don't have the serious but rare side effect of increased blood clots. On the downside, they can cause depression or breast tenderness. Their effectiveness can also be greatly reduced when your daughter is taking certain other medicines at the same time.

Reminder pills are the same color as hormone pills, so your daughter just takes a pill every day without paying attention to which type she is taking.

It is very important that your daughter take the mini-pill at the same time each day. She can be a few hours late with the combined pill without much worry. But if your daughter misses one mini-pill, she should take it right away and then take the next pill at the regular time. If she is more than three hours late, she should use backup contraception for the next forty-eight hours. If she misses two or more consecutive pills, she should restart immediately and take two pills a day for two days. Because the mini-pill is so unforgiving of relatively short delays, only the most organized and conscientious adolescents should use it.

The mini-pill costs about the same as combined OCs, one hundred to three hundred dollars per year.

The Injectables, Implant, Patch, and Ring

OCs are not the only hormone-based contraceptives. There are several others, and they are most notable for not needing to be taken daily. Two are injected (Depo-Provera and Lunelle); one is an implant (Norplant); one is inserted into the vagina (NuvaRing); and the last one is a patch (Ortho Evra). These are among the most effective methods of contraception for your child to consider, and because nothing has to be done on the day your teenager has sex, they are nearly foolproof for pregnancy prevention. However, none of them provides STD protection, so they should be used in conjunction with condoms.

Depo-Provera

Depo-Provera is given as a shot every twelve weeks. It contains only progestin, and works by inhibiting ovulation and probably by affecting other reproductive functions.

Your daughter is unlikely to become pregnant if she is a few weeks late for her repeat injection, but of course, it's best not to take chances. If she decides she wants to have a child, she may want to stop getting shots about a year or so before she would like to get pregnant and switch to some other form of contraception for the interim. Some girls will not ovulate until nine or ten months after the shot, while other girls can get pregnant much sooner.

Depo costs about thirty to seventy-five dollars per injection (one hundred twenty to three hundred dollars per year), plus the cost of the medical visits.

Upsides

Depo-Provera is easy to use perfectly, and is highly effective at preventing pregnancy.

It can reduce menstrual cramps, menstrual pain, mittleschmerz, and endometriosis pain. It also decreases the risk of endometrial cancer, ovarian cancer, and PID.

Downsides

One of the main complaints women have about Depo-Provera is that it can cause irregular periods. Your daughter may stop menstruating, or she may have frequent periods. Because Depo has an ongoing effect for at least three months, treating side effects is not as easy as with the Pill (which she can stop at any time). With Depo, she'll need to ride those side effects out.

Depo-Provera can cause depression and mood swings. It can also cause breast tenderness. Depo can cause weight gain, probably by increasing the girl's appetite, although weight gain not caused by Depo is also sometimes attributed to it.

Females who use Depo-Provera long-term may develop decreased bone density. This is still being researched, but your daughter can ask her clinician for the latest information when making her decision.

Lunelle

Lunelle is injected each month, and is like combined OCs in that it has both estrogen and progestin (unlike Depo-Provera, which only has progestin). It prevents pregnancy the same way that combined OCs do. The first shot is usually given within five days of the start of a period.

The cost is around thirty to forty dollars per shot, although the cost of the medical visit may make it higher.

Upsides

For a girl who might not remember to take a pill each day, Lunelle can be easier to use than OCs, and it's highly effective at preventing pregnancy.

Additional benefits are similar to those of combined OCs.

Downsides

Girls may forget to go in for their shot each month.

Potential side effects include headache, breast pain, acne, and infection at the injection site, as well as other side effects that occur with combined OCs.

Norplant

As we go to press, Norplant is no longer being produced by its original manufacturer. However, many females are still using it, and another manufacturer may take over the product, so we are including a description here.

Norplant consists of six small rod-shaped capsules that are implanted under the skin. The capsules contain a drug called levonorgestrel (a type of progestin), which inhibits ovulation and fertilization. One administration of Norplant generally works for three to five years.

The capsules are inserted under the skin through a small incision above the inside of the elbow. (Local anesthesia is used.) They can sometimes be detected as a subtle bulge. After five years (or sooner if your daughter wants to stop using them), the capsules are removed. The effects are immediately reversible once that happens, so your daughter needs to use another form of contraception if she doesn't want to get pregnant.

The cost is around four hundred dollars for the rods, although prices vary. The price of insertion tends to be somewhere around five hundred to seven hundred dollars, and the price of removal tends to be higher. Spread over five years, the cost may be somewhere around three hundred fifty dollars per year.

Upsides

Girls like the fact that Norplant is convenient and long-lasting and that they don't need to remember to do anything (except use condoms to prevent STDs). Norplant is particularly appealing to those who want a hormonal form of contraception but cannot remember to take pills on a regular basis or go to the clinician for periodic injections. Many benefits and side effects are similar to those of the mini-pill and Depo-Provera, which also contain only progestin and not estrogen.

Downsides

If your daughter develops some of the side effects we describe above and wants to put an end to them, she will need to have the Norplant removed.

Some girls are afraid to use Norplant. The insertion of little rods that keep releasing "chemicals" can seem much more nefarious than a pill or injection, even if the chemicals work the same way. Girls may also dislike the feeling that they are not in control because the Norplant is working continuously in their body for such a long time. Even though it can be removed, the idea that it can stay for five years creates the potential for fantastical thinking about highly exaggerated consequences. We have heard rumors of massive hair loss, weight gain of twenty or forty pounds, cancer, alcoholism, depression, and sterility.

Adding to these fears, there were some questions about the effectiveness of some specific lots of Norplant a few years ago. Although those lots were later found to be fine, some girls may have doubts about using Norplant at all.

Some girls think it's too visible. They worry that people will see the rods under their skin, which is certainly a possibility, and that it will send a signal that they are "promiscuous." As quoted in a study of Norplant users, "[One guy said to me,] 'Hey hey, baby you have Norplant. Wanna fuck?' "

Some medications reduce Norplant's effectiveness.

NuvaRing

NuvaRing, also called the vaginal ring, is a doughnut-shaped plastic ring, about two and a quarter inches in diameter, that fits into the vagina around or near the cervix and releases the type of hormones found in combined OCs, estrogen and progestin. It is kept in place for three weeks, and then removed by the girl for the fourth week, when menstruation occurs. After the fourth week, she inserts a new ring for the next cycle.

The girl inserts the ring herself. It is flexible and so can be folded for insertion, and the exact location in the vagina is not important for it to work. If she removes it early or if it comes out (which is uncommon) and she doesn't re-insert it within three hours, she needs to use other contraception until the ring has been re-inserted for seven days so that the hormone levels in her body are high enough again to provide contraception.

Upsides

Because the ring releases a constant flow of hormones, the daily dose isn't as high as with OCs, so side effects are expected to be less frequent.

It provides greater flexibility than some hormonal contraceptives because once a girl obtains the ring, she can insert it on her own when she is ready and she can stop using it if she is having side effects or decides she doesn't need it.

Downsides

Side effects, which are uncommon, include vaginal discharge, infection, and irritation. There is also the possibility of other side effects that can occur with combined OCs. More information about side effects will become available once the ring has been on the market for a while.

Some girls may not like inserting the ring in their vagina.

Ortho Evra

The patch contains the same pair of hormones used in combined OCs, except they are absorbed through the skin. A girl wears one patch non-stop for a week for three weeks in a row, and then goes for a week without a patch, during which time she menstruates. It is a square about one and three-quarters of an inch on a side, and the girl can wear it on her lower belly, butt, upper arm, or upper back or chest, but not on her breasts. The patch usually sticks to her skin for the full week, even during bathing and swimming; if it comes off, another one can be put on, but she should still change to a new patch on the same day each week.

The initial studies showed pregnancy rates similar to those with OCs, although women who weighed two hundred pounds or more were much more likely than other women to get pregnant.

Upsides

The patch provides similar pregnancy prevention to OCs without the need to remember to take a daily pill. Its effects can be stopped more quickly than those of the injectable and the implant.

The hormones are still absorbed even if the girl is ill with vomiting or diarrhea, which is not always the case with OCs.

Downsides

Your daughter may not like having the patch visible when her clothes are off.

Side effects include breast tenderness, headaches, skin reactions where the patch is placed, nausea and vomiting, painful menstruation, and belly pain.

The patch may be similar to combined OCs in potentially causing deep vein thrombosis (a blood clot) and other heart or circulatory system diseases like strokes or heart attacks. However, it's likely that as with OCs, these complications would be rare among adolescents. Smoking could increase the chances of these complications. More information about side effects will become available once the patch has been on the market for a while.

Spermicide

Spermicides contain agents that, as the name suggests, kill sperm. They come in creams, films, foams, jellies/gels, suppositories, and tablets. Nonoxynol-9 is the most commonly available spermicide in the United States, although others are available in other parts of the world and at times in the States.

Gels and foams may create a direct barrier that keeps the sperm from reaching the cervix. And gels, foams, and creams can also function as sexual lubricants. Female barrier methods such as the diaphragm and cervical cap are designed to hold a spermicide in place against the cervix.

A girl inserts the spermicide into her vagina with her hand, with an applicator, or in the cup of a diaphragm or cap. However she puts it in, the spermicide needs to make contact with her cervix. Suppositories and vaginal contraceptive film should be inserted ten to fifteen minutes before intercourse, depending on the product, to allow time for it to dissolve. Unless used with a diaphragm or cap, a spermicide should be placed in the vagina less than one hour prior to intercourse. If more time has passed, additional spermicide should be added, and extra should be added with each additional act of intercourse.

A girl should not remove the spermicide until at least six hours after intercourse. This includes douching, which can wash out the spermicide before it has done its job. Douching solutions that contain spermicide are not effective as contraceptives because the sperm have generally already swum through the cervix by the time the girl is able to douche. Indeed, many clinicians advise against douching because routine douching has been associated with an increased risk of PID and ectopic pregnancy.

Nonoxynol-9 used to be recommended for prevention of HIV and some other STDs, but that recommendation has been discontinued. Newer research on HIV, gonorrhea, and chlamydia has found that nonoxynol-9 does not reduce their spread. Rather, there is some evidence that it can irritate the vagina or anus and make it easier to become infected with HIV or possibly another STD when exposed. Irritation may be more of a problem for people who use nonoxynol-9 very frequently (more than twice a day). Less is known about the effect of other spermicides on HIV and STDs.

Because research into spermicides is ongoing, your child should talk to a clinician or check the CDC website for the latest information if she's considering using one. At the moment, though, she would do better to rely on a contraceptive method that does not require she also use a spermicide (which in the United States almost always contains nonoxynol-9, although this too may change). That means choosing a hormonal method rather than a diaphragm or cap; the latter two don't prevent pregnancy nearly as well unless they are used with a spermicide. Using a condom with a hormonal method provides protection against both pregnancy and STD transmission without the potential increased risk of infection that comes with nonoxynol-9.

Multi-use applicator kits for foam and gel cost ten to twenty dollars, and refills cost five to ten dollars. Films and suppositories cost five to twenty dollars per pack.

Upsides

Spermicides are one of the forms of contraception that a girl can take charge of and use without her partner's participating or perhaps even knowing. Adolescents do not need a prescription to purchase them.

Downsides

Spermicides are principally designed to prevent pregnancy. However, their failure rate is high enough that they should generally be used along with other methods such as condoms, diaphragms, and caps.

They aren't useful for HIV and STD prevention, as discussed above, and they may increase the chances of becoming infected.

Some people find them messy. Some people have allergies to permicides or get vaginal or penile irritation from them. Some do not like the taste if they perform oral sex after the spermicide has been inserted.

The Diaphragm

The diaphragm is made of rubber and looks like a disk with the edge curled in, something like a cross between a small Frisbee and a yarmulke, with a metal spring in the rim. The cup of the diaphragm (the concave side) holds a spermicide, and your daughter inserts the diaphragm with the spermicide against her cervix. She should also spread some of the spermicide around the edges of the diaphragm. The diaphragm is held in place by the spring, her pubic bone, and her vaginal muscles. Once it is in place, she should not be able to feel it. The diaphragm itself blocks the sperm from entering her cervix, and the spermicide kills the sperm.

Diaphragms come in various styles with different shapes and spring mechanisms and in a range of sizes. If your daughter decides to use a diaphragm, her clinician will measure her for the proper size and style. Sometimes a girl's cervix and uterus have a particular shape or position that makes it hard to fit a diaphragm for her.

Your daughter can insert the diaphragm into her vagina up to six hours before intercourse and leave it in for at least six hours afterwards. (This means she can insert it before going to the movies with her boyfriend.) If it remains in longer than six hours, she should add additional spermicide with an applicator without removing the diaphragm. It is fine to have vaginal intercourse more than once before removing the diaphragm, but she should insert more spermicide before each act of intercourse. She should not leave it in more than twenty-four hours or use it during menstruation because of the risk of toxic shock syndrome (see Chapter 6 for symptoms). Her clinician can discuss risks and how to reduce them.

A diaphragm costs twenty to fifty dollars, plus the charge for the clinical visit and the spermicidal cream or jelly.

Diaphragms and cervical caps (discussed next) have a lot in common, so we discuss upsides and downsides of both barriers here.

Upsides

Barriers are methods your daughter can control without the need for the boy's involvement.

Unlike most female-controlled methods, barriers have the advantages of not causing serious side effects and not affecting the girl's hormonal patterns (we discussed hormonal methods above).

Girls who expect to be having intercourse only intermittently or who do not want to take oral contraceptives may find barriers a good choice.

The diaphragm and the cap are generally quite safe.

Downsides

Diaphragms and caps increase the risk of urinary tract infections, bacterial vaginosis, and vaginal candidiasis, possibly due to the spermicide. The allergic reactions we discussed in relation to latex condoms can occur with a latex diaphragm or cap as well. Likewise, oil-based lubricants that can wear out a latex condom should also be avoided and water-based spermicides used instead.

Toxic shock syndrome is a rare complication—it occurs about two times in 1 million uses of diaphragms and caps.

Diaphragms can be knocked off the cervix during intercourse. If your daughter and her partner become aware that this has occurred, they can use emergency contraception. If they are using another type of contraception along with the diaphragm, such as a condom for STD protection, they should be fine.

Nonoxynol-9, the major spermicide available in the United States, does not protect against HIV or other STDs, and may increase their transmission (see discussion above).

Diaphragms and other female barrier methods have not been as popular with teenagers as with adult women, in part because some teenagers feel uncomfortable with the idea of inserting them into their vagina.

The Cervical Cap

The cervical cap looks like a large rubber thimble that holds spermicide in the cup. The cap fits over the base of the cervix and is held in place by suction. As with a diaphragm, the cap acts as a barrier, and the spermicide kills the sperm.

Your daughter should keep it in for at least eight hours after intercourse. She can keep it in for up to forty-eight hours at a time without adding additional spermicide, but she should not use it for longer than that because of the possible risk of toxic shock syndrome.

Her clinician will fit her for the cap. She should use an additional method of contraception when she first uses the cap until it's clear it stays in properly. The cap hasn't been popular with teens in the United States, partly because it can be difficult to insert and also because it hasn't been widely available in the U.S.

The cap is less effective for girls who have given birth because of changes in the cervix.

A cap is about the same price as a diaphragm, twenty to fifty dollars, plus the charge for the medical visit and the cost of the contraceptive cream or jelly.

See the above discussion of the diaphragm for other upsides and downsides.

Withdrawal

The Latin name for it, coitus interruptus, pretty much says it all. The boy withdraws his penis from the girl's vagina before ejaculating. The same approach can apply to interrupted anal or oral intercourse for STD prevention.

This is a contraceptive technique where the girl needs to have complete trust in the boy, and the boy needs to be certain he deserves that trust. He needs to take full responsibility for knowing when he is close to ejaculation and for withdrawing before he ejaculates. There is little the girl can do, because she will typically not have enough advance warning to take charge.

Even if the boy always withdraws before ejaculating, the girl can still get pregnant, because his pre-ejaculate can contain some sperm from a prior ejaculation (although in much lower quantities than in ejaculate). Similarly, withdrawal does not prevent STD transmission.

Clearly, successful use of the withdrawal technique requires enormous willpower and self-control. Teenage boys may not have much experience sensing when they are about to ejaculate, and even the most responsible boy may have trouble withdrawing, especially given evidence that both males' and females' thinking can get fuzzy as orgasm approaches. The risk of an unintended pregnancy can seem more and more remote with the rising anticipation of imminent pleasure.

For this reason, we discourage adolescents from relying on withdrawal.

Periodic Abstinence

Periodic abstinence (also called the rhythm method or the fertility awareness method) depends on a couple's refraining from vaginal intercourse while the girl is ovulating. The egg survives for about twelve to twenty-four hours after ovulation (which occurs about fourteen days before menstruation), and the sperm survive in the vagina and uterus for up to five days, so the goal is to make sure to avoid intercourse for a six-day span—the five days prior to ovulation as well as the day after ovulation.

Most techniques for determining the start and end of the fertile period involve watching for physical changes in the body controlled by the same hormones that control the ovulatory cycle. These hormones and the changes they cause are imprecise, so it is best to add several days to the start and end of the fertile period when using this method—this will come out to a period of ten to fourteen days each menstrual cycle when a girl should consider herself most likely to get pregnant. The main methods for assessing the fertile period include:

Basal Body Temperature Method. The basal body temperature refers to the "resting" body temperature, which is best measured upon awakening. The temperature is generally lower during the first part of the menstrual cycle, and then it rises around the time of ovulation; the change—usually less than half a degree Fahrenheit—isn't high enough for most girls to notice. When using this method, girls should assume they are fertile from just after their menses until their temperature has remained elevated for at least three days. Studying how to take one's temperature properly and how much of a rise to look for are necessary to use this method properly. The temperature pattern can be disrupted by illness, stress, travel, or lack of sleep, so it is not always a reliable indicator. Temperature kits cost five to ten dollars.

Calendar Method. In the 1930s, a calendar was developed to estimate the fertile period using the length of prior menstrual cycles. The calendar takes into account that there are variations from cycle to cycle, so it designates a fertile period that is longer than the girl's actual fertile period. The girl needs to track her cycles (from the first day of bleeding to the day before the first day of the next bleeding) so that she knows the shortest and longest in the past six to twelve months. She will need this information to use the calendar to estimate the beginning and end of her potential fertile period. A calendar can be obtained from a clinician, a family planning clinic, or a religious institution.

Cervical Position and Feel Method. At the beginning of the fertile period, the cervix moves up higher and the cervical opening widens and becomes softer. After ovulation, the cervix moves lower and the opening closes and becomes harder. The girl can learn to feel these changes with her fingers.

Cervical Secretions Method (Cervical Mucus Method, Ovulation Method). Cervical secretions appear at the beginning of the fertile period and are initially sticky, thick, and cloudy. They then become clear, stretchy, and slippery, which is when they are best able to help the sperm reach the egg. As the fertile period is ending, the secretions dry up and block up the opening of the cervix, so that sperm can't swim into the uterus. Secretions remain scant or absent when the girl is not in her fertile period. Medications, spermicides, lubricants, douching, a vaginal infection, semen in the vagina, and the normal lubrication of sexual arousal can all make it difficult to notice changes in cervical secretions. When a girl is first learning to judge her secretions, it can be very helpful to get feedback from a clinician, family member, or someone else to determine whether she is interpreting her secretions correctly.

These methods can be used in combination—a typical combination being the cervical secretions method and basal body temperature method (which together are called the *sympto-thermal method*), sometimes with the cervical position and feel method or the calendar method as a backup.

Confusing, eh? Although it doesn't require any pills or any little

latex Frisbees, this method may actually be the most complex. It is estimated that it takes four to six hours to teach the necessary skills, which
are probably best learned in more than one session. With good training,
concentration, and commitment, this method can be made to work
well, but because of its complexity, the willpower required, and the
irregularity of young women's cycles, we don't generally recommend this
method for adolescents.

Intrauterine Devices

The intrauterine device (IUD) is a small T-shaped object that is inserted
into the uterus. IUDs have generally not been recommended for adolescents, in part because they tend to fit less well in the uterus of a
woman who has not carried a pregnancy and in part because of concerns
over a possible increased risk of PID, especially in the first several
months after insertion. However, at least one recent study of copper
IUDs found no increased risk of infertility, which is often caused by
PID. Some clinicians are now recommending the IUD as a reasonable
choice for certain adolescents, especially for those who have given birth.

The IUD is one of the most effective methods of contraception. It
appears to work by preventing fertilization or implantation. The copper
T 380 IUD (ParaGard) can remain in the uterus for up to ten years. The
Progestasert IUD contains progesterone and is replaced every year. The
Mirena IUD contains a similar hormone, levonorgestrel, and remains
effective for five to seven years. Each month the woman checks a thin
cord hanging down from the IUD to make sure the IUD is still in place.
A clinician can provide the latest information about side effects.

The IUD costs 100 to 400 dollars depending on the type, plus the
medical charges for insertion and removal. If the IUD is left in for two
years, the per year cost, of course, decreases to half.

Sterilization

Even on a bad day, you wouldn't consider this for your adolescent.

Appendix B

SEXUALLY TRANSMITTED DISEASES

IN THIS APPENDIX, we describe each of the major sexually transmitted diseases (STDs) along with their symptoms, diagnosis, and treatment.

We also discuss prevention. Clearly, complete abstinence from partnered sexual activity is the most effective way to prevent sexual transmission of all STDs. Similarly, engaging in sexual activity only within a monogamous relationship in which neither person has an STD at the start of the relationship also prevents the spread of STDs. But for those in other circumstances, there are ways to reduce (although not completely eliminate) the chances of contracting or spreading an infection, and we list these with each disease.

Latex condoms are the mainstay for reducing STD transmission during sexual activity. Although their effectiveness has not been demonstrated conclusively for each STD, studies with people who are using condoms as well as studies in laboratories have shown them to provide substantial protection against some diseases (especially HIV). Scientists infer from these studies that condoms similarly protect against other diseases and so recommend condom use against them as well. Plastic condoms and female condoms may be effective against most STDs, but research is still being conducted. Animal-skin condoms are not recommended for disease prevention because most bacteria and viruses are small enough to pass through them. For more detail, see Appendix A. Of course, condoms only protect against STD transmission involving the penis. Many STDs can also be transmitted through other routes, such as between the vagina and mouth.

Methods of diagnosis and treatment are continually being improved, so always consult your child's clinician for the most comprehensive and up-to-date information. You can also find recent information on the website of the federal Centers for Disease Control and Prevention (www.cdc.gov). The CDC hotline provides information as well as referrals for confidential diagnosis and treatment of STDs (1-800-227-8922 or 1-800-342-2437).

Chlamydia

Chlamydia, a type of bacteria, is the number one preventable cause of infertility and ectopic pregnancy in the United States.

Symptoms. Both females and males usually have no noticeable symptoms from their chlamydia infection.

Females may develop a discharge from their cervix (called mucopurulent cervicitis), but it may look like their normal vaginal fluid. They might also have vaginal bleeding after intercourse. But because chlamydia doesn't cause any pain (at least not right away), most infected females have no idea they've got an STD. Meanwhile, it can be working its way through their reproductive system, causing damage and also spreading to sex partners.

Like females, males often have no noticeable symptoms, which means they can also spread the disease for quite a while without knowing they have it. Chlamydia sometimes causes a condition in males called non-gonococcal urethritis (NGU), which results in frequent or painful urination and a discharge from the urethra that may look like clear mucus or white pus. It may be most noticeable as a stain in their underwear. Although chlamydia is the most common cause of NGU, other diseases, including herpes and trichomoniasis, can cause similar symptoms. Your son's clinician can help figure out which infection is causing his symptoms.

Chlamydia can infect other areas of the body as well, such as the rectum, where the infection will sometimes cause inflammation (with burning, pain, itching, or discharge) but can, again, be completely silent.

Complications. Males can develop a urethral stricture, a narrowing of the tube in the penis through which urine and semen pass. They can also get epididymitis, an infection of the organ in which sperm are stored near each testicle in the scrotum. The symptoms include pain and tenderness near the testicle and sometimes fever. Both of these complications can eventually cause infertility for males. Females can get pelvic inflammatory disease (PID), which can also cause infertility and is described on page 367.

Diagnosis. Chlamydia can be diagnosed with a urine test. Or a swab (like a long Q-tip) can be inserted into the female's cervical os (the opening of the cervix) or the male's urethra. A swab is also used to check for rectal chlamydia.

Because chlamydia usually has no symptoms, adolescents engaging in partnered sexual activity are advised to have an annual screening for chlamydia, even if they do not have symptoms. (If your child is having multiple partners, screening more often—perhaps every six months—is recommended.)

Treatment. Antibiotics are the standard treatment. Many people with chlamydia also have gonorrhea, so the clinician will usually test and treat your child for gonorrhea as well.

Contacts. Sexual partners should be informed that they could be infected and that they should go for testing and treatment even if they don't have symptoms. It's not clear how far back to go, but many clinicians recommend that partners from four to six months prior to the start of symptoms should be contacted (or if there are no symptoms, from four to six months prior to the time of diagnosis). If there have been no partners during those months, then the most recent partner should be contacted. Until treatment is complete (for people who receive only one dose of antibiotics, this means seven days later because it takes time to work), infected persons should assume they can still spread the disease. Pregnant females can transmit chlamydia to the baby during vaginal birth, potentially causing an eye infection or pneumonia.

As is true for most STDs, both males and females can transmit chlamydia without having had any symptoms.

Prevention. When used properly, latex condoms can reduce the chances of catching or spreading chlamydia.

Epidemiology. Estimates range from 3 to 8 million new cases of chlamydia each year in the United States. It is reported four times as often in females as males, and the difference between the sexes is even larger among adolescents.

Pelvic Inflammatory Disease (PID)

PID is a very serious inflammation that can affect a female's uterus, fallopian tubes, ovaries, and related areas. It is quite common in sexually active female adolescents. PID is generally caused by chlamydia, gonorrhea, or other types of bacteria, or by several bacteria at once. As we discuss in Chapters 6 and 11, the tissue of the cervix takes time to mature, so the adolescent's cervix is initially less protective against chlamydia and gonorrhea than the mature adult cervix.

Symptoms. Many females have subtle symptoms that are not severe enough to prompt them to seek medical attention, giving the disease more time to cause damage to the reproductive organs. They may feel pain and tenderness in the lower belly where the reproductive organs are. They might also have fever, chills, abnormal vaginal bleeding, pain with vaginal intercourse, vaginal discharge, or cervical discharge (which they probably cannot distinguish from vaginal discharge).

Complications. PID can lead to infertility, ectopic pregnancies, or chronic pelvic pain. Nearly one in ten females becomes infertile after her first episode of PID, and the rate increases rapidly with successive episodes. PID and chlamydia infections are thought to have been major contributors to the dramatic increase in ectopic pregnancies during the last quarter of the twentieth century.

Diagnosis. PID can be difficult to diagnose because other disorders, such as appendicitis or an ectopic pregnancy, can cause the same symptoms. The clinician will usually perform a pelvic exam and may also conduct laboratory tests.

Treatment. Antibiotics are the standard treatment.

Prevention. When used properly, latex condoms can reduce the chances of contracting or spreading the infections that cause PID. Also, proper and timely treatment of STDs will prevent PID.

Epidemiology. Over one million females per year are estimated to develop PID, with the infection rate highest among teenagers.

Gonorrhea

Gonorrhea is caused by a type of bacteria and, like chlamydia, can cause serious problems.

Symptoms. Most males do not get any symptoms, but if symptoms are going to develop, they will usually appear within three to five days of exposure. Symptoms in males include having pain when they urinate and needing to urinate more often than usual. They may also have a discharge from their urethra that is like pus (often called "the drip"). Females are even less likely to have recognizable symptoms. When symptoms occur, they usually begin in the first week after exposure and may include pain with urination as well as an abnormal vaginal discharge, abnormal menstruation, or pain during vaginal intercourse. Females may also develop mucopurulent cervicitis, described in the chlamydia section. Both males and females can get gonorrhea in the anus, which can cause discharge, burning, pain, and itching, or in the throat, which may feel like a regular sore throat—or they can be completely asymptomatic.

Complications. Males can get complications like epididymitis or a urethral stricture, which are described in the chlamydia section and which can result in infertility. However, males usually get symptoms before complications, so they typically seek treatment and are cured before the complications cause permanent damage. By contrast, females may not have serious symptoms until the complications have already caused serious damage. About 40 percent of females with untreated cervical infections will get PID, which is discussed later in this appendix. Gonorrhea can also spread through the blood system to the joints, liver, heart, and brain, but such dissemination is rare in the United States.

Diagnosis. The clinician may collect some of the discharge or urine, or culture a specific area such as the throat, to make the diagnosis.

Treatment. Antibiotics are the standard treatment. Strains of the bacteria are starting to develop that are resistant to regular antibiotics and need high-powered antibiotics. Once gonorrhea has spread through the blood system, treatment is more complicated and generally requires hospitalization. Until treatment is complete, infected persons should assume they can still spread the disease. Over one-quarter of people with gonorrhea also have chlamydia, so the clinician will usually test and treat your child for chlamydia as well.

Contacts. It is easier for females to get gonorrhea from males than vice versa. Most females who have sex with an infected male become infected, whereas only about one in four males who have sex with infected females becomes infected. It's recommended that sex partners from the two months prior to the development of symptoms or prior to diagnosis (if there were no symptoms) should be tested and treated. If there were no sex partners during those months, the most recent partner should be tested and treated.

Females can pass gonorrhea to their baby during vaginal birth. That's why the clinician puts an ointment in all babies' eyes right after birth, to kill any gonorrhea that may be there, although the baby would need additional treatment if the mother is infected.

Prevention. When used properly, latex condoms can reduce the chances of catching or spreading gonorrhea.

Epidemiology. There are an estimated 650,000 new cases each year in the United States. Among teens, females account for about twice as many cases as males.

Hepatitis B Virus

Among the various types of hepatitis, the one that is most often transmitted sexually is hepatitis B.

Symptoms and Complications. Most people have no symptoms, but if symptoms occur, they usually appear between six weeks and six months after infection. Those who have symptoms may get jaundice (yellowing of the skin and eyes), dark urine, fatigue, loss of appetite, nausea, vomiting, headache, fever, rash, hives, joint aches, and belly tenderness. Symptoms usually resolve within three to six months.

Some people become chronic carriers of the virus and will always be at risk for spreading the disease to sexual partners and others with whom they have close contact, including their babies before, during, and after birth. They will also have an increased chance of getting cirrhosis or cancer of the liver, both of which can be fatal.

Diagnosis. The diagnosis is made by a blood test.

Treatment. There is no specific treatment for hepatitis B infection. Most people will recover on their own, though some measures can be taken to make the recovery process more comfortable.

Contacts. A clinician can advise on how far back to go in informing sexual partners and others.

If your child has been exposed and has not previously been vaccinated, contact a clinician. Immune globulins can help prevent developing the disease. He or she should receive this therapy within fourteen days of exposure, and should also get vaccinated. Nonsexual household contacts should also be vaccinated, and if they have been exposed to the infected person's blood (for example, they shared a toothbrush or razor blade), they should get the immune globulins as well.

Prevention. A series of vaccines is available that prevents infection with hepatitis B. It is recommended for all infants, but not all receive it, so it is also recommended for unvaccinated adolescents.

When used properly, latex condoms can reduce the chances of catching or spreading hepatitis B through intercourse.

Epidemiology. About 77,000 new cases are estimated to occur each year in the United States, and about 750,000 people are thought to have the infection at any one time. About one half to two-thirds of all hepatitis B cases are attributed to sexual transmission.

Herpes Simplex Virus (HSV)

Symptoms and Complications. Genital herpes consists of vesicles (small fluid-filled bumps, also called blisters) that typically appear on the head of the penis or in the vagina and can be very painful. People can become infected with herpes not only in their genitals, but also in their mouth (often called cold sores or fever blisters), rectum, or eye, and on their skin. Herpes is not always transmitted sexually, although genital herpes usually is. There are two viruses that cause herpes, HSV-1 and HSV-2. Most genital cases are caused by HSV-2, although HSV-1, which usually causes oral (mouth) herpes, can also infect the genitals. Many people do not know they have the infection because they have a very mild form, or they do not know when they are having an outbreak because the vesicles are in the vagina or rectum and so are not visible.

The disease is spread by direct contact between the site of an outbreak (or impending outbreak) on a person's body and another person's mucous membranes (for example, the walls of the vagina) or broken skin (for example, a cut on a finger). The actual vesicles are particularly infective, with about one-third to two-thirds of exposed sexual partners becoming infected.

The initial outbreak (called the primary infection) can be extremely painful. It usually occurs between three to seven days after exposure. It may start with itching or extra sensitivity to touch and then develop into painful vesicles up to about 3 millimeters in diameter (about the size of a chicken pox). The vesicles may break down and leave behind an ulcer. They can last for up to two weeks (sometimes longer), but they heal without scarring. Infection in the vagina may also cause a cervicitis with a discharge similar to that in chlamydia. The person may also have pain with urination. People often get flu-like symptoms, with fever, fatigue, headache, and large, tender lymph nodes. Vesicles may spread to other body parts as well.

Many people feel odd sensations such as itching, tingling, or burning before a recurrence. Recurrences do not usually last as long as the initial outbreak.

The genital ulcers caused by herpes (as well as those caused by syphilis and chancroid) are problematic not only because of associated pain and other problems, but also because they make it easier to become infected with HIV.

Diagnosis. The diagnosis is generally made by the visual appearance of the vesicles, but laboratory studies of the vesicles or blood tests may also be performed.

Treatment. The virus remains in the body indefinitely and can cause recurrent outbreaks throughout the rest of the person's life. Oral medications can reduce the frequency and duration of outbreaks. However, there is no cure for HSV. Treatment should be started when the person first senses an impending outbreak and certainly within one day of the outbreak. If people have six or more recurrences per year, daily therapy can reduce recurrences by 70 percent to 80 percent. Because the rate of recurrence usually decreases with time, the clinician may recommend that your child stop daily medication after a year to see if he or she still needs it. People receiving therapy may still be able to transmit the virus, although further research is needed. Intravenous medication may also be used for people who have unusually severe cases, such as when the disease has spread to internal organs.

Contacts. One of the challenges of preventing the spread of herpes is that people can transmit it without even knowing they have it or, if they do know they have it, without knowing that they are currently infectious. Transmission without symptoms is more common for HSV-2 than HSV-1 and for people who have had genital herpes for less than a year.

Herpes can also cause severe problems for a baby who is infected when passing through the birth canal. If your daughter has ever had herpes and is pregnant, she should tell her clinician.

Prevention. When used properly, latex condoms can reduce the chances of contracting or spreading HSV in areas that are covered (the penis) or protected (such as the vagina or rectum) by the condom, but condoms do not provide protection against HSV in other areas (such as the skin around the genitals).

Epidemiology. An estimated 500,000 to 1 million new cases occur in the United States each year, with between 30 and 60 million people estimated to be infected overall.

Human Immunodeficiency Virus (HIV)

Symptoms and Complications. HIV is a virus that typically does not cause immediate symptoms (except for Acute Retroviral Syndrome, described below); rather, it weakens the immune system over time, leading to Acquired Immunodeficiency Syndrome (AIDS) and its associated symptoms and diseases (such as pneumocystis, toxoplasmosis, and tuberculosis), which can lead to death.

In the first few weeks after infection, people may develop Acute Retroviral Syndrome, with fever, fatigue, enlarged lymph nodes, and a rash. Subsequent signs of disease progression include fever, weight loss, diarrhea, cough, shortness of breath, and thrush (a pasty white yeast that clings to the inside of the mouth). People can also get various infections and other diseases because their immune system isn't working well. The time of progression from infection with HIV to development of AIDS for someone who is not getting treatment can be as short as a few months or as long as seventeen years or more, with about half of untreated infected people developing AIDS within about ten years.

The HIV that is prevalent in the United States is actually called HIV-1. A related virus, HIV-2, is mostly found in central Africa and acts more slowly than HIV-1.

Diagnosis. Early diagnosis is important because treatment can slow the deterioration of the immune system and protect against getting various infections (for example, pneumocystis pneumonia). Also, a diagnosis of HIV affects how clinicians diagnose and treat other diseases and how they care for pregnant females.

Most people with HIV infection will have a positive test within three months of infection, although special tests may be able to detect infection within several days of exposure. A blood test is typically used to test for HIV, although newer tests that use saliva are available. Some communities provide anonymous testing, where your child does not need to tell his or her name or give any other identifying information. Clinicians who provide testing should provide counseling before and after the test to discuss the full range of implications of different test results.

Treatment. There are various medications available for people with HIV. Dramatic advances over the past decade have made a huge difference in the quality and length of life for people infected with the virus. However, your child should not assume that these medications mean that HIV is no longer a concern. The medications do not work for everyone, they have side effects, they are expensive, and they may stop working after a while.

Although counseling is appropriate for anyone who has (or is tested for) an STD, it is particularly important for people with HIV, who may want help in coping with the implications of the diagnosis, dealing with the reactions of others, getting good health care, taking care of themselves, and preventing transmission to others.

Contacts. HIV can enter the body through sexual activity; by sharing needles, syringes, or other injection equipment; and during blood transfusions. It can also spread from mother to child before or during birth or through breastfeeding. Among sexual activities, receptive anal and vaginal intercourse are particularly risky for getting infected, but insertive anal and vaginal intercourse can also transmit the disease. The disease can also spread through oral sex, although this is a much less common route. Even when an infected person has no symptoms, he or she can spread the virus to others. Genital infections (such as those described in this appendix) increase the chances of contracting or spreading HIV.

Following exposure to HIV (for example, when the condom breaks during intercourse with someone who is HIV-positive), so-called post-exposure prophylaxis, usually consisting of one month's worth of some of the same medications taken by people with HIV infection, can reduce the risk of getting an infection. To have the best chance of working, these medications should be started within 72 hours of the exposure.

Prevention. When used properly, latex condoms can greatly reduce the chances of contracting or spreading HIV.

Epidemiology. Although rates of diagnosis of HIV infection and AIDS have been relatively low in adolescents, it is believed that many are infected but don't find out until they are older. Given the typical length of time between infection and symptoms, many adults with HIV were probably infected as teenagers. About 20,000 people in the United States are estimated to become infected each year, and about half a million are estimated to have the infection at present. It has been estimated that about one-quarter of new HIV infections occur in people twenty-two or younger. Although HIV was initially diagnosed in many more males than females (in part because of its emergence in the gay male community), studies of adolescents show less gender imbalance, with both males and females becoming infected during adolescence.

Human Papillomavirus (HPV)

HPV is a virus. Among the more than one hundred types of HPV, most of which are harmless and cause regular skin warts, about thirty can be spread by sexual contact, and even most of these are harmless. Some can cause genital warts (also called venereal warts or condylomata acuminata), but some can cause cervical cancer or other cancers.

Symptoms and Complications. Genital warts can develop on or around the penis or labia, in the urethra, in the vagina, on the cervix, or around or inside the anus. They can sometimes appear in the mouth or throat. Warts can appear alone or in groups; they can be tiny or grow large enough to be quite noticeable, sometimes looking like little cauliflowers. The virus may also appear as flat lesions that are more subtle than typical warts. Sometimes, warts can be painful or itchy. Although females may sometimes have symptoms of vaginitis or painful intercourse, by and large, warts are not a major problem—the main reason to treat them is that people don't like the way they look. Not everyone who has warts even notices them.

The reason HPV gets so much attention is that some types of HPV (types that don't cause warts) can cause cervical cancer and other genital cancers. Over 90 percent of cervical cancers come from HPV, but less than 1 percent of HPV develops into cervical cancer.

The adolescent cervix is particularly susceptible to HPV infection because the protective tissue of the adult cervix has not fully formed. There is some evidence that the younger a female is when she first becomes infected with HPV, the more likely it will progress to a potentially cancerous lesion (assuming it's the type of HPV that can progress to cancer). However, the chances that it will progress are still very, very low.

Without treatment, warts often go away within three to five years. It's generally believed that most adolescents (some estimate as many as 70 percent) who have engaged in partnered sexual activity have been infected with HPV at some point, that it goes away within a few years, and that very few develop cancer from it. Although cervical cancer is extremely rare among adolescents, they can get squamous intra-epithelial lesions (SIL), which can be detected with a Pap smear. Some types of SIL (called low-grade) usually go away on their own without treatment; another type (high-grade SIL) also usually goes away, but may progress to cancer (again, rarely in adolescents). Cervical cancer appears to be more likely among middle-aged women who have had cervical HPV infection that has persisted for many years. HPV and its relationship to cancer are the subjects of a lot of ongoing research, and new information is likely to emerge over the next few years. If your child has HPV, her clinician can explain to her the implications in more detail. She can also check the CDC website for recent information.

Diagnosis. Of course, visible warts can be diagnosed just by looking at them. But even when there are no visible warts, SIL can be detected on a Pap smear. If your daughter's Pap smear is positive for SIL, she will probably have a colposcopy, where the clinician uses a special microscope to look at the cervix. A chemical called acetic acid (pretty much the same as regular vinegar) can make affected areas of the cervix more visible so that they can be biopsied. The Pap smear will not detect high-grade SIL in all females who have it. There are also new tests that can detect certain types of HPV infection, and even better tests are anticipated over the next several years.

Treatment. Although warts will often go away on their own, treatments are available to remove warts. These include, among other techniques, applying medicine to the warts, freezing them with liquid nitrogen, or using laser surgery or other types of surgery. The choice depends on such characteristics as the size, location, and number of lesions. Removing warts does not eliminate the virus from the body, although it is believed the virus will usually go away on its own.

Low-grade SIL is usually not treated but rather just checked with regular Pap smears to make sure it goes away. High-grade SIL is usually treated by removing or freezing the lesion or by other methods.

Contacts. It doesn't seem to be as critical that sex partners be examined as it is with most other STDs—a couple is unlikely to re-infect each other and the partner may very well be infected already—but it is typically a good idea so partners can have any visible warts removed and get checked for other STDs.

About two-thirds of people who are sexually exposed to the virus become infected. Warts can appear within three weeks to twenty months after exposure, with an average of two to three months. Many people never develop visible warts and have no idea they are infected. It can take from months to years for HPV infection to develop into SIL, and it may take years to decades for cervical cancer to develop.

Prevention. When used properly, latex condoms can reduce the chances of catching or spreading HPV in areas that are covered (most of the penis) or protected (such as the vagina or rectum) by the condom, but condoms do not provide protection against HPV in other areas (such as the skin around the genitals). The female condom may provide more protection because it covers a wider area, but not much research has been done at this time. Although the role of condoms in reducing the spread of HPV is less well understood than for many other STDs, condom use has been associated with a reduction in cervical cancer.

Epidemiology. An estimated 5.5 million new HPV cases occur in the United States each year, with 20,000,000 people thought to be infected at any one time.

Pubic Lice (Pediculosis Pubis)

Pubic lice (also called crabs) are tiny insects that are akin to the lice that children often get in the hair on their head, except that pubic lice are usually located in the pubic hair (and sometimes as far away as the eyelashes and underarm hair). They are typically spread by sexual contact, although they can also be spread by sharing clothing or bedsheets.

Symptoms. Pubic lice cause intense itching.

Diagnosis. The lice or their tiny eggs (called nits) are visible on the pubic hair. If your child removes a louse from his hair, he may be able to see it moving, especially if he uses a magnifying glass.

Treatment. Treatment is with a medicated cream or shampoo that is applied to the affected areas and then washed off after it's had enough time to work. It's also necessary to kill lice and nits in the bedding and clothes. Washable material should be washed in hot water and dried in a hot dryer, or dry-cleaned. Materials that cannot be washed can be set aside without body contact for seventy-two hours. If symptoms persist, another course of treatment may be necessary.

Contacts. Sex partners and household contacts from the prior month should be treated.

Epidemiology. An estimated 3 million people are infected each year in the United States.

Scabies

Scabies is caused by a mite (a type of insect) that burrows into the skin.

Symptoms. Scabies can appear as small red bumps, sometimes in a surprisingly straight line and often scratched open because they itch a lot. The bumps may be located in various places on the body where there has been contact with an infected person or where the mite has spread. The first time someone is infected with scabies, it takes several weeks to a month to develop symptoms, but future infections may take only twenty-four hours to produce symptoms. A person can spread scabies before the symptoms appear. Scabies can be spread by nonsexual contact and by sharing clothes and sheets.

Diagnosis. Diagnosis may be made by examining the appearance of the rash or by scraping a lesion from the body and looking at it under a microscope.

Treatment. Treatment is with a cream or lotion that is left on the body for eight to twenty-four hours. Bedding and clothes should be treated as described for pubic lice. Itching may persist for several weeks. Some clinicians will recommend another course of treatment in a week if itching persists, while others will recommend this only in certain circumstances.

Contacts. Sex partners and household contacts from the prior month should be treated.

Syphilis

Syphilis is caused by an organism called a spirochete. It is much less common in the United States than it once was.

Symptoms and Complications. There are several stages of syphilis. Primary syphilis manifests as a chancre, a painless ulcer at the place where the person was exposed to syphilis that appears an average of three weeks, but as long as three months, after exposure. The chancre will usually heal within two months and leave no scar. Because it is painless, the infected person might not even notice it and might unwittingly spread the disease. Many people do not get a chancre. If people with primary syphilis do not receive treatment, they may develop secondary syphilis in one to two months or longer. Secondary syphilis can cause a rash on the palms and soles, enlarged lymph nodes, hair loss, and a whole list of other symptoms. Patients may also have condylomata lata, which are fleshy, moist tissue growths. Latent syphilis can occur at any time and refers to a period when the person has no symptoms but still has the infection.

Up to a third of people who have untreated secondary syphilis go on to develop tertiary syphilis, which has many serious consequences, such as problems of the heart and blood vessels, and nodules in the skin called gumma. The disease can affect the central nervous system (for example, the brain) during any of the three stages.

Diagnosis. Laboratory tests for syphilis can be performed on blood or on material from a lesion or lymph node. A physical exam is also useful in making the diagnosis.

Treatment. Antibiotics are the standard treatment.

Contacts. Sexual spread of syphilis occurs only when skin lesions such as a chancre are present, which is generally limited to the first year of infection. But sex partners of people with untreated syphilis at any stage should also see a clinician. If your child is diagnosed with syphilis, the clinician can advise how far back to go in telling prior sex partners, because the probable length of infectivity will vary with the stage of illness. Pregnant females can pass syphilis on to the developing fetus, with serious consequences.

Prevention. When used properly, latex condoms can reduce the chances of contracting or spreading syphilis in areas that are covered (the penis) or protected (such as the vagina or rectum) by the condom, but condoms do not provide protection against syphilis in other areas (such as the skin around the genitals).

Epidemiology. There are an estimated 70,000 new cases each year in the United States.

Vaginitis

The symptoms of vaginitis usually involve an abnormal vaginal discharge or vulvar itching and irritation, sometimes with an atypical odor. There may also be burning with urination. The most common causes of discharge are bacterial vaginosis, trichomoniasis, and candidiasis. The cervical discharge of chlamydia or gonorrhea may appear similar to the discharge of vaginitis.

Bacterial Vaginosis

Symptoms. Bacterial vaginosis is the most common reason for abnormal vaginal discharge or odor, but many females who have vaginosis do not have any symptoms. Several types of bacteria, including gardnerella, can cause it. Although it is rare in females who have never had intercourse and more common in females with multiple sex partners, it is not clear whether it is actually transmitted through sexual activity or whether there is something that occurs during sexual activity that predisposes to the condition. The bacteria that cause it normally live in the vagina and don't cause any problems until something happens to disturb the balance, at which point these bacteria grow and disrupt the microscopic peaceable kingdoms living in the body. The bacteria that cause bacterial vaginosis may also be a major cause of PID.

Complications. Bacterial vaginosis during pregnancy has been associated with problems such as premature delivery.

Diagnosis. The clinician can examine the discharge or a swab of fluid from inside the vagina with laboratory testing and by looking at it under a microscope.

Treatment. Antibiotics, sometimes in the form of a vaginal cream, are the standard treatment.

Contacts. Sex partners do not need treatment.

Prevention. Latex condoms may help prevent bacterial vaginosis, but it's not clear. Check with your daughter's clinician or the CDC website for the latest recommendations.

Epidemiology. Cases of bacterial vaginosis are not officially counted, but the disease appears to be fairly prevalent.

Trichomoniasis

Trichomoniasis is caused by an organism called a protozoan.

Symptoms. Females tend to have symptoms—usually an unpleasant-smelling, yellow-green, frothy discharge with irritation of the vulva—but a number of females do not. Infected males usually do not have symptoms, although some have NGU (see section on chlamydia).

Complications. Trichomoniasis can cause problems during pregnancy, such as premature delivery.

Diagnosis. Diagnosis can be made with laboratory testing of vaginal fluid or by looking at it under a microscope.

Treatment. Antibiotics are the standard treatment. Treatment is not always effective the first time, so if symptoms do not resolve, the infected person should return to the clinician to see if she (or he) needs additional treatment. Females who have trichomoniasis often have other STDs as well, so the clinician should screen for other STDs and provide treatment when needed.

Contacts. Current sex partners should be treated, and they should abstain from sex until treatment is complete and symptoms are gone. Your child's clinician can help her decide how far back to go in contacting prior partners about the infection.

Prevention. When used properly, latex condoms can reduce the chances of catching or spreading trichomoniasis.

Epidemiology. There are an estimated 5 million new cases each year in the United States.

Vulvovaginal Candidiasis

Candidiasis is caused by a yeast (also called a fungus). It is not strictly an STD (it is usually not transmitted by sexual intercourse), but the symptoms are so similar to those caused by STDs that we describe it here.

Symptoms. Candidiasis can cause vaginal discharge and itching, as well as burning and soreness and pain with vaginal intercourse. Some females will have cottage-cheese-like discharge sticking to the walls of their vagina.

Diagnosis. Diagnosis can be made with laboratory testing of vaginal fluid or by looking at it under a microscope.

Treatment. The treatment is with an anti-yeast medication that can be applied in the vagina. The medication is usually oil-based and so should not be used with latex contraceptives such as condoms.

Contacts. Sex partners usually do not need treatment.

Epidemiology. It is estimated that three-quarters of women will get vulvovaginal candidiasis at some time during their lives.

Index

About the Authors

JUSTIN RICHARDSON, M.D., is an assistant clinical professor of psychiatry at Columbia University and Cornell University. He received a B.A. in biology with honors, an M.A. in social anthropology, and an M.D. all from Harvard University. He trained in psychiatry at McLean Hospital/Harvard Medical School, where he was the chief resident. His achievements there were acknowledged with awards from the American Medical Association, the American Psychoanalytic Association, and the Group for the Advancement of Psychiatry.

Over the past several years, Dr. Richardson has advised dozens of independent schools throughout the eastern United States on the subject of the sexual development of children. His work at these schools earned him a profile in the *New York Times* in 1997.

Dr. Richardson has been a contributing editor of the *Harvard Review of Psychiatry* for nearly ten years. He maintains a private practice in psychiatry and psychoanalysis in Manhattan.

MARK A. SCHUSTER, M.D., Ph.D., is an associate professor of pediatrics and public health at the University of California, Los Angeles (UCLA), and codirector of the Center for Research on Maternal, Child, and Adolescent Health at RAND, the Santa Monica think tank. Dr. Schuster obtained his B.A. summa cum laude from Yale, his M.D. from Harvard, his M.P.P. from the Kennedy School of Government, and his Ph.D. from the RAND Graduate School. His pediatric internship and residency training were at Harvard's Boston Children's Hospital, and his fellowship training was at the UCLA Robert Wood Johnson Clinical Scholars Program.

As founding director of the CDC-sponsored UCLA/RAND Center for Adolescent Health Promotion, he researches the role of parents in promoting children's health. He conducted a groundbreaking study on the sexual practices of adolescent virgins and one of the first evaluations of a high school condom availability program. He is currently leading an NIH-funded project that helps parents learn communication skills for talking with their kids about sexual matters.

Dr. Schuster is the author of many articles in academic journals on child and adolescent health issues, and he is an editor of the book *Child Rearing in America: Challenges Facing Parents with Young Children* (Cambridge University Press, 2002). He has served as a member of the Clinical Practice Committee of the California State Office of Family Planning, has advised the Kaiser Family Foundation on HIV prevention for adolescents in South Africa, and is consulting with the Los Angeles County Department of Health Services on increasing parent involvement in promoting healthy adolescent sexual development. He practices pediatrics at the Mattel Children's Hospital at UCLA.